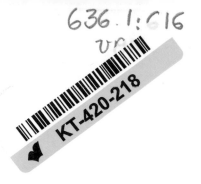

INFECTIOUS DISEASES

HORSE *of the*

Diagnosis, pathology, management, and public health

J. H. van der Kolk
DVM, PhD, dipl ECEIM
Department of Equine Sciences–Medicine
Faculty of Veterinary Medicine
Utrecht University, the Netherlands

E. J. B. Veldhuis Kroeze
DVM, dipl ECVP
Department of Pathobiology
Faculty of Veterinary Medicine
Utrecht University, the Netherlands

MANSON PUBLISHING / THE VETERINARY PRESS

Copyright © 2013 Manson Publishing Ltd
ISBN: 978-1-84076-165-8

A CIP catalogue record for this book is available from the British Library.

For full details of all Manson Publishing Ltd titles please write to:
Manson Publishing Ltd, 73 Corringham Road, London NW11 7DL, UK.
Tel: +44(0)20 8905 5150
Fax: +44(0)20 8201 9233
Email: manson@mansonpublishing.com
Website: www.mansonpublishing.com

Commissioning editor: Jill Northcott
Project manager: Kate Nardoni
Copy editor: Ruth Maxwell
Layout: DiacriTech, Chennai, India
Colour reproduction: Tenon & Polert Colour Scanning Ltd, Hong Kong
Printed by: Grafos SA, Barcelona, Spain

CONTENTS

INTRODUCTION

In equine medicine one of the most important areas is the field of infectious diseases. This field is very dynamic and ever evolving with emerging and fading diseases. Many professionals are dedicated to equine infectious diseases ranging from clinicians via laboratory diagnosticians to pathologists. This book is the outcome of close collaboration between a clinician and a pathologist and as such positively affected the selection of colour plates provided. Rapid development of molecular biology techniques has greatly improved diagnostic possibilities in equine infectious diseases, and facilitates epidemiological as well as zoonotic studies. In this book the majority of equine infectious diseases are arranged based on the various microbes and parasites involved, using Fauquet *et al.* (2005) for the classification of viruses, Garrity *et al.* (2004) for the classification of the prokaryotes, and Kassai (1999) for the classification of the helminths. In the individual sections the opportunities available for diagnosis of various causative agents using molecular biology have been described. However, these opportunities are usually limited by the options provided by local diagnostic laboratories and of course they should be contacted prior to sample submission. Nevertheless, the mere presence of a microbe and/or parasite in or on an animal cannot be considered adequate evidence that it is the aetiological agent of a disease that may exist. Diagnostic aids must be used to supplement, not supplant, clinical observations.

In order to support clinicians, a list of differential diagnoses has been provided in Appendix 1. Furthermore, Appendix 2 has been provided in an attempt to update the current view on zoonotic aspects of equine infectious diseases. Appendix 3 emphasizes the importance of clinical pathology in the diagnosis of infectious diseases.

The authors hope that this book will be helpful for anyone dealing with equine infectious diseases and suggestions to improve future issues are more than welcome.

We sincerely acknowledge the contributions of M. Aleman, C.M. Butler, A. van Dijk, G.C.M. Grinwis, E. Gruys, M. Heinrichs, D. Kersten, B. Malmhagen, K. Matiasek, G. Uilenberg, E. Smiet, E. Teske, and V.M. van der Veen.

References and further reading
Coles EH 1986. *Veterinary Clinical Pathology*, 4th edn. WB Saunders, London.

Fauquet CM, Mayo MA, Maniloff J, Desselberger U, Ball LA (eds) 2005. *Virus Taxonomy*. 8th Report of the International Committee on Taxonomy of Viruses. Academic Press, Elsevier, Amsterdam.

Garrity GM, Bell JA, Lilburn TG 2004. Taxonomic outline of the prokaryotes. In: *Bergey's Manual of Systematic Bacteriology*, 2nd edn. Springer, New York.

Kassai T 1999. *Veterinary Helminthology*. Butterworth-Heinemann, Oxford.

DISCLAIMER

ABBREVIATIONS

ABL	Australian bat lyssavirus		EMG	electromyography
ABV	avian bornavirus		EPA	epidemic polyarthritis
ADV	Aujeszky's disease virus		EPE	equine proliferative enteropathy
AGID	agar gel immunodiffusion		EPM	equine protozoal myeloencephalitis
AHS	African horse sickness		ERAV	equine rhinitis A virus
AHSV	African horse sickness virus		ERBV	equine rhinitis B virus
AI	antibody index		ETBF	enterotoxigenic *Bacteroides fragilis*
AIDS	aquired immune deficiency syndrome		ExPEC	extraintestinal pathogenic *Escherichia coli*
AST	aspartate aminotransferase		FAT	fluorescent antibody test
BAL	bronchoalveolar lavage		FEI	Fédération Equestre Internationale
BCG	bacillus Calmette–Guérin		FMDV	foot-and-mouth disease virus
BDV	Borna disease virus		γ–GT	γ-glutamyl transferase
bid	twice daily		GALT	gut-associated lymphoid tissue
BoNT	botulinum neurotoxin		GGT	gamma-glutamyltransferase
BPV	bovine papillomavirus		GI	gastrointestinal
BW	body weight		GLDH	glutamate dehydrogenase
CA-MRSA	community-associated methicillin-resistant *Staphylococcus aureus*		HA-MRSA	hospital-associated methicillin-resistant *Staphylococcus aureus*
CDC	complement-dependent cytotoxicity (assay)		H&E	haematoxylin and eosin
CEM	contagious equine metritis		HeV	Hendra virus
CF	complement fixation		HI	haemagglutination inhibition
CFT	complement fixation test		HIV	human immunodeficiency virus
CK	creatine kinase		HJV	Highlands J virus
CNF	cytotoxic necrotizing factor		HYPP	hyperkalaemic periodic paralysis
CNS	central nervous system		IAD	inflammatory airway disease
CPXV	cowpox virus		IFA	immunofluorescence assay
CSF	cerebrospinal fluid		IFAT	indirect fluorescent antibody test
CT	computed tomography		IFT	immunofluorescence test
CTA	cell cytotoxicity assay		IgG(T)	immune globulin G induced by tetanus toxoid
DDSP	dorsal displacement of the soft palate		IM	intramuscular
EAV	equine arteritis virus		IPMA	immunoperoxidase monolayer assay
EcPV	equine papillomavirus		IV	intravenous
EDTA	ethylenediaminetetraacetic acid		JEV	Japanese encephalitis virus
EEV	equine encephalomyelitis virus		KUN	Kunjin virus
EEEV	eastern equine encephalomyelitis virus		LAMP	loop-mediated isothermal amplification
EGS	equine grass sickness		LDH	lactate dehydrogenase
EHV	equine herpesvirus		LPS	lipopolysaccharide
EIA	equine infectious anaemia, enzyme immunoassay		LTR	long terminal repeat
EIAV	equine infectious anaemia virus		MAC	IgM antibody capture
EIPH	exercise-induced pulmonary haemorrhage		MAT	microscopic agglutination test
			MIC	minimum inhibitory concentration
EL	(equine) epizootic lymphangitis		MLST	multilocus sequence typing
(c)ELISA	(competitive) enzyme-linked immunosorbent assay		MPXV	monkeypox virus
EM	electron microscopy		MRI	magnetic resonance imaging

MRSA	methicillin-resistant *Staphylococcus aureus*
MVA	modified vaccinia Ankara
MVE	Murray Valley encephalitis (virus)
NA	North America
NASBA	nucleic acid sequence based amplification
NiV	Nipah virus
NSAID	nonsteroidal anti-inflammatory drug
OPV	orthopoxvirus
PAGE	polyacrylamide gel electrophoresis
PAS	periodic acid-Schiff
PCR	polymerase chain reaction
PDD	proventricular dilatation disease
PEP	post-exposure prophylaxis
PFGE	pulsed-field gel electrophoresis
PFU	plaque-forming unit
PMT	*Pasteurella multocida* toxin
PO	per os
PPIA	pituitary pars intermedia adenoma
PRNT	plaque reduction neutralization test
PRV	pseudorabies virus
RAO	recurrent airway obstruction
RAPD	random amplified polymorphic DNA
RFLP	restriction fragment length polymorphism
RLB	reverse line blot
RRV	Ross River virus
RT	reverse transcription
SC	subcutaneous
SCCmec	staphylococcal cassette chromosome element carrying the *mecA* gene
SCID	severe combined immune deficiency
SDS-PAGE	sodium dodecyl sulphate polyacrylamide gel electrophoresis
SHI	synergistic haemolysis inhibition
sid	once a day
SNT	serum neutralization test
spa	encoding gene of protein A
SRAP	sequence-related amplified polymorphism
SRH	single radial haemolysis
SSCP	single-strand conformation polymorphism
TB	tuberculosis
TCE	transarterial coil embolization
TMP/S	trimethoprim-potentiated sulphonamide
TMP/SDZ	trimethoprim/sulphadiazine
USUV	Usutu virus
VACV	vaccinia virus
VEE	Venezuelan equine encephalomyelitis
VEEV	Venezuelan equine encephalomyelitis virus
VN	virus neutralization
VSIV	vesicular stomatitis Indiana virus
VSNJV	vesicular stomatitis New Jersey virus
VSV	vesicular stomatitis virus
WBC	white blood cell
WEEV	western equine encephalomyelitis virus
WNV	West Nile virus

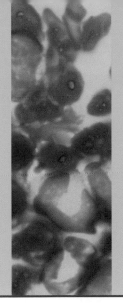

Chapter 1
Bacterial diseases

Anaplasma phagocytophilum: EQUINE ANAPLASMOSIS

Phylum BXII Proteobacteria
Class I Alphaproteobacteria/Order II Rickettsiales/Family II Anaplasmataceae/Genus I *Anaplasma*

Definition/Overview

Equine anaplasmosis is a noncontagious infectious disease of horses caused by *Anaplasma phagocytophilum* (formerly named *Ehrlichia phagocytophila* and *Ehrlichia equi*) identified as emerging in Europe (Vorou *et al.* 2007).

Aetiology

Equine anaplasmosis is caused by the obligate intracellular bacterium *A. phagocytophilum*. Cross-species differences in pathogenicity and ecologically separate strains within this bacterial species appear to exist (Franzén *et al.* 2005, Foley *et al.* 2009), as two unique genetic variants infecting horses in the Czech Republic were identified (Zeman & Jahn 2009). Horses inoculated with the human-derived *A. phagocytophilum* agent results in clinical disease largely indistinguishable from equine anaplasmosis (Madigan *et al.* 1995). The mode of transmission is unknown (but it is most likely a tick), although co-infection with *Borrelia burgdorferi* is attributed to their common vector. Ticks of the *Ixodes ricinus* complex also act as vectors in the spread of *B. burgdorferi* and co-infections of *A. phagocytophilum* and *B. burgdorferi* have been confirmed in horses (Chang *et al.* 2000, Magnarelli *et al.* 2000).

Epidemiology

Equine anaplasmosis was first described in the USA in 1969 (Gribble 1969), and has since been reported in other countries, including Switzerland, Sweden, France, Germany, Italy, the UK, the Czech Republic, and the Netherlands (Gerhards *et al.* 1987, Butler *et al.* 2008, Zeman & Jahn 2009). Most infections develop during the late fall, winter, and spring (Madigan & Gribble 1987). *I. ricinus* is one of the vectors of *A. phagocytophilum* in Europe, in which rates of infection range from 1.9 to 34%. In 1997 only 0.4% of equine blood samples examined were found positive for antibodies to *A. phagocytophilum* in the Latium region (Lillini *et al.* 2006). However, the rate of *A. phagocytophilum* antibody prevalence in healthy horses on USA farms enzootic for equine anaplasmosis can be as high as 10% (Madigan *et al.* 1990), whereas 9.8% of horses with fever of unknown origin tested positive for *A. phagocytophilum* in the Netherlands (Butler *et al.* 2008).

Transmission and propagation of *A. phagocytophilum* occur in large mammals such as horses, cattle, sheep, goats, dogs, and cats. Small mammals and not ticks are the reservoirs of anaplasmosis (Lillini *et al.* 2006). Roe deer are the main reservoir for *A. phagocytophilum* in central Europe and Scandinavia, with a high seroprevalence of about 95% and a variable rate of polymerase chain reaction (PCR)-proven infection ranging from 12.5% in the Czech Republic to 85.6% in Slovenia (Skarphedinsson *et al.* 2005).

The role of migrating birds in long-range tick transfer may be important since the same *A. phagocytophilum* gene sequences were detected in infected ticks on migrating birds and in humans and domestic animals in Sweden (Bjoersdorff *et al.* 2001).

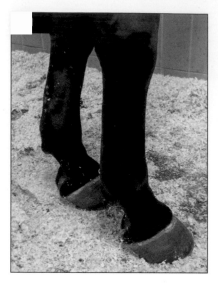

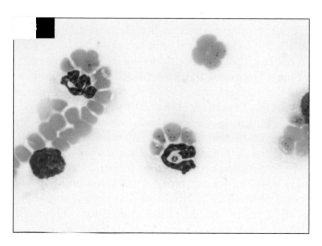

1 Clinical signs seen in equine anaplasmosis include distal limb oedema.

2 Equine anaplasmosis. The integument is irregular due to generalized urticaria or hives (variably sized oedematous bumps) especially apparent on thorax, neck, and proximal extremities. A hypersensitivity reaction is implicated; this feverish horse proved positive for *Anaplasma phagocytophilum*.

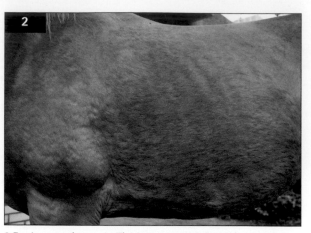

3 Granulocytic anaplasmosis (ehrlichiosis). Equine blood smear. The central neutrophil contains a cytoplasmic ring-shaped inclusion consistent with *Anaplasma phagocytophilum*. Inclusions may be detected in granulocytes and are polymorphic, round, irregular to ring-shaped, ranging from 0.75 to 3.5 µm in diameter. Round to ovoid morulae (2.5–3.5 µm in diameter) are composed of small granules. Single initial bodies measure approximately 0.5 µm in diameter. (May–Grünwald–Giemsa stain.)

Incubation period

The incubation period in experimentally infected horses varies from 1 to 9 days (Stannard *et al.* 1969, Franzén *et al.* 2005). One of two horses receiving high dosage of infective blood (20 × 10⁶ infected neutrophils) died suddenly and unexpectedly 2 days into clinical illness (Franzén *et al.* 2005).

Clinical presentation

Clinical signs include high fever, depression, inappetence, petechiation, icterus, ataxia, rhabdomyolysis, and distal limb oedema (**1**) associated with lymphopenia, neutropenia, thrombocytopenia, and anaemia (Gribble 1969, Madigan & Gribble 1987, Gerhards *et al.* 1987, Madigan 1993, Franzén *et al.* 2005, Butler *et al.* 2008, Hilton *et al.* 2008). Extensive urticaria may also be associated with equine anaplasmosis (**2**). The disease can be self-limiting when untreated, and the clinical signs abated and disappeared without specific treatment 7–14 days after onset of the disease (Gerhards *et al.* 1987, Gribble 1969). By 22 days after infection, in one study, all abnormal signs associated with equine anaplasmosis had fully abated in all surviving horses (Franzén *et al.* 2005). However, infection with *A. phagocytophilum* can persist in the horse for at least 129 days although the continued presence of the organism is not associated with detectable clinical or pathological abnormalities (Franzén *et al.* 2009). It is unclear whether horses younger than 3–4 years of age generally experience less severe clinical disease (Gribble 1969, Madigan & Gribble 1987, Butler *et al.* 2008). Occasionally euthanasia is required because of deterioration despite treatment (Butler *et al.* 2008).

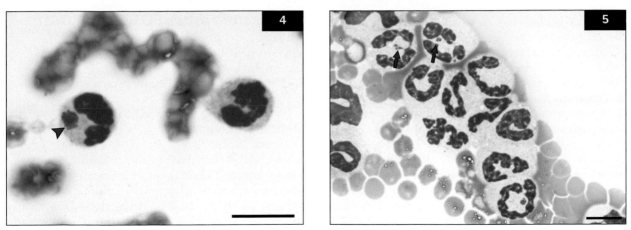

4, 5 Granulocytic anaplasmosis (ehrlichiosis), cytology specimen from a blood smear containing several small bacterial polymorphic cytoplasmic morulae (**4**, arrowhead) or single initial bodies (**5**, arrows) within neutrophils. *Anaplasma phagocytophilum*. (May–Grünwald–Giemsa stain. Bars 10 μm.)

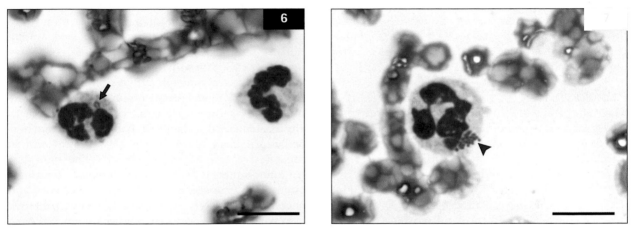

6, 7 Granulocytic anaplasmosis (ehrlichiosis), cytology specimens from a blood smear with infected neutrophils, containing an intracytoplasmic ring form (**6**, arrow) and clustered initial bodies (**7**, arrowhead) of *Anaplasma phagocytophilum*. (May–Grünwald-Giemsa stain. Bars 20 μm.)

Differential diagnosis

Clinical signs are similar to those caused by infections with other pathogens such as *B. burgdorferi*, *B. caballi*, *Theileria equi*, equine herpesvirus, equine infectious anaemia virus, equine arteritis virus, viral encephalitides and Leptospiraceae (Butler *et al.* 2008).

Diagnosis

Diagnosis of equine anaplasmosis is usually based on the detection of characteristic cytoplasmic inclusion bodies in peripheral blood (3–7); either morulae or elementary bodies are seen. In the neutrophilic and occasionally eosinophilic granulocytes on a Wright–Giemsa- or haematoxylin and eosin (H&E)-stained smear of peripheral blood (8) obtained during days 3–5 of fever during peak ehrlichiaemia (Gribble 1969, Madigan & Gribble 1987, Madigan

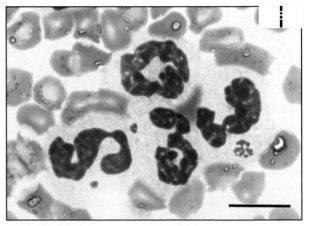

8 Granulocytic anaplasmosis (ehrlichiosis), cytology specimen from a blood smear with three infected neutrophils each containing different forms of *A. phagocytophilum* inclusions. (May–Grünwald–Giemsa stain. Bar 20 μm.)

1993). Morulae (<4 µm in diameter) consist of elementary bodies (<1 µm in diameter). Microscopic interpretation of a buffy coat smear of H&E-stained peripheral blood is a sensitive and practical diagnostic tool for the veterinarian considering possible infection with *A. phagocytophilum* in horses with pyrexia, but some cases may require PCR testing for diagnosis (Butler *et al.* 2008, Hilton *et al.* 2008). In addition, the PCR signal was consistently detected 2–3 days before appearance of clinical signs and persisted 4–9 days beyond abatement of clinical signs, whereas diagnostic inclusion bodies (varying from 0.5–16% of neutrophils) were first noted on average 2.6±1.5 days after onset of fever (Franzén *et al.* 2005).

Horses seroconverted by 12–16 days after inoculation, reaching maximal indirect immunofluorescence assay (IFA) titres (up to 1:5,120) within 3–7 days from when seropositivity was identified (Franzén *et al.* 2005). The indirect fluorescent antibody titre to *A. phagocytophilum* persists for approximately 300 days after inoculation of the organism (Nyindo *et al.* 1978).

Pathology

Macroscopically, oedema of the ventrum and limbs may be present including subcutaneous petechiae. Histologically there is evidence of vasculitides in the affected subcutis (Jubb *et al.* 2007). During fever rickettsial inclusions can be detected in granulocytes of a blood smear, and are polymorphic, round, irregular to ring-shaped, ranging from 0.75 to 3.5 µm in diameter. Round to ovoid morulae (2.5–3.5 µm in diameter) are composed of small granules. Single initial bodies measure approximately 0.5 µm in diameter (Jubb *et al.* 2007).

Management/Treatment

The treatment of choice is oxytetracycline 7 mg/kg BW IV sid for 3–7 days to hasten recovery and alleviate clinical signs (Madigan & Gribble 1987). Clinical immunity in experimental horses was shown to last 2 years (Gribble 1969).

Public health significance

Although five Anaplasmataceae members, including *A. phagocytophilum, E. chaffeensis, E. ewingii, E. canis,* and *Neorickettsia sennetsu* infect humans, only the first three species have been investigated fully. All forms of human ehrlichiosis share many clinical and laboratory manifestations, including fever, headache, myalgia and malaise, thrombocytopenia, leucopenia, and indices of hepatic injury (Dumler *et al.* 2007).

Neorickettsia risticii: POTOMAC HORSE FEVER

Phylum BXII Proteobacteria
Class I Alphaproteobacteria/Order II Rickettsiales/Family II Anaplasmataceae/Genus V *Neorickettsia*

Definition/Overview

Potomac horse fever (also known as equine monocytic ehrlichiosis) is an acute and potentially fatal equine disease associated with depression, anorexia, fever, dehydration, laminitis, abortion, and watery diarrhoea (Holland *et al.* 1985, Rikihisa *et al.* 1985) caused by *Neorickettsia risticii* (formerly *Ehrlichia risticii*).

Aetiology

N. risticii is an obligate intracellular bacterium of the Anaplasmataceae family in the order Rickettsiales. The organism has an unique affinity for monocytes and during the course of the disease and among horses, monocyte counts are variable, but they increase to 13% in some horses (Dutta *et al.* 1988). Characteristic cytoplasmic inclusion bodies (either morulae or elementary bodies) occur in the monocytes from peripheral blood during peak ehrlichiaemia. Morulae (less than 4 µm in diameter) consist of elementary bodies (less than 1 µm in diameter) (Holland *et al.* 1985). The complete genome sequence of *N. risticii* consists of a single circular chromosome of 879, 977 base pairs and encodes 38 RNA species and 898 proteins. Comparison with its closely related human pathogen *N. sennetsu* showed that 758 (88.2%) of protein-coding genes are conserved between *N. risticii* and *N. sennetsu* (Lin *et al.* 2009).

Epidemiology

It has been shown that the trematode *Acanthatrium oregonense* is a natural reservoir and probably a vector of *N. risticii*, as *N. risticii* is vertically transmitted (from adult to egg) in *A. oregonense* (Gibson *et al.* 2005). In addition, caddisflies were reported as second intermediate hosts of *N. risticii*-infected trematodes by carrying infected metacercariae (Madigan *et al.* 2000, Mott *et al.* 2002). Furthermore, *N. risticii* can also be transmitted horizontally from trematode to bats (Gibson *et al.* 2005). *N. risticii* has not been reported outside the USA.

Incubation period

The incubation period varies from 3 to 9 days. Major clinical and haematological features of induced *N. risticii* infection are biphasic increase in rectal temperature (with peak increases to 38.9°C and 39.3°C on post-inoculation days 5 and 12, respectively), depression, anorexia, decreased white blood cell (WBC) count (maximal decrease of 47% on post-inoculation day 12), and diarrhoea from post-inoculation days 14 to 18. Increased WBC count was an inconsistent feature with a maximal increase of 52% on post-inoculation day 20 (Dutta *et al.* 1988).

Clinical presentation

Under field conditions, *N. risticii* infection is characterized by increased rectal temperature, anorexia, depression, leucopenia, and then diarrhoea (**9**).

Occasionally horses develop profound ileus and severe colic (**10**) (Whitlock & Palmer 1986, Palmer *et al.* 1986). Diarrhoea developed in 73% of horses and mortality was 9% (Dutta *et al.* 1988). Laminitis and limb oedema are often seen as a sequel to *N. risticii* infection, and mortality is 10–20% (Whitlock & Palmer 1986). However, clinically undetectable infections exist (Ristic *et al.* 1986). *In utero* infection (Dawson *et al.* 1987) has also been reported as well as abortion (81 days post-infection) with recovery of the organism from the bone marrow of a fetus on the 200th day of gestation (Long *et al.* 1992).

Differential diagnosis

The differential diagnosis includes various causes of acute diarrhoea (see p. 263).

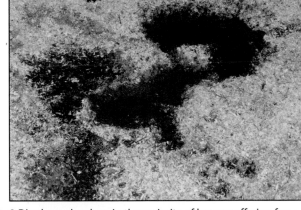

9 Diarrhoea develops in the majority of horses suffering from Potomac horse fever.

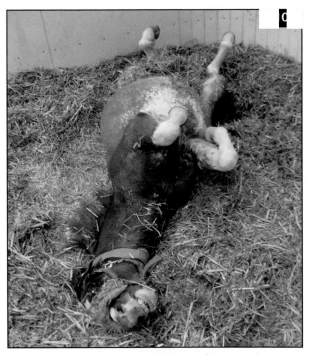

10 Colic can be noticed as an initial sign of Potomac horse fever.

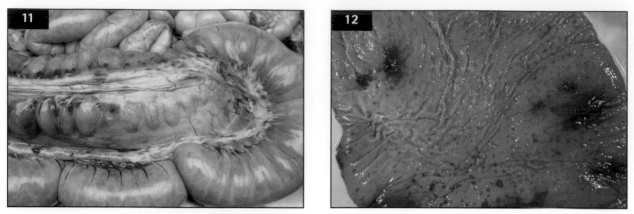

11, 12 Ulcerative colitis. The colon is severely congested with prominent distended mesocolonic lymph vessels (**11**). The mucosa is thickened and oedematous with multiple mucosal ulcerations and haemorrhages (**12**). These lesions may be indicative of Potomac horse fever.

Diagnosis

Using mice inoculation, *N. risticii* was first detected in the blood on post-inoculation day 10, peaked on post-inoculation day 19, and was not detectable after post-inoculation day 24. The *N. risticii* titre was maximal during the peak increase in rectal temperature, and infected horses seroconvert as detected by IFA assay and enzyme-linked immunosorbent assay (ELISA) with antibody titres between 1:160–1:640 and >1:5,000, respectively (Dutta *et al.* 1988).

For diagnosis, preference is given to culture or PCR. PCR was successfully used to detect the organism directly from the blood buffy coat cells of infected horses. It was estimated that buffy coat cells obtained from less than 1 ml of blood from infected horses was adequate for the detection of *N. risticii* (Biswas *et al.* 1991). *N. risticii* was detected in the blood by nested PCR in 81% of the culture-positive clinical specimens, indicating that the nested PCR is as sensitive as culture for detecting infection with *N. risticii* (Mott *et al.* 1997). However, characteristic cytoplasmic inclusion bodies (either morulae or elementary bodies) can be visualized in the monocytes on a Wright–Giemsa- or H&E-stained smear of peripheral blood obtained during peak ehrlichiaemia (Holland *et al.* 1985).

Pathology

Pathological features usually observed are mild to moderate typhlitis and colitis, with congested and ulcerated mucosae (**11, 12**), most prominent in the right dorsal colon, and mesenteric lymphadenopathy. Similar less grave lesions may be present in the stomach and small intestine. Subcutaneous oedema and laminitis may be accompanying gross features. Microscopically, intestinal lesions are composed of mucosal congestion and haemorrhages with superficial epithelial erosive to necrotizing lesions and fibrin deposits. Furthermore, crypt abscesses and mixed inflammatory hypercellularity of the lamina propria may be present. Rickettsial clustered organisms of <1 μm can be identified in special silver stains within the apical cytoplasm of cryptal enterocytes and in macrophages in the lamina propria (Jubb *et al.* 2007).

Management/Treatment

The only effective treatment is the administration of tetracycline in the early stages of the disease as there is no truly effective vaccine available (Dutta *et al.* 1998, Rikihisa *et al.* 2004). IV administration of oxytetracycline (6.6 mg/kg BW sid for 5 days) is an effective treatment when given early in the clinical course (Palmer *et al.* 1992). There is protective immunity against *N. risticii* infection, as evidenced by clinical resistence to reinfection for as long as 20 months after the initial infection (Palmer *et al.* 1990). Despite treatment with oxytetracycline (6.6 mg/kg BW bid IV beginning 14 hours before inoculation and continuing for 10 days) before inoculation, the antigenic stimulation was sufficient to induce such protective immunity (Palmer *et al.* 1988).

Public health significance

Not convincing as yet.

Bartonella henselae: BARTONELLOSIS

Phylum BXII Proteobacteria
Class I Alphaproteobacteria/Order VI
Rhizobiales/Family III Bartonellaceae/Genus I
Bartonella

Definition/Overview

Bartonella spp. are associated with an extended animal host range (including equines) and are identified as emerging in Europe (Vorou *et al.* 2007).

Aetiology

Bartonella (formerly *Rochalimaea* species) spp. are members of the α-proteobacteria group that includes the genera *Rickettsia, Ehrlichia, Brucella,* and the plant pathogen *Agrobacterium tumefaciens*. They are fastidious, Gram-negative short-to-spirillar bacteria that occur in the blood of man and other mammals; they are usually vector borne but can also be transmitted by animal scratches and bites from haematophagous insects, such as sandflies (*Lutzomyia* spp.), fleas, and lice (Maguiña *et al.* 2009).

Incubation period

Not established in the equine species yet.

Clinical presentation

B. henselae was isolated from the blood of a horse with chronic arthropathy and a horse with presumptive vasculitis (Jones *et al.* 2008).

Diagnosis

Blood samples can be tested for the presence of *Bartonella* spp. by a combination of multiplex real-time PCR and enrichment culture technique (Jones *et al.* 2008).

Pathology

B. henselae infection caused abortion of a foal exhibiting necrosis and vasculitis in multiple tissues, with intralesional Gram-negative short-to-spirillar bacteria (Johnson *et al.* 2009).

Management/Treatment

Human *Bartonella* isolates are highly susceptible to antibiotics, including most of the beta-lactams, the aminoglycosides, the macrolides, doxycycline, and rifampicin (rifampin) (Maurin *et al.* 1995).

Public health significance

The bartonelloses of medical importance comprise Carrión's disease, trench fever, cat-scratch disease, bacillary angiomatosis, and peliosis hepatis. The *Bartonella* spp. are considered emerging human pathogens (Maguiña *et al.* 2009). *B. henselae* has been identified as the causative agent of cat-scratch disease. On the other hand *B. quintana* which causes the body lice-mediated trench fever in humans and had no known animal reservoir, was shown to infect a domestic cat (Vorou *et al.* 2007). Furthermore, *Bartonella* spp. were first recognized to cause endocarditis in humans in 1993 when cases caused by *B. quintana, B. elizabethae,* and *B. henselae* were reported. Since the first isolation of *B. vinsonii* subsp. *berkhoffii* from a dog with endocarditis, this organism has emerged as an important pathogen in dogs and an emerging pathogen in people (Chomel *et al.* 2009).

Brucella spp.: BRUCELLOSIS

Phylum BXVII Spirochaetes
Class I Alphaproteobacteria/Order VI
Rhizobiales/Family IV Brucellaceae/Genus I
Brucella: Gram-negative aerobic rods and cocci

Definition/Overview

Coincidental infection in horses caused by various bacteria of the genus *Brucella* is especially associated with abortion and fistulous withers. Brucellosis has important public health significance and is a reportable disease.

Aetiology

Brucellae are facultative intracellular, Gram-negative, partially acid-fast coccobacilli. The bacterium is 0.5–0.7 µm in diameter and 0.6-1.5 µm in length. They are oxidase, catalase, and urease positive. *Brucella* species considered important agents of human disease include *B. melitensis*, *B. abortus*, and *B. suis* (Ekers 1978, Mohandas *et al.* 2009). Isolation of *B. suis* biotype 1 (Cook & Kingston 1988) and *B. abortus* biotypes 1, 2, and 4 (Ekers 1978, Carrigan *et al.* 1987) was reported from horses.

Epidemiology

The epidemiology of human brucellosis, the commonest zoonotic infection worldwide, has drastically changed over the past decade because of various sanitary, socioeconomic, and political reasons, together with the evolution of international travel. Several areas traditionally considered to be endemic, such as France, Israel, and most of Latin America, have achieved control of the disease. On the other hand, new foci of human brucellosis have emerged, particularly in central Asia, while the situation in certain countries of the near East (e.g. Syria) is rapidly worsening (Pappas *et al.* 2006). *B. melitensis* biovar 3 is the most commonly isolated species from animals in Egypt, Jordan, Israel, Tunisia, and Turkey (Refai 2002). The seroprevalence of *Brucella* species among horses in Jordan was 1% and 8.5% in donkeys. Contact with small ruminant herds with a history of brucellosis was associated with a high odds ratio (20 and 81 for horses and donkeys, respectively) for *Brucella* seropositivity in equids (Abo-Shehada 2009). It has been suggested that equines with a seroprevalence rate of 0.2% are not a reservoir of brucellosis and do not play an important role in the epidemiological patterns of this disease in northeastern Mexico (Acosta-González *et al.* 2006), with horses in Latin America mainly infected with *B. abortus* and *B. suis* (Lucero *et al.* 2008).

In horses admitted for evaluation of fistulous withers, 38% tested for antibody to *B. abortus* were seropositive. Horses that tested seropositive were significantly more likely to have been pastured with cattle that were seropositive for *B. abortus*, and were also significantly more likely to have had radiographic evidence of vertebral osteomyelitis than were horses that tested seronegative (Cohen *et al.* 1992).

Pathophysiology

These bacteria do not produce classical virulence factors, and their capacity to survive and replicate successfully within a variety of host cells underlies their pathogenicity. Extensive replication of the Brucellae in placental trophoblasts is associated with reproductive tract pathology in natural hosts, and prolonged persistence in macrophages leads to the chronic infections that are a hallmark of brucellosis in both natural hosts and humans (Roop *et al.* 2009).

Incubation period

Experimental intraconjunctival infection of horses with *B. abortus* revealed no appreciable clinical signs up to 30 months except mild pyrexia (MacMillan *et al.* 1982, MacMillan & Cockrem 1986).

Clinical presentation

The clinical signs of the disease are variable, but include fistulous withers (Cohen *et al.* 1992), abortion (Shortridge 1967, McCaughey & Kerr 1967), arthritis (Carrigan *et al.* 1987), and vertebral osteomyelitis (Collins *et al.* 1971).

Differential diagnosis

The differential diagnosis predominantly includes various causes of abortion and fever (see p. 263).

Diagnosis

The diagnosis is based on a positive culture of the bacterium and/or seroconversion as assessed by a complement fixation test eventually combined with a positive reaction to the intradermal skin test. However, an intradermal skin test was positive in infected adults only, and negative in all foals tested (MacMillan & Cockrem 1986).

Antibodies to *B. abortus* became detectable from the second week after inoculation. Titres in the serum agglutination and complement fixation tests declined substantially after 6–8 weeks but reactions to the Coombs antiglobulin, 2-mercaptoethanol, and immunodiffusion tests were maintained (MacMillan *et al.* 1982). Of interest, genus-specific real-time PCR assays, e.g. based on the bcsp31 gene, will lead to an early diagnosis but for the purpose of epidemiological surveillance a species-specific real-time PCR deriving from the conventional AMOS (AbortusMelitensisOvisSuis)-PCR is necessary (Al Dahouk *et al*. 2004).

Pathology

Post-mortem examination of a foal suffering from brucellosis disclosed granulomatous lesions in the lungs, liver, testes, and metatarsophalangeal synovial membranes. *B. abortus* identical with strain 544 was recovered from lymphoid and other tissues (MacMillan & Cockrem 1986).

Management/Treatment

Horses with a tentative diagnosis of brucellosis should be isolated to prevent possible human exposure. Treatment should not be attempted as the pathogen has important public health significance and brucellosis is a reportable disease. The most commonly used veterinary vaccines are *B. abortus* S19 and *B. melitensis* Rev.1 vaccines. *B. abortus* RB51 vaccine is used in some countries on a small scale. Vaccination is limited to cattle and small ruminants (Refai 2002). Five horses that were seropositive for *B. abortus* were administered strain 19 *Brucella* vaccine SC (n = 1) or IV (n = 4). The horse treated by SC injection of vaccine improved during hospitalization, but was lost to follow-up evaluation. Three of four horses treated by IV injection died, but one horse recovered within 4 weeks of treatment (Cohen *et al*. 1992).

Public health significance

Brucellosis has important public health significance. Brucellosis, especially caused by *B. melitensis* particularly biovar 3 (Refai 2002), remains one of the most common zoonotic diseases worldwide with more than 500,000 human cases reported annually (Seleem *et al*. 2010). Involvement of the musculoskeletal system is the most common complication of human brucellosis, while neurobrucellosis (like meningitis) and endocarditis are life-threatening complications (Ranjbar *et al*. 2009).

Cardiovascular complications occur in <2%, but account for most of the mortality. *Brucella* endocarditis usually involves normal native aortic valves in 75% of cases. A combination of antibiotics and valve replacement is the most acceptable treatment (Mohandas *et al*. 2009). Cutaneous manifestations including erythema nodosum are not specific and affect 1–14% of patients with brucellosis (Mazokopakis *et al*. 2003). Uveitis is also seen (Rolando *et al*. 2009). The standard treatment for acute and chronic brucellosis is a combination of doxycycline with a second drug such as rifampicin or gentamicin, in order to treat and to prevent complications and relapse (Sakran *et al*. 2006).

Burkholderia mallei: 'GLANDERS'

Phylum BXVII Spirochaetes
Class II Betaproteobacteria/Family
Burkholderiaceae/Genus I *Burkholderia*: Gram-
negative aerobic rods and cocci

Definition/Overview

Glanders is an ancient, highly fatal, and usually chronic respiratory disease of solipeds caused by *Burkholderia mallei* (formerly *Pseudomonas mallei*) with humans being accidental hosts. The diagnosis is based on the presence of characteristic stellate scars in the nasal septum and a positive reaction to the mallein test, combined with a positive culture of *B. mallei*. Human infections are often fatal if untreated.

Aetiology

B. mallei is a facultative rod-shaped Gram-negative nonspore-forming, nonmotile, intracellular pathogen that can invade, survive, and replicate in epithelial and phagocytic cell lines (Ribot & Ulrich 2006). It is an obligate animal pathogen whose natural hosts are horses, donkeys, and mules, but infections can also occur in felines, camels, and goats. Virulence in *B. mallei* is multifactorial and several virulence determinants have been identified and characterized (Schell *et al*. 2007). Seventeen distinct ribotypes were identified from human and equine infections (Harvey & Minter 2005).

Epidemiology

Glanders is endemic in Africa, Asia, the Middle East, and Central and South America. Carriers that have made an apparent recovery from the disease are the most important source of infection, as the pathogen does not survive for more than 6 weeks outside the host (Lehavi *et al*. 2002).

Pathophysiology

Equines are generally infected orally (Schell *et al*. 2007). Following penetration of the mucosae, the pathogen is spread via the lymphatic tissues.

Incubation period

The incubation period varies from 1 to 2 days following intratracheal deposition, with rectal temperatures increased to above 40°C (Lopez *et al*. 2003).

Clinical presentation

Clinical signs include febrile episodes, cough, blood-encrusted material on nostrils, inflammatory nodules and ulcers developed in the nasal passages with a sticky yellow discharge, characteristic stellate scars in the nasal septum, purulent nasal discharge, enlargement of submaxillary lymph nodes, chronic lymphangitis, skin abscessation, progressive debility, orchitis, and dyspnoea associated with interstitial pneumonia. Furthermore, apparent neurological degeneration is seen in acute glanders (Lopez *et al*. 2003). Life expectancy was judged likely to have been less than 12 hours in *B. mallei* inoculated horses due to subsequent pulmonary oedema (Lopez *et al*. 2003).

Differential diagnosis

The differential diagnosis includes various causes of fever and dyspnoea (see p. 262).

Diagnosis

The presence of stellate scars in the nasal septum is regarded as pathognomonic. *B. mallei* can be cultured easily from purulent nasal discharge and the complement fixation test can be used for serology. Furthermore, the mallein test can also be used to identify infected horses; purulent exudate in the eye associated with blepharospasm of a glanderous animal 24–48 hours following subconjunctival inoculation is regarded as a positive test result. Alternatively, the intracutaneous mallein test can be used with an increase in rectal temperature and a swelling at the point of injection regarded as a positive test result (Arun *et al*. 1999). When tested comparatively with Dutch PPD mallein as standard, trichloroacetic acid-precipitated proteins were comparable to Dutch PPD mallein in potency and innocuity, whereas ammonium sulphate-precipitated proteins elicited nonspecific reactions (Verma *et al*. 1994).

Competitive enzyme-linked immunosorbent assay (cELISA) test specificity for *B. mallei* was 99%. Concordance and kappa value between the complement fixation (CF) and the cELISA procedures for the serodiagnosis of *B. mallei* infection in experimentally exposed horses were 70% and 0.44, respectively (Katz *et al*. 2000). The cELISA offers the possibility for automatization, can be applied to noncomplement fixing sera, and used for various host species although the complement fixation test (CFT) is internationally mandatory for testing of equine sera for the absence of glanders to date (Sprague *et al*. 2009).

13 Hypopyon, suppurative uveitis. The anterior eye chamber is blurred with specks of a fibrinopurulent exudate. From this foal *Burkholderia cepacia* was isolated. Members of the *B. cepacia* complex are regarded as opportunistic pathogens.

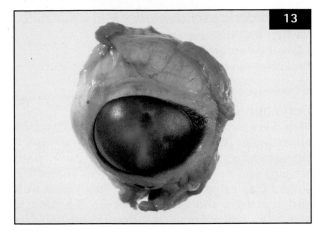

Hydrolysis probe-based real-time PCR using the uneven distribution of type III secretion system genes afforded considerable improvements in the specificity and rapidity of the diagnosis of *B. pseudomallei*, *B. mallei*, and *B. thailandensis*, and allows rapid discrimination from opportunistic pathogens such as members of the *B. cepacia* complex (**13**), that routine diagnostic laboratories are more likely to encounter (Thibault *et al.* 2004).

Pathology

B. mallei infection results in pyogranulomatous and necrotic pulmonary nodules, and ulcerative nodular skin and respiratory mucosal lesions with characteristic white stellate scars in the nasal septum. Histologically, lung lesions comprise liquefactive necrosis including neutrophils and surrounding epithelioid macrophages and fibrosis. The dermal disease of ulcerations including lymphangitis is named 'farcy' (Jubb *et al.* 2007). Remarkably, *Streptococcus equi* subsp. *zooepidemicus* was isolated from the brain of all *B. mallei* inoculated horses (Lopez *et al.* 2003).

Management/Treatment

Horses with a tentative diagnosis of glanders should be isolated to prevent possible human exposure. Treatment should not be attempted as the pathogen has important public health significance and glanders is a reportable disease.

Public health significance

Humans are accidental hosts of *B. mallei* and the majority of cases have been the result of occupational contact with infected horses. Whereas equines are generally infected orally, the primary route of infection in humans is contamination of skin abrasions or mucous membranes with nasal discharge or skin lesion exudate from an infected animal (Schell *et al.* 2007). Person-to-person spread of *B. mallei* is extremely rare. In humans, glanders is characterized by initial onset of fever, rigors and malaise, culminating in a rapid onset of pneumonia, bacteraemia, pustules and abscesses, leading to death in 7–10 days without antibiotic treatment. The course of infection is dependent on the route of exposure. Direct contact with the skin can lead to a localized cutaneous infection. Inhalation of aerosol or dust containing *B. mallei* can lead to septicaemic, pulmonary, or chronic infections of the muscle, liver, and spleen. The disease has a 95% case fatality rate for untreated septicaemia infections and a 50% case fatality rate in antibiotic-treated individuals (Mandell *et al.* 1995). *Burkholderia* infections are difficult to treat with antibiotics and no vaccine exists (Whitlock *et al.* 2007).

Burkholderia pseudomallei: MELIOIDOSIS

Phylum BXVII Spirochaetes
Class II Betaproteobacteria/Family
Burkholderiaceae/Genus I *Burkholderia*: Gram-negative aerobic rods and cocci

Definition/Overview

Melioidosis is a rare disease caused by *Burkholderia pseudomallei* (formerly *Pseudomonas pseudomallei*) characterized by an intracellular life cycle. Both humans and animals (including birds, crocodiles, and kangaroos) are susceptible to melioidosis with both latency and a wide range of clinical manifestations. Some species may develop melioidosis only if immunocompromised. Sheep, goats, and horses are particularly susceptible, but zoonotic transmission to humans is extremely unusual (Neubauer *et al.* 1997, Choy *et al.* 2000). Melioidosis has important public health significance and is a reportable disease.

Aetiology

B. pseudomallei is a Gram-negative, bipolar-staining, pleomorphic, motile bacillus, which is principally an environmental saprophyte responsible for melioidosis.

Epidemiology

This saprophyte inhabitant of telluric environments is mainly encountered in southeast Asia and northern Australia, but is sporadically isolated in subtropical and temperate countries (White 2003). Melioidosis has become an increasingly important disease in endemic areas such as northern Thailand and Australia (Currie *et al.* 2000*a*). In endemic areas, the positive rates of antibodies against *B. pseudomallei* in humans, horses, oxen, and pigs were 4–15%, 9–18%, 7–33%, and 35%, respectively (Li *et al.* 1994).

Pathophysiology

Following ingestion via contaminated soil or faeces, a diverse assortment of virulence factors (quorum sensing, type III secretion system, lipopolysaccharide and other surface polysaccharides) allows *B. pseudomallei* to become an effective opportunistic pathogen; its intracellular life cycle also allows it to avoid or subvert the host immune system (Adler *et al.* 2009, Wiersinga & van der Poll 2009). The BoaA and BoaB genes specify adhesins that mediate adherence to epithelial cells of the human respiratory tract. The BoaA gene product is shared by *B. pseudomallei* and *B. mallei*, whereas BoaB appears to be a *B. pseudomallei*-specific adherence factor (Balder *et al.* 2010).

Incubation period

This is not established in the equine species yet. The incubation period in man from defined inoculating events was previously ascertained as 1–21 (mean 9) days (Currie *et al.* 2000*b*).

Clinical presentation

Clinical signs include fever, septicaemia, oedema, colic, diarrhoea, and lymphangitis of the legs. A case of acute meningoencephalomyelitis caused by infection with *B. pseudomallei* has been described associated with inability to stand, opisthotonus, facial paralysis (**14**) and nystagmus, rapidly progressing to violent struggling (Ladds *et al.* 1981).

Differential diagnosis

The differential diagnosis includes various causes of internal abscessation (without characteristic stellate scars in the nasal septum as seen in *B. mallei*) (see p. 262). Listeriosis should be considered in a case of meningitis.

Diagnosis

B. pseudomallei can be cultured easily from purulent nasal discharge. The diagnosis is based on a positive reaction to the mallein test combined with a positive culture.

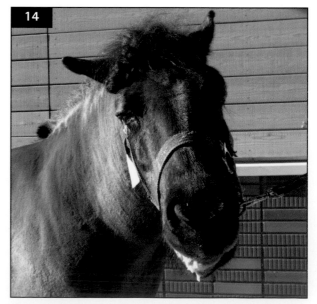

14 Facial paralysis is associated with equine melioidosis.

Hydrolysis probe-based real-time PCR methods using the uneven distribution of type III secretion system genes afford considerable improvements in the specificity and rapidity of the diagnosis of *B. pseudomallei*, *B. mallei*, and *B. thailandensis* and allow rapid discrimination from opportunistic pathogens, such as members of the *B. cepacia* complex (**15, 16**), that routine diagnostic laboratories are more likely to encounter (Thibault *et al.* 2004).

Pathology

Multiple abscesses in most organs are characteristic of the disease. The encapsulated nodules with caseous centres are composed of necrosis, neutrophils, lymphocytes, and epithelioid macrophages. In a case of acute meningoencephalomyelitis gross examination revealed malacia and haemorrhage in the medulla oblongata and adjacent spinal cord. Microscopically there were disseminated focal neutrophilic accumulations in affected areas, perivascular cuffing with mononuclear cells and lymphocytes, and marked oedema. Intracellular bacteria were identified in sections stained by the Giemsa method (Ladds *et al.* 1981).

Management/Treatment

Horses with a tentative diagnosis of melioidosis should be isolated to prevent possible human exposure. Treatment should not be attempted as the disease has important public health significance. Furthermore, the ubiquitous bacterium is characterized by remarkable insensitivity to antimicrobial drugs. For instance, *B. pseudomallei* is intrinsically resistant to aminoglycosides and macrolides, mostly due to AmrAB-OprA efflux pump expression (Trunck *et al.* 2009).

Immunization with heat-inactivated *B. pseudomallei* cells provided the highest levels of protection against either melioidosis or glanders, indicating longer-term potential for heat-inactivated bacteria to be developed as vaccines against melioidosis and glanders (Sarkar-Tyson *et al.* 2009).

Public health significance

Melioidosis has important public health significance and is a reportable disease. It is a life-threatening disease that is mainly acquired through skin inoculation or pulmonary contamination, although other routes have been documented (Neubauer *et al.* 1997). Primary skin melioidosis occurred in 12% of human patients. Secondary skin melioidosis (multiple pustules from haematogenous spread) was present in 2%. Patients with primary skin melioidosis were more likely to have chronic presentations (duration of a minimum of 2 months)

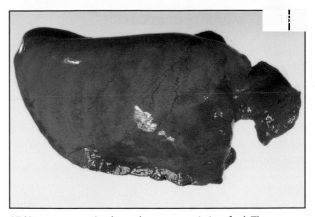

15 Necrosuppurative bronchopneumonia in a foal. The cranioventral lung field is hyperaemic, consolidated, and firm. Lesions resemble pulmonary lesions in melioidosis. From this foal *Burkholderia cepacia* was isolated.

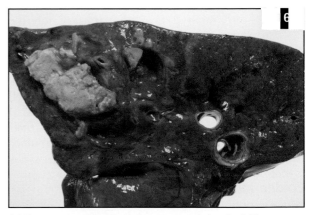

16 Necrosuppurative bronchopneumonia in a foal. The cranioventral lung lobes show on cut section a well-delineated hyperaemic area enclosing pale yellow, variably sized, caseating, coagulative, necrosuppurative sequesters of remnant pulmonary parenchyma. Lesions resemble pulmonary lesions in melioidosis. From this foal *Burkholderia cepacia* was isolated.

(Gibney *et al.* 2008). Severe septicaemia secondary to melioidosis carries a high mortality. Although melioidosis can involve most tissues and organs, pericardial involvement is rare (De Keulenaer *et al.* 2008). Of human cases, 46% were bacteraemic and 19% died (Currie *et al.* 2000*a*).

Bordetella bronchiseptica

Phylum BXVII Spirochaetes
Class II Betaproteobacteria/Family
III Alcanigenaceae/Genus III *Bordetella*: Gram-negative aerobic rods and cocci

Definition/Overview

The opportunistic bacterium *Bordetella bronchiseptica* is a rare cause of acute respiratory disease and abortion/infertility.

Aetiology

Pasteurellaceae are Gram-negative bacteria with an important role as primary or opportunistic, mainly respiratory, pathogens in domestic and wild animals. Some species of Pasteurellaceae cause severe diseases with high economic losses in commercial animal husbandry and are of great diagnostic concern (Dousse *et al.* 2008). Sixteen distinct ribotypes were identified in *B. bronchiseptica* strains (Register *et al.* 1997). Four main types of variation of the *B. bronchiseptica* lipopolysaccharide (LPS) are apparent: (1) heterogeneity of the core, (2) presence or absence of 0-chains, (3) differences at the level of the hinge region between the 0-chain and the core, and (4) differences in the association with other cell surface constituents. Isolates from different animal species did not show significant differences in their patterns of reactivity with monoclonal antibodies (LeBlay *et al.* 1997).

Epidemiology

Glucose nonfermenting Gram-negative bacilli have been recognized as opportunistic pathogens of humans. The most common veterinary glucose nonfermenting Gram-negative bacilli were *Pseudomonas aeruginosa*, *Acinetobacter calcoaceticus*, *B. bronchiseptica*, and *Pseudomonas pseudoalcaligenes*. Of all clinical veterinary specimens submitted for cultures, 10% contained nonfermenters (Mathewson & Simpson 1982). *B. bronchiseptica* was isolated from bronchial lavage specimens in distal respiratory tract disease (nasal discharge, cough, pneumonia) in 13% of foals (1–8 months old) (Hoffman *et al.* 1993).

Pathophysiology

Either *B. bronchiseptica* does not persist inside animals or susceptible animals possess specific receptors for smooth-type LPSs, in contrast to man (Le Blay *et al.* 1997).

Incubation period

Not established in the equine species yet.

Clinical presentation

Clinical presentation includes respiratory disease in foals (**17**) (Koehne *et al.* 1981), coughing in Thoroughbred racehorses (Christley *et al.* 2001), bronchopneumonia (Saxegaard *et al.* 1971), abortion (Mohan & Obwolo 1991), and infertility (Mather *et al.* 1973). *B. parapertussis* did not grow in tracheobronchial washing from a horse (Porter & Wardlaw 1994).

Differential diagnosis

The differential diagnosis includes various causes of fever and dyspnoea (see p. 262).

Diagnosis

Diagnosis primarily depends on culture of the bacterium from tracheobronchial washing samples combined with clinical signs. Analysis of tracheobronchial washing samples for known *Bordetella* nutrients revealed concentrations of amino acids and nicotinic acid averaging 0.35 mM and 0.56 μg/ml, respectively (Porter & Wardlaw 1994).

Pathology

Common lesions caused by *B. bronchiseptica* include a catarrhal to suppurative bronchopneumonia and a (sero)fibrinous pleuropneumonia. These are usually opportunistic secondary infections preceded by viral infections in juvenile animals.

Management/Treatment

Treatment of diseased animals is supportive and specific treatment should be based on *in-vitro* antimicrobial susceptibility testing.

Public health significance

The absence of smooth-type LPSs appears to be rather frequent in human isolates, since long-chain LPSs were detectable in only 52% of human isolates, whereas 94% of animal isolates contained molecules of that type (Le Blay *et al.* 1997). *B. bronchiseptica* might have some public health significance and its zoonotic risk should be minimized.

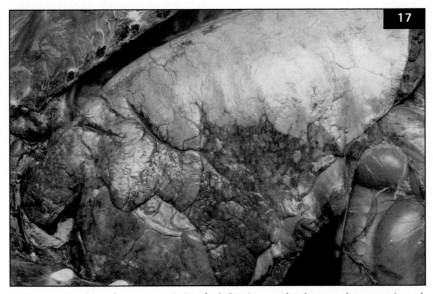

17 Suppurative bronchopneumonia in a foal. Cranioventral pulmonary hyperaemia and consolidation. A primary viral respiratory infection (herpesvirus, influenza virus) can be complicated by opportunistic bacteria like *Streptococcus* spp., *Escherichia coli*, *Klebsiella pneumoniae*, *Rhodococcus equi*, and *Bordetella bronchiseptica*.

Taylorella equigenitalis: CONTAGIOUS EQUINE METRITIS

Phylum BXVII Spirochaetes
Class II Betaproteobacteria/Family III
Alcanigenaceae/Genus XI *Taylorella*: Gram-negative, microaerophilic, fastidious slow-growing coccobacilli

Definition/Overview

Contagious equine metritis (CEM) caused by *Taylorella equigenitalis* is a highly contagious disease that is transmitted venereally. The carrier state occurs in the mare and the stallion and carrier animals are frequently the source of infection for new outbreaks (Timoney 1996).

Aetiology

T. equigenitalis is a Gram-negative, microaerophilic, fastidious slow-growing coccobacillus with streptomycin-sensitive and -resistant biotypes (Timoney 1996). Isolates of *T. equigenitalis* obtained from European horses analysed by pulsed-field gel electrophoresis (PFGE) were classified into 18 genotypes (Kagawa *et al.* 2001). High sequence similarity (99.5% or more) was observed throughout isolates from Japan, Australia, and France, except from nucleotide positions 138 to 501 where substitutions and deletions were noted (Matsuda *et al.* 2006). A phylogenetic analysis revealed a position of *T. equigenitalis* in the beta subclass of the class Proteobacteria apart from the position of *Haemophilus influenzae*, which belongs in the gamma subclass of Proteobacteria. A close phylogenetic relationship among *T. equigenitalis*, *Alcaligenes xylosoxidans*, and *Bordetella bronchiseptica* was detected (Bleumink-Pluym *et al.* 1993). Lipopolysaccharide O-PS could be a specific marker for identification and differentiation of *T. equigenitalis* and *T. asinigenitalis*, and provide the basis for the development of specific detection assays for *T. equigenitalis* (Brooks *et al.* 2010).

Epidemiology

CEM has given rise to international concern since it was first recognized as a novel venereal disease of equids in 1977. The first known outbreak of CEM in the USA was in Kentucky in 1978. For some time none of the subsequent outbreaks impacted significantly on the horse industry. That changed dramatically in 2008, however, after the discovery of some 1,005 exposed and carrier stallions and mares in 48 states. Neither clinical evidence of CEM nor decreased pregnancy rates were reportedly a feature in infected or exposed mares. In light of these findings, the question arose as to whether or not the considerable expense incurred in investigating the latest CEM occurrence was warranted (Timoney 2011). Among stallions examined in Slovenia, 92% were negative to *T. equigenitalis* by either PCR or culture (Zdovc *et al.* 2005). In comparison, from 1999 through 2001, four out of 120 imported European stallions tested positive for CEM at a quarantine facility in Darlington, MD, USA (Kristula & Smith 2004). Samples from mares with no clinical signs of CEM submitted for conventional culture were negative for *T. equigenitalis*, but in the PCR assay 49% were positive for *Taylorella* DNA. The high incidence of *Taylorella* in horse populations without apparent clinical signs of CEM, the occurrence of incidental clinical cases, and the known variability between strains indicate that *Taylorella* was endemic in the horse population (Parlevliet *et al.* 1997).

Pathophysiology

CEM is transmitted by direct or indirect venereal contact. The invasiveness of *T. equigenitalis* strains seemed to be associated with the contagiousness of the infection, whereas the replication index seemed to be associated with the severity of the symptoms of contagious equine metritis (Bleumink-Pluym *et al.* 1996).

Incubation period

Horses challenged with *T. equigenitalis* showed seroconversion from day 11 post-inoculation (Katz & Geer 2001).

Clinical presentation

CEM can be the cause of short-term infertility sometimes associated with mucopurulent discharge and, very rarely, abortion in mares (Fontijne *et al.* 1989). Unlike the mare, stallions exposed to *T. equigenitalis* do not develop clinical signs of disease (Timoney 1996). It has been concluded that *T. equigenitalis* is of limited significance in horse breeding (Parlevliet *et al.* 1997).

Differential diagnosis

Atypical (donkey-origin) *Taylorella* spp. infections should be considered as a differential diagnosis of equine infertility in mares (Katz *et al.* 2000). *T. asinigenitalis*, resembling *T. equigenitalis*, was recently isolated from the urethral fossa, urethra, and penile sheath of a 3-year-old stallion of the Ardennes breed when it was routinely tested for CEM. However, the colony appearance, the slow growth rate, and the results in the API ZYM test differed slightly from those of *T. equigenitalis*. Sequence analysis of 16S rRNA genes was shown to be a reliable tool for differentiation of donkey-related *T. asinigenitalis* from *T. equigenitalis*, as well

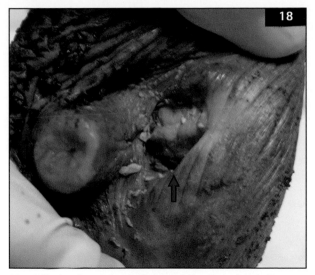

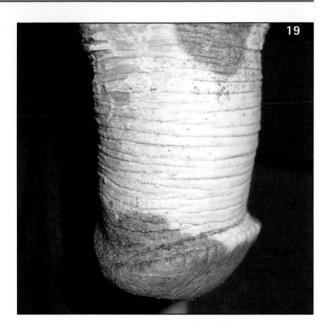

18, 19 *Taylorella asinigenitalis* resembling *T. equigenitalis* might be isolated from the urethral fossa (arrow) in horses.

as for identification of these species. The *T. asinigenitalis* strain had a low minimum inhibitory concentration (MIC) of gentamicin (≤1 μg/ml) but a high MIC of streptomycin (>16 μg/ml) (Båverud *et al.* 2006).

Diagnosis

Diagnosis is based primarily on culture of the bacterium from its predilection sites in the reproductive tract of the mare and the stallion (**18, 19**) (Timoney 1996). However, the rate of *T. equigenitalis* detection was higher with PCR than with the classic bacteriological examination. PCR is especially valuable in cases of intensive bacterial and fungal contamination of swabs where the isolation of *T. equigenitalis* usually fails (Zdovc *et al.* 2005). A direct-PCR assay was developed for the rapid detection of *T. equigenitalis* in equine genital swabs without need for a preliminary step of DNA extraction or bacterial isolation (Duquesne *et al.* 2007). The assay is also able to discriminate between *T. equigenitalis* and *T. asinigenitalis* (Wakeley *et al.* 2006).

In chronically infected mares, the organism was detectable in the clitoral swabs of nearly 93%, but in the cervical swabs of only 31%. In contrast, in acutely infected mares, the organism was detectable in the clitoral swabs of nearly 69%, but in the

cervical swabs of 84% (Wood *et al.* 2005).

There was close agreement between CFT and ELISA methodologies during the post exposure time period used to detect CEM serodiagnostically in regulatory animal health testing programmes. Unlike the CFT, which requires an overnight incubation step, the ELISAs are more convenient and can be completed in 3 hours (Katz & Geer 2001).

Pathology

Macroscopically no vaginal lesions are apparent; the endometrial mucosa may be swollen and corrugated with a scant mucopurulent exudate. Histology of uterine biopsies might reveal a mild endometritis, characterized by interstitial mucosal oedema and a mild inflammatory infiltrate composed of neutrophils; later plasma cells may be more evident (Jubb *et al.* 2007).

Management/Treatment

Aggressive systemic antibiotic therapy accompanied by routine topical therapy might be required to treat CEM-positive stallions (Kristula & Smith 2004).

Public health significance

Not convincing yet.

Francisella tularensis: TULAREMIA

Phylum BXII Proteobacteria
Class III Gammaproteobacteria/Order
V Thiotrichales/Family II Francisellaceae/Genus I
Francisella: Gram-negative aerobic rods and cocci

Definition/Overview

Tularemia caused by *Francisella tularensis* (formerly *Pasteurella tularensis*) is identified as emerging in Europe (Vorou *et al.* 2007) although the pathogenicity of *F. tularensis* for the horse appears to be extremely low.

Aetiology

F. tularensis is a Gram-negative arthropod-borne coccobacillus (Petersen *et al.* 2009).

Epidemiology

The serological response in burros and horses to the viable LVS strain of *F. tularensis* generated high-titred agglutinating antisera and fluorescent antibody conjugates in both groups of animals. Maximum titres were obtained in horses 14–21 days (up to 1:1,024 and 1:360, respectively) and in burros 21–28 days (up to 1:1,024 and 1:160, respectively) after the start of vaccination. The use of so-called Woodhour's adjuvants or booster inoculations did not result in increased titres (Green *et al.* 1970).

Pathophysiology

Free-living amoebae feed on bacteria, fungi, and algae. However, some microorganisms have evolved to become resistant to these protists. These amoeba-resistant microorganisms include established pathogens, such as *F. tularensis*, *Legionella* spp., *Chlamydophila pneumoniae*, and *Listeria mono-cytogenes*. Free-living amoebae represent an important reservoir of amoeba-resistant micro-organisms and may, while encysted, protect the internalized bacteria from chlorine and other biocides. On the other hand, free-living amoebae may act as a 'Trojan horse', bringing hidden amoeba-resistant microorganisms within the human or animal 'Troy', and may produce vesicles filled with amoeba-resistant microorganisms, increasing their transmission potential (Greub & Raoult 2004).

Incubation period

Not established in the equine species yet.

Clinical presentation

Not established in the equine species yet.

Pathology

Not established in the equine species yet.

Public health significance

Tularemia is regarded as an important (tickborne) zoonosis with two primary disease manifestations, ulceroglandular and glandular. Two subspecies of *F. tularensis* cause most human illness, namely subspecies *tularensis*, also known as type A, and subspecies *holarctica*, referred to as type B. The equine species is not regarded as a main reservoir for human infection in contrast with rodents and lagomorphs (Petersen *et al.* 2009).

Legionella pneumophila

Phylum BXII Proteobacteria
Class III Gammaproteobacteria/Order VI
Legionellales/Family I Legionellaceae/Genus I
Legionella: Gram-negative aerobic rods and cocci

Definition/Overview

Febrile lymphadenopathy can be experimentally induced by *Legionella pneumophila*. It has been concluded that there is no evidence to support a role for the horse in the maintenance of these organisms in nature (Cho *et al.* 1983).

Aetiology

The pathogenicity of *L. pneumophila* serogroups 1 and 3 for the horse appears to be low (Cho *et al.* 1983).

Epidemiology

Seroconversions in horses provided additional evidence that horses become naturally exposed to *Legionella* spp. Nineteen percent of horses seroconverted to at least one serogroup (out of 4) of *L. pneumophila* (Cho *et al.* 1984). With 58% of the sera tested negative, 35% had end-point titres of 1:2, 7% end-point of 1:16 and 0.3% an end-point of 1:256. South African serological results revealed a much lower exposure rate than that reported in the USA (Wilkins & Bergh 1988). In addition, a high percentage of seropositivity suggested that horses are commonly infected with *L. pneumophila* or related organisms, and the age-specific rates of occurrence indicated that infection was related directly to duration of exposure. The occurrence of positive (1:64) equine sera (31%) was significantly higher than the occurrence of positive sera in cattle (5%), swine (3%), sheep (2%), dogs (2%), goats (0.5%), wildlife (0%), and humans (0.4%) as assessed by means of microagglutination. The highest titre measured in horses was 1:512. Of the positive sera in horses, 44% reacted to a single serogroup (III or I most commonly), and 56% reacted to multiple serogroups (II and III or I, II, and III most commonly) (Collins *et al.* 1982).

Pathophysiology

Not established in the equine species yet.

Incubation period

A transient decrease in circulating lymphocytes occurred 2 days after inoculation (Cho *et al.* 1983).

Clinical presentation

Signs of clinical illness were restricted to a transient febrile response and lymphadenopathy (Cho *et al.* 1983).

Diagnosis

Agglutinating antibodies persisted at least 4 months after infection (Cho *et al.* 1983) with a high correlation (r = 0.89) found between titres measured by either the indirect fluorescent antibody test or the microagglutination test (Cho *et al.* 1984). All horses exhibited a marked increase in agglutinating antibodies to *L. pneumophila* serogroups 1 and 3 as early as 4 days after experimental challenge (Cho *et al.* 1983).

Pathology

At necropsy, only moderate generalized lymphadenopathy was noted with lymph nodes showing evidence of reactive hyperplasia. Histologically, the lungs contained evidence of a low-grade inflammatory response characterized by focal proliferation of alveolar lining cells, with few neutrophils and eosinophils (Cho *et al.* 1983).

Management/Treatment

Not appropriate yet.

Public health significance

Not convincing yet as it has been stated that the horse could not be considered to be a source of infection but that both humans and animals were probably exposed to a common source of infection. Serological testing of people closely associated with horses showed that out of 22 people, three had a positive end-point titre of 1:64 and only one person showed an end-point titre of 1:256 (Wilkins & Bergh 1988).

Coxiella burnetii: Q FEVER
Phylum BXII Proteobacteria
Class III Gammaproteobacteria/Order VI
Legionellales/Family II Coxiellaceae/Genus I
Coxiella

Definition/Overview
Coxiella burnetii, the causative agent of Q fever, is not currently reported to affect horses. Only seropositivity was mentioned in horses ranging from 5.5–21.7% in Uruguay (Somma-Moreira *et al.* 1987).

Moraxella spp.
Phylum BXII Proteobacteria
Class III Gammaproteobacteria/Order IX
Pseudomonadales/Family II Moraxellaceae/Genus I
Moraxella: Gram-negative aerobic rods and cocci

Definition/Overview
Moraxella spp. are a frequent isolate in ocular and pharyngeal flora of clinically normal horses and horses suffering from lymphoid follicular hyperplasia and conjunctivitis.

Aetiology
A Gram-negative, aerobic, oxidase-positive diplococcus, that may colonize the conjunctiva and the pharynx in horses. In ocular flora of clinically normal horses (20), *Corynebacterium* spp., *Staphylococcus* spp., *Bacillus* spp., and *Moraxella* spp. are the bacteria most frequently isolated (Andrew *et al.* 2003), with *Moraxella* spp. comprising 28% of Gram-negative bacteria involved (Gemensky-Metzler *et al.* 2005).

Epidemiology
There were no significant differences between the number or type of organisms cultured during the sampling seasons in ocular flora of clinically normal Florida horses, whereas the likelihood of detecting an organism depended on the horse's age (Andrew *et al.* 2003).

Pathophysiology
Unknown in the equine species yet.

Incubation period
Not established in the equine species yet.

Clinical presentation
Moraxella spp. are associated with lymphoid follicular hyperplasia (21) (Hoquet *et al.* 1985) and conjunctivitis (Hughes & Pugh 1970, Huntington *et al.* 1987), although their clinical significance remains unclear in the equine species.

Diagnosis
Diagnosis primarily depends on culture of the bacterium in diseased animals combined with clinical signs compared to negative controls.

Pathology
Moraxella spp. were isolated in 88% of horses with pharyngitis of grades III and IV, followed by *Streptococcus equi* subsp. *zooepidemicus*, *Pseudomonas aeruginosa*, coagulase-negative staphylococci, and *Enterobacter* spp. (Hoquet *et al.* 1985).

Management/Treatment
Treatment of diseased animals is supportive.

Public health significance
Not convincing yet. *Moraxella catarrhalis* is an exclusively human pathogen and is a common cause of otitis media in infants and children, causing 15–20% of acute otitis media episodes. *M. catarrhalis* causes an estimated 2–4 million exacerbations of chronic obstructive pulmonary disease in adults annually in the USA. Most strains produce beta-lactamase and are thus resistant to ampicillin but susceptible to several classes of oral antimicrobial agents (Murphy & Parameswaran 2009).

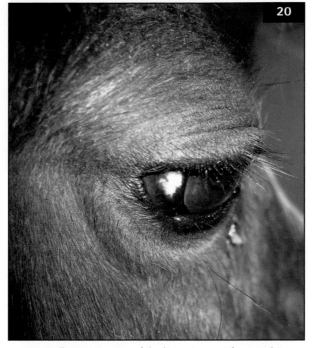

20 *Moraxella* spp. are one of the bacteria most frequently isolated in ocular flora of clinically normal horses with the likelihood of detecting it depending on the horse's age.

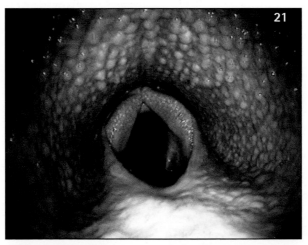

21 The isolation of *Moraxella* spp. and *S. equi* subsp. *zooepidemicus* in large numbers is frequent in horses with lymphoid follicular hyperplasia grades III and IV. However, *Moraxella* spp. are one of the bacteria also most frequently isolated in pharyngeal flora of clinically normal horses. Illustration shows lymphoid follicular hyperplasia grade IV associated with dorsal displacement of the soft palate (DDSP).

Escherichia coli

Phylum BXII Proteobacteria
Class III Gammaproteobacteria/Order XIII
Enterobacteriales/Family I Enterobacteriaceae/
Genus I *Escherichia*: Facultatively anaerobic Gram-negative rods

Definition/Overview

Escherichia coli can cause acute, highly fatal septicaemia of newborn foals. *E. coli* is the most common pathogen isolated from foals with sepsis (**22**) (Wilson & Madigan 1989). In foals, enteropathogenic *E. coli* and subsequent neonatal diarrhoea are very rare (in contrast with pigs and calves) as compared with extraintestinal pathogenic *E. coli* (ExPEC). In the near future, real-time PCR might facilitate fast confirmation of a diagnosis of septicaemia, thereby improving the therapeutic management of neonatal foals.

Aetiology

E. coli are Gram-negative rods belonging to the family Enterobacteriaceae. ExPEC strains carrying distinct virulence attributes are known to cause diseases in humans and animals and infect organs other than the gastrointestinal (GI) tract (**23–25**) (DebRoy *et al.* 2008).

Epidemiology

Gram-positive isolates, predominantly *Streptococcus/Enterococcus* spp., were obtained in 41% of foals·less than 7 days of age admitted to an intensive care unit. Gram-negative isolates were predominantly of the Enterobacteriaceae family, in particular *E. coli* (Russell *et al.* 2008). *E. coli* was also the organism most commonly isolated (in 44% of cases) from foals with bacteraemia in another report, followed by *Actinobacillus* spp. (25%), of which 62% were *A. equuli* (Corley *et al.* 2007). Furthermore, *E. coli* was consistently isolated most frequently in bacteraemic neonatal Thoroughbreds (Sanchez *et al.* 2008). In addition, the most common intraoperative culture isolates from horses undergoing abdominal surgery were *E. coli*, *Streptococcus* spp., and *Enterococcus* spp. (Rodriquez *et al.* 2009).

For horses, there was not a significant interaction between populations of the indicator organisms and manure type (fresh versus dry). The population size of faecal streptococci (5.47 and 6.14 log10/g in fresh and dry, respectively) in horse manure was higher than the population size of *E. coli* (4.79 and 5.08 log10/g in fresh and dry, respectively) (Weaver *et al.* 2005). However, *E. coli* of equine faecal origin are commonly resistant to antibiotics used in human and veterinary medicine (Ahmed *et al.* 2010).

Pathophysiology

A carbohydrate metabolic operon (frz) that is highly associated with extraintestinal pathogenic *E. coli* strains promotes bacterial fitness under stressful conditions, such as oxygen restriction, late stationary phase of growth, or growth in serum or in the intestinal tract (Rouquet *et al.* 2009).

Incubation period

Not established in the equine species yet, but may be as short as several hours.

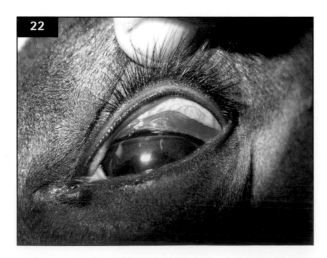

22 Marked episcleral haemorrhage and conjunctivitis secondary to endotoxaemia in a foal.

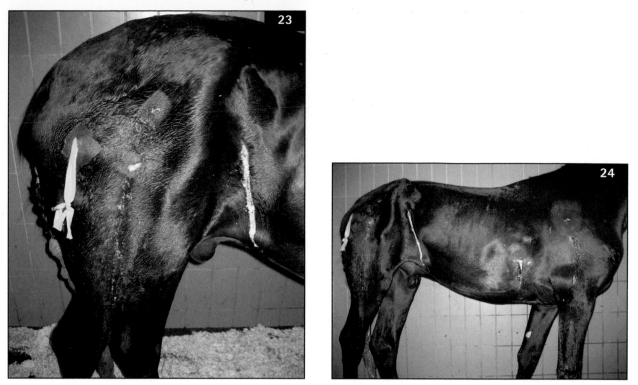

23, 24 External abscessation associated with *E. coli* in a yearling Friesian stallion. Note the yellow drain in one of the abscesses.

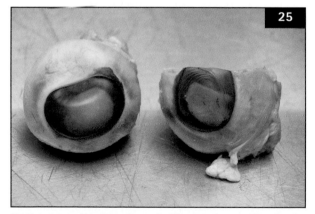

25 Hypopyon, *E. coli* septicaemia. The anterior eye chamber is filled with a pale yellowish purulent exudate due to a suppurative uveitis. (Formalin fixed specimens.)

Clinical presentation

Clinical signs include fever (or hypothermia associated with shock), anorexia, and depression/coma. Polyarthritis, polyserositis (including meningoencephalitis) and pneumonia might develop as the most important sequelae in neonatal foals, reflecting a poor prognosis. Foals with Gram-negative bacteraemia had lower total WBC and lymphocyte counts at admission than did those from which only Gram-positive bacteria were cultured. Mixed organism bacteraemia was associated with tachycardia, increased serum concentrations of sodium, chloride, and urea nitrogen, acidosis, respiratory distress, recumbency on admission, and nonsurvival (Corley *et al.* 2007). *E. coli* was not associated with diarrhoea in foals (Netherwood *et al.* 1996).

ExPEC might also occur in other opportunistic settings in the immunocompromised host. For instance, ExPEC O2H21 has been associated with fatal bronchopneumonia in a 12-year-old Quarter Horse mare in association with *Enterococcus* sp., and *Klebsiella pneumoniae* (DebRoy *et al.* 2008).

Differential diagnosis

The differential diagnosis includes other causes of foal septicaemia (see p. 262).

Diagnosis

Bacterial culture of blood is the current goldstandard test with which to diagnose sepsis in foals. Detection frequency of *E. coli* from equine blood was significantly greater by use of the resin-containing blood culture system (61%) than that achieved by use of the conventional blood culture system (30%) or the lysis–centrifugation-based blood culture system (0%) (Lorenzo-Figueras *et al.* 2006). Furthermore, culturing endometrial biopsy tissue or uterine fluids is a more sensitive method for identifying *E. coli* than culture swab, while endometrial cytology identifies twice as many mares with acute inflammation than uterine culture swab (LeBlanc 2010). Comparison between conventional blood culture and real-time PCR in septic foals revealed a sensitivity of 82%, a specificity of 99%, a positive predictive value of 90%, and a negative predictive value of 97% for real-time PCR (results for the universal bacterial 16S rRNA gene including *E. coli* in broth). However, for the foreseeable future, PCR-based testing (able to detect as few as 15 colony-forming units) will not replace conventional culture due to the requirement for purified culture isolates in antimicrobial susceptibility testing (Pusterla *et al.* 2009).

With the increasing prevalence of Gram-positive microorganisms and their unpredictable sensitivity patterns, blood cultures remain important in the diagnosis and treatment of equine neonatal septicaemia (Russell *et al.* 2008).

Pathology

Usually *E. coli* infections induce a suppurative and fibrinous inflammation such as in placentitis, pyometra (**26**), cholangitis (**27, 28**), and (neonatal) septicaemic (lepto)meningitis, serositis, uveitis, and (poly)arthritis.

Management/Treatment

Treatment of diseased foals is supportive (including antibiotic therapy) with special reference to improvement of antibody status by means of the administration of hyperimmune serum. In addition, it is of importance to provide good hygiene including antiseptic treatment of the umbilical cord stump in neonatal foals.

The MIC of ceftiofur required to inhibit growth of 90% of isolates of *E. coli*, *Pasteurella* spp., *Klebsiella* spp., and beta-haemolytic streptococci was < 0.5 μg/ml. Intravenous administration of ceftiofur sodium at the rate of 5 mg/kg BW every 12h would provide sufficient coverage for the treatment of susceptible bacterial isolates (Meyer *et al.* 2009).

Both hospitalization and antimicrobial drug administration were associated with prevalence of antimicrobial resistance among *E. coli* strains isolated from the faeces of horses. Resistance to sulfamethoxazole and to trimethoprim–sulfamethoxazole was most common, followed by resistance to gentamicin and resistance to tetracycline. Use of a potentiated sulphonamide, aminoglycosides, cephalosporins, or metronidazole was positively associated with resistance to one or more antimicrobial drugs, but use of penicillins was not associated with increased risk of resistance to antimicrobial drugs (Dunowska *et al.* 2006).

Public health significance

Its potential zoonotic risk should be minimized.

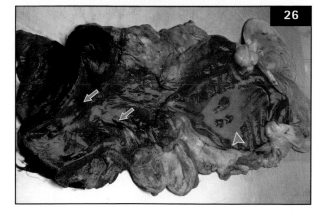

26 *E. coli* pyometra in a Shetland pony mare. The incised enlarged hyperaemic uterus contains a moderate amount of seropurulent exudate (arrowhead). Usually a pyometra is a sequela of a heavy parturition, as in this case evidenced by the vaginal and cervical haemorrhages (arrows). Other reported bacterial invaders include: *Streptococcus equi* subsp. *zooepidemicus, Actinomyces* spp., *Pasteurella* spp., and *Pseudomonas* spp.

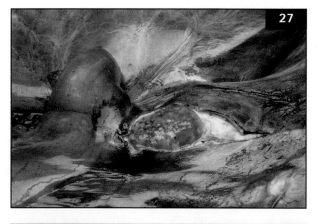

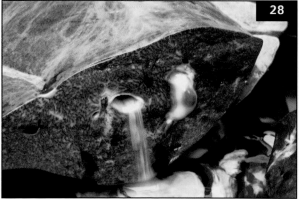

27, 28 Choledocholithiasis, hepatolithiasis, and suppurative cholangitis. Both extra- and intrahepatic bile ducts are obstructed by gallstones or choleliths and profuse accompanying suppuration due to bacterial infections. Implicated in this case was *Escherichia coli*.

Salmonella spp.: SALMONELLOSIS

Phylum BXII Proteobacteria
Class III Gammaproteobacteria/Order XIII
Enterobacteriales/Genus XXXIV *Salmonella*:
Facultatively anaerobic Gram-negative rods

Definition/Overview

Colitis/typhlitis associated with diarrhoea in adult horses or neonatal septicaemia is caused by various *Salmonella* species. The detection of latent carriers remains a challenge. Equine clinics and veterinary teaching hospitals are at risk of becoming repositories for salmonellosis, despite an existing infection control program (Dallap Schaer *et al.* 2010), underlining the need for the prudent use of antimicrobials.

Aetiology

Salmonella spp. are Gram-negative, facultatively anaerobic, intracellular rods belonging to the family Enterobacteriaceae. Salmonellosis is caused by a great variety of serovars classified as members of the genus *Salmonella* within the species *S. enterica*, with serovar *typhimurium* usually being most prevalent. The immune response to most somatic 'O' antigens of different *Salmonella* groups is not (A, B, C2) or little (C1, D) affected by antigenic competition (Singh *et al.* 2006). Integron-positive *S. typhimurium* isolates from horses with clinical disease belong to distinct strains, demonstrating the capability of *S. typhimurium* to acquire additional antibiotic resistance determinants, so underlining the need for the prudent use of antimicrobials (Vo *et al.* 2007).

Epidemiology

Various *Salmonella* species show a worldwide distribution with a reported prevalence of 2% (House *et al.* 1999). Hospitalized foals over 1 month of age with diarrhoea were significantly more likely to have *Salmonella* spp. (OR = 2.6, 95% CI = 1.2–6.0), rotavirus (OR = 13.3, 95% CI = 5.3–33), and parasites (OR = 23, 95% CI = 3.1–185) detected compared with younger foals. However, the type of infectious agent identified in the faeces or bacteraemia was not significantly associated with survival (Frederick *et al.* 2009).

Horses that were parenterally treated with antimicrobials for other reasons than salmonellosis were found to be at 6.4 times greater risk of developing salmonellosis, and those treated orally and parenterally were at 40.4 times greater risk, compared to horses that did not receive antimicrobial treatment (Hird *et al.* 1986). In addition, abdominal surgery was identified as a risk factor for nosocomial *Salmonella* infections in horses. Horses that underwent abdominal surgery

required enhanced infection control and preventative care (Ekiri *et al.* 2009). Furthermore, for a horse with salmonellosis, the odds of developing thrombophlebitis were 68 times those for a similar horse without salmonellosis (Dolente *et al.* 2005).

It has been suggested that there is a highly epidemiological relationship between equine *S. typhimurium* phage type 104 isolates and certain multidrug-resistant bovine isolates in the same area (Niwa *et al.* 2009). Ceftiofur resistance in *S. enterica* rose from 4.0% in 1999 to 18.8% in 2003. Isolates from diagnostic laboratories had higher levels of resistance (18.5%), whereas levels in isolates from on-farm (3.4%) and slaughter (7.1%) sources were lower. Animals with a higher than average proportion of ceftiofur-resistant *Salmonella* included cattle (17.6%), horses (19.2%), and dogs (20.8%) (Frye & Fedorka-Cray 2007). In addition, swine *Salmonella* isolates displayed the highest rate of resistance, being resistant to at least one antimicrobial (92%), followed by those recovered from turkey (91%), cattle (77%), chicken (68%), and equines (20%) (Zhao *et al.* 2007).

An outbreak of salmonellosis caused by *S. newport* multidrug-resistant-AmpC at a large animal veterinary teaching hospital was associated with a case fatality rate of 32% in equines (Dallap Schaer *et al.* 2010).

Pathophysiology

Following oral infection, invasion of the host usually takes place via the intestinal wall progressing into the mesenteric lymph nodes. In adult horses, progression beyond the mesenteric lymph nodes and associated sepsis seldom occur, whereas diarrhoea is most common due to hypersecretion and malabsorption predominantly in the large colon and caecum. Protein-losing enteropathy may result in hypoproteinaemia associated with oedema formation (Plummer 2006). Septicaemia is most prominent in neonatal foals.

Equine DEFA1 is an enteric alpha-defensin exclusively produced in Paneth cells showing an activity against a broad spectrum of horse pathogens (Bruhn *et al.* 2009).

Incubation period

Not established in the equine species yet, but may be as short as 24 hours.

Clinical presentation

Clinical salmonellosis in adult horses is usually due to uptake from an asymptomatic carrier or associated with previous stress. Clinical signs include fever, anorexia, depression, and eventually colic followed by more or less obvious (haemorrhagic) diarrhoea (29, 30) and weight loss. Sometimes abortion, laminitis, or limb and ventral oedema develop as sequelae in adult horses. In neonatal foals sepsis with or without diarrhoea is seen and sequelae like meningoencephalitis, polyarthritis, polyserositis, omphalitis, and (rib) osteomyelitis occur (Neil *et al.* 2010).

Differential diagnosis
The differential diagnosis includes various causes of acute diarrhoea and causes of foal septicaemia (see p. 262, 263).

Diagnosis
The diagnosis should be based on the demonstration of the bacterium in blood (in the septicaemic stage in foals) or faeces using either enriching media and/or PCR, combined with the presence of characteristic clinical signs. Eventually a biopsy of rectal mucosa might be used (Duijkeren & Houwers 2000, Pusterla *et al.* 2009). A quantitative real-time PCR assay targeting the Salmonella *invA* gene had an overall relative accuracy of 98%, a relative sensitivity of 100%, and a relative specificity of 98%, when compared to conventional culture (Pusterla *et al.* 2009).

It is important to realize that an infected animal may become a latent carrier or an active carrier, passing the bacteria intermittently via the faeces. The criterion to evaluate the elimination of *Salmonella* should be that cultures of three stool samples obtained at least 2 weeks apart are negative for the original strain (Duijkeren & Houwers 2000). Nevertheless, the detection of latent carriers remains a challenge.

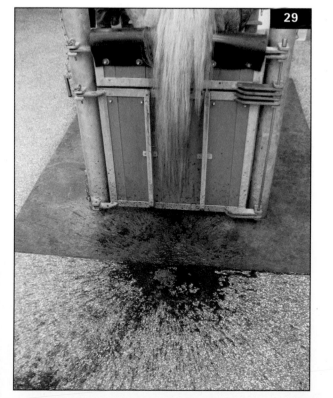

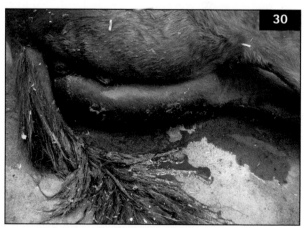

29, 30 Haemorrhagic diarrhoeic colitis in an 18-year-old Warmblood gelding (**29**) and a 4-month-old Warmblood filly (**30**).

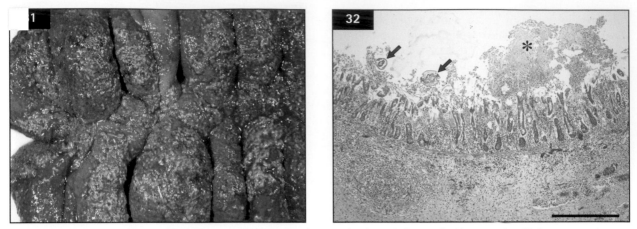

31, 32 Fibrinonecrotic colitis. **31**: The colon mucosa is swollen, haemorrhagic, and ulcerated with a covering fibrinosuppurative pseudomembrane; **32**: the corresponding micrograph (pseudomembrane indicated by the asterisk). Note the two sections of coexisting small strongyles (arrows). *Salmonella typhimurium*. (H&E stain. Bar 500 μm.)

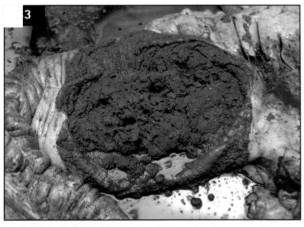

33 Colonic sand obstruction. Right dorsal colon ascendens overfilled and obstructed by ingested impacted greenish stained sandy contents. This condition frequently coincides with diarrhoeic colitis due to cyathostominosis and salmonellosis.

Pathology

In septicaemic cases multiple serosal and mucosal petechial haemorrhages are noticed at necropsy. There may be a haemorrhagic gastroenterocolitis with especially an intense fibrinohaemorrhagic inflammation of the large intestine with ulcerations and a covering fibrinopurulent pseudomembrane (**31**). Typical in chronic cases are raised fibrinous button-like ulcers. Moreover, on histology congestion and oedema of mucosa and submucosa with mixed inflammatory infiltrates and intravascular fibrin thrombi in the lamina propria may be evident (**32**).

Management/Treatment

Treatment of diseased horses is supportive (including transfaunation). According to most veterinary sources the use of antimicrobials is only indicated for patients with systemic *Salmonella* infections or in *Salmonella*-infected immunocompromised patients. Antimicrobial treatment of patients with uncomplicated *Salmonella* enteritis is even considered to be contraindicated, with the exception of animals younger than 6 months (Duijkeren & Houwers 2000). In addition, given the association between salmonellosis and cyathostominosis it is important to combine good hygiene (**33**) with prudent use of anthelmintics.

Public health significance

Horses with a tentative diagnosis of salmonellosis should be isolated to prevent possible human exposure. The pathogen has important public health significance and salmonellosis is a reportable disease. Human salmonellosis presents as two clinical entities. The first, enteric fever, is caused by *S. typhi* or *S. paratyphi A, B*, or *C*. These infections are generally transmitted from person to person without animal involvement. The second, 'non-typhoid salmonellosis' is caused by other *Salmonella* serotypes that reside primarily in animals and have zoonotic potential (Humphrey *et al.* 1998). The fluoroquinolones are the drugs of choice in human medicine for severe *Salmonella* infections and for the elimination of the carrier state (Duijkeren & Houwers 2000).

Pasteurella spp.

Phylum BXII Proteobacteria
Class III Gammaproteobacteria/Order XIV
Pasteurellales/Family I Pasteurellaceae/Genus I
Pasteurella: Gram-negative aerobic rods and cocci

Definition/Overview

Pasteurella spp. are Gram-negative bacteria (including *Mannheimia* [formerly *Pasteurella*] *haemolytica*) predominantly associated with pneumonia, pleuropneumonia, and endocarditis in horses. It is well-known as an opportunistic equine pathogen of the respiratory tract following transport stress.

Aetiology

P. multocida is an important veterinary (**34**) and opportunistic human pathogen. The species is diverse and complex with respect to antigenic variation, host predilection, and pathogenesis. Certain serological types are the aetiological agents of severe pasteurellosis, such as fowl cholera in domestic and wild birds, bovine haemorrhagic septicaemia, and porcine atrophic rhinitis (Hunt *et al.* 2000). However, tracheobronchial aspirates from clinically normal foals revealed *Actinobacillus/ Pasteurella* spp. (Crane *et al.* 1989).

Epidemiology

Following transportation by road for 12 h, transtracheal aspirates showed an accumulation of purulent respiratory tract secretions with increased numbers of bacteria, particularly beta-haemolytic *Streptococcus* spp. and members of the Pasteurellaceae family. As a consequence, bacterial contamination of the lower respiratory tract occurs as a routine consequence of transportation of horses and is likely to be an important determinant in the development of transport-associated respiratory disease (Raidal *et al.* 1997a). In addition, acute death occurred in a racehorse with pneumonia after long-distance transportation associated with a mixed infection of *P. caballi*, *Streptococcus suis*, and *Streptococcus equi* subsp. *zooepidemicus* (Hayakawa *et al.* 1993).

Pathophysiology

The dermonecrotic toxin from *P. multocida* (PMT) disrupts G-protein signal transduction through selective deamidation. The C3 deamidase domain of PMT has no sequence similarity to the deamidase domains of the dermonecrotic toxins from *Escherichia coli* (cytotoxic necrotizing factor [CNF]1–3), *Yersinia* (CNFY) and *Bordetella* (dermonecrotic toxin). PMT-C3 belongs to a family of transglutaminase-like proteins, with active site

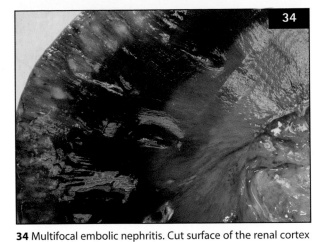

34 Multifocal embolic nephritis. Cut surface of the renal cortex contains multiple pale necrosuppurative foci. Bacterial culture yielded *Mannheimia* (*Pasteurella*) *haemolytica*.

Cys–His–Asp catalytic triads distinct from *E. coli* CNF1 (Wilson & Ho 2010). Gq family members of heterotrimeric G protein activate beta isoforms of phospholipase C that hydrolyzes phosphatidyl-inositol phosphate to diacylglycerol and inositol triphosphate, leading to protein kinase C activation and intracellular Ca^{2+} mobilization, respectively. PMT is regarded as a Gq signalling activator (Mizuno & Itoh 2009).

Incubation period

Not yet established in the equine species.

Clinical presentation

Of bacterial isolates from horses with evidence of lower airway disease, 51% were *Actinobacillus equuli*, 18% were *A. suis*-like, 11% were *Pasteurella pneumotropica*, 8% were *A. lignieresii*, 7% were *M. haemolytica*, and 5% were *P. mairii*, indicating that a range of *Actinobacillus* and *Pasteurella* species can be isolated from the lower airways of horses (Ward *et al.* 1998). In comparison, among the facultatively anaerobic isolates involved in lower respiratory tract or paraoral bacterial infections, *S. equi* subsp. *zooepidemicus* accounted for 31% of isolates, followed by *Pasteurella* spp. 19%, *Escherichia coli* 17%, *Actinomyces* spp. 9%, and *Streptococcus* spp. 9% (Bailey & Love 1991).

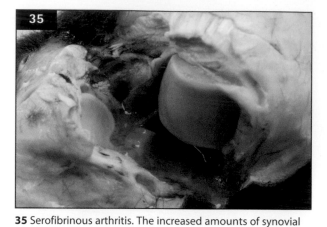

35 Serofibrinous arthritis. The increased amounts of synovial fluid show slightly increased turbidity. Note the hyperaemic synovial membranes. Bacterial culture yielded *Mannheimia* (*Pasteurella*) *haemolytica*.

The aerobic bacteria most frequently isolated from horses with pneumonia or pleuropneumonia were beta-haemolytic *Streptococcus* spp., *Pasteurella* spp., *Escherichia coli*, and *Enterobacter* spp. The anaerobic species most frequently isolated were *Bacteroides* spp. and *Clostridium* spp. (Sweeney *et al.* 1991).

Pasteurella/Actinobacillus-like spp. in tracheal washes were associated with an increasing risk of clinically apparent respiratory disease in racehorses in training (Chapman *et al.* 2000, Newton *et al.* 2003). However, infection of the airways with even large numbers of *Streptococcus equi* subsp. *zooepidemicus* or *Pasteurella*-like spp. did not facilitate the occurrence of exercise-induced pulmonary haemorrhage (EIPH) (Newton & Wood 2002).

Clinical signs also included polyarthritis (35) associated with *P. canis* (Bourgault *et al.* 1994) and pneumonia associated with *M. haemolytica* (Saxegaard & Svenkrud 1974) in foals. Furthermore, ulcerative lymphangitis caused by *M. haemolytica* (Miller & Dresher 1981) and endocarditis (Maxson & Reef 1997) associated with *P. caballi* (Church *et al.* 1998) were reported.

Differential diagnosis
The differential diagnosis includes various causes of fever and dyspnoea (see p. 262).

Diagnosis
Diagnosis depends on the detection of bacteria combined with appropriate clinical signs.

Pathology
Vegetative lesions were found most frequently on the mitral valve and secondarily on the aortic valve, with *Pasteurella/Actinobacillus* spp. and *Streptococcus* spp. most commonly cultured from horses with bacterial endocarditis (Maxson & Reef 1997, Church *et al.* 1998).

Management/Treatment
Treatment with procaine penicillin (up to 40,000 IU/kg BW) prior to or during confinement with head elevation had no effect on the systemic leucocyte response or on the accumulation of inflammatory lower respiratory tract secretions (Raidal *et al.* 1997*b*).

Bimodal populations were observed for ampicillin, kanamycin, and oxytetracycline susceptibility among various Gram-negative bacterial isolates, especially those of equine origin. This observation indicates a probable lack of added response to increased antimicrobial dosages, such that a poor response to initial treatment with a nominal dosage would require a change in antimicrobial rather than increased dosage (Burrows *et al.* 1993).

The MIC of cefpodoxime required to inhibit growth of 90% of isolates for *Salmonella enterica*, *Escherichia coli*, *Pasteurella* spp., *Klebsiella* spp., and beta-haemolytic streptococci was 0.38, 1.00, 0.16, 0.19, and 0.09 µg/ml, respectively. Oral administration of cefpodoxime at a dosage of 10 mg/kg BW every 6–12 h would appear appropriate for the treatment of equine neonates with bacterial infections (Carrillo *et al.* 2005).

Public health significance
P. multocida meningitis might be caused by kissing animals (Kawashima *et al.* 2010), especially other than horses. For example, a human patient suffering from type 2 diabetes mellitus developed peritonitis induced by *P. multocida*. Pulsed-field gel electrophoresis (PFGE) showed that the *P. multocida* isolated from the patient was completely identical to the strain isolated from his domestic cat (Satomura *et al.* 2010).

Yersinia enterocolitica: YERSINIOSIS
Phylum BXII Proteobacteria
Class III Gammaproteobacteria/Order XIII
Enterobacteriales/ Family I
Enterobacteriaceae/Genus XLIII *Yersinia*: Gram-
negative aerobic rods and cocci

Definition/Overview
Yersinia enterocolitica is among putative pathogens
found at very low prevalence in diarrhoea and/or
pneumonia predominantly in foals. *Y. enterocolitica*
is the most common species causing human enteric
yersiniosis, which is still the third most frequently
reported foodborne gastroenteritis in Europe (Bucher
et al. 2008).

Aetiology
Yersinia spp. are Gram-negative, rod-shaped
facultative anaerobes. *Y. enterocolitica, Y. pseudotuberculosis,* and *Y. pestis* are human pathogens.
Bacteria of the genus *Yersinia* have been isolated
commonly from the environment, including water
supplies of various types. Environmental strains
therefore should be differentiated from serotypes
O:3, O:9, O:5, O:27, and O:8 of *Y. enterocolitica,*
which are the ones most frequently associated with
human infections in Europe, Japan, Canada, and the
USA. These pathotypes are psychrotrophic, and
hence can multiply in fresh waters and could
constitute a major hazard to drinking water.
Epidemiological data concerning waterborne
yersiniosis, however, are scarce (Leclerc *et al.* 2002).
The pathogenicity of *Y. enterocolitica* for the horse
appears to be extremely low.

Epidemiology
Atypical environmental *Y. enterocolitica* was isolated
from a horse faecal sample (1%) (Wooley *et al.*
1980) and *Y. enterocolitica* was found in a similar
very low prevalence in horse/mule manure (Derlet &
Carlson 2002). No pathogenic strains were isolated
from tonsils of slaughter horses (Bucher *et al.* 2008).
Y. enterocolitica was not associated with diarrhoea
in foals (Netherwood *et al.* 1996), but the prevalence
of *Y. enterocolitica* was similar in normal and
diarrhoeic foals (Browning *et al.* 1991).

Pathophysiology
Pathogenic *Yersinia* spp. (*Y. pestis,
Y. pseudotuberculosis,* and *Y. enterocolitica*) harbour
a 70-kb virulence plasmid (pYV) that encodes a type
III secretion system and a set of at least six effector
proteins (YopH, YopO, YopP, YopE, YopM, and
YopT) that are injected into the host cell cytoplasm.
Yops (*Yersinia* outer proteins) disturb the dynamics
of the cytoskeleton, inhibit phagocytosis by
macrophages, and downregulate the production of
proinflammatory cytokines, which makes it possible
for *Yersinina* spp. to multiply extracellularly in
lymphoid tissue (Trülzsch *et al.* 2004).

Incubation period
Not established in the equine species yet.

Clinical presentation
Watery diarrhoea and pneumonia were observed in
foals at a stud-farm with 10% of foals dying due to
suppurative lesions (Czernomysy-Furowicz 1997).

Fatigue, anaemia, fever, abnormal breath sound,
anorexia, and weight loss were associated with
mixed *Histoplasma* sp. and *Y. enterocolitica*
infection of the lungs in a 4-year-old Thoroughbred
racehorse (Katayama *et al.* 2001).

Differential diagnosis
The differential diagnosis includes other causes of
foal diarrhoea (see p. 262).

Diagnosis
Rapid identification of enteropathogenic bacteria in
faecal samples is critical for clinical diagnosis and
antimicrobial therapy. Diagnosis should depend on
the detection of *Y. enterocolitica* (in bacterial culture)
combined with clinical signs.

Of interest, a multiplex PCR with hybridization
to a DNA microarray allows the rapid detection of
Y. enterocolitica (Kim *et al.* 2010).

Pathology
Y. enterocolitica was associated with granuloma
formation in the duodenum, lung, liver, and
abdominal lymph nodes (Katayama *et al.* 2001).

Management/Treatment
Treatment of diseased foals is supportive (including
fluid and antibiotic therapy) with special reference
to improvement of antibody status by means of the
administration of hyperimmune serum.

Public health significance
Y. enterocolitica generally causes sporadic human
(enteric) infections but outbreaks are rare (Bucher *et
al.* 2008). *Yersinia* sp. has been associated with a
horse bite (Räisänen & Alavaikko 1989).

Actinobacillus lignieresii: ACTINOBACILLOSIS ('WOODEN TONGUE')

Phylum BXII Proteobacteria
Class III Gammaproteobacteria/Order XIV
Pasteurellales/Family I Pasteurellaceae/Genus II
Actinobacillus: Gram-negative aerobic rods and
cocci

Definition/Overview

Actinobacillosis is a syndrome identical to 'wooden
tongue' in cattle caused by *Actinobacillus lignieresii*.

Aetiology

Actinobacillus lignieresii is a small Gram-negative
rod. Equine isolates of *A. lignieresii* include the type
strain of *A. lignieresii* and genomospecies 1
(Christensen *et al.* 2002). The groupings of cultures
resulting from different testing methods had little
relation to each other and to the anatomic source of
the strains except the strains comprising API-CH
biotype II, which originated in the equine respiratory
tract, and the *A. lignieresii* cluster (Samitz &
Biberstein 1991).

Epidemiology

Among bacterial isolates from horses with and
without evidence of lower airway disease, 8% were
A. lignieresii (Ward *et al.* 1998).

Incubation period

Not established in the equine species yet.

Clinical presentation

Clinical signs include dysphagia and salivation,
chronic nasal cellulitis, a 'wooden tongue' (**36, 37**),
lower airway inflammation, and chronic mastitis
(Baum *et al.* 1984, Ward *et al.* 1998, Carmalt *et al.*
1999).

Diagnosis

The definitive diagnosis is based on cytological
examination and culture (Baum *et al.* 1984).

Pathology

Examination of biopsy specimens revealed
diffuse dermal fibrosis, micropustule formation, and
vascular thrombosis; large numbers of *A. lignieresii*
were isolated in pure culture (Carmalt *et al.* 1999).
On histopathology, pyogranulomatous inflammatory foci are typically centred on the coccobacilli
which are embedded in eosinophilic proteinaceous
radiating or asteroid club-shaped aggregates
(morphologically aspecific aspect known as
Splendore–Hoeppli phenomenon). Extensive accompanying fibrosis is the cause of the firm 'wooden
tongue' characteristic of the affected tissues.

Management/Treatment

If actinobacillosis is suspected, immediate treatment
with sodium iodide should be instituted along with
supportive therapy. In one study it responded rapidly
to ampicillin combined with 150 ml of 20% sodium
iodide solution IV. Within 24 hours of the sodium
iodide administration, the tongue was markedly
reduced in size. By 36 hours, the 13-year-old
Connemara could retract the tongue and was able to
eat and drink (Baum *et al.* 1984). Prolonged
treatment with IV administration of sodium iodide
and oral administration of trimethoprim–
sulfamethoxazole caused regression of the swelling
and did not induce abortion in a 10-year-old
pregnant Norwegian Fjord horse, and treatment
with oral administration of rifampicin (rifampin)
and trimethoprim–sulfamethoxazole resulted in
complete resolution of clinical signs in a 5-month-
old American Paint filly (Carmalt *et al.* 1999).

Public health significance

A. lignieresii is found in infected wounds of humans
bitten by horses (Dibb *et al.* 1981, Peel *et al.* 1991,
Benaoudia *et al.* 1994).

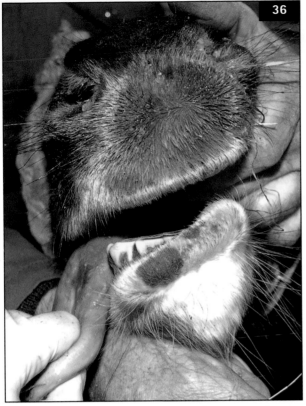

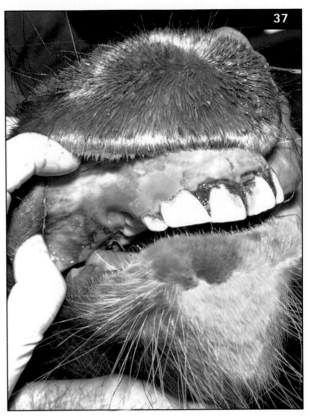

36 *Actinobacillus lignieresii*. Chronic granulomatous and ulcerative glossitis in a 10-month-old pony. The mid-section of the pulled-out tongue is very firm, thickened, and painful. Note the focal dorsal greenish hyperkeratosis partly covering the affected area. (Courtesy of Dr V.M. van der Veen.)

37 *Actinobacillus lignieresii*. Chronic pyogranulomatous and ulcerative stomatitis and gingivitis. Focally the exposed oral soft tissues are hyperaemic and swollen with ulcerations. These lesions resolved shortly after two intravenous sodium iodide infusions. (Courtesy of Dr V.M. van der Veen.)

Actinobacillus equuli: 'SLEEPY FOAL DISEASE'

Phylum BXII Proteobacteria
Class III Gammaproteobacteria/Order XIV
Pasteurellales/Family I Pasteurellaceae/Genus II
Actinobacillus: Gram-negative aerobic rods and cocci

Definition/Overview

An acute, highly fatal septicaemia of newborn foals is caused by *Actinobacillus equuli* (formerly named *Shigella equirulis*), also known as sleepy foal disease (38).

Aetiology

Actinobacillus equuli is a Gram-negative pleomorphic rod-shaped bacterium and has recently been subdivided into nonhaemolytic (subspecies *equuli*) and haemolytic (subspecies *haemolyticus*) strains (Kuhnert *et al.* 2003).

Epidemiology

Both *A. equuli* strains seem to be part of the normal flora of the equine oral cavity (Kuhnert *et al.* 2003) and oesophagus (Meyer *et al.* 2010). As a consequence, in affected foals organisms are proposed to originate from the mare (Baker 1972, Raisis *et al.* 1996).

Pathophysiology

Infections develop after transmission of bacteria through the placenta prior to birth, or contamination of the umbilicus, inhalation into the respiratory system, or ingestion into the GI tract of the foal after birth (Baker 1972, Raisis *et al.* 1996).

Incubation period

Not established in the equine species yet, but may be as short as several hours.

Clinical presentation

A. equuli is reported to be a common cause of acute septicaemia and enteritis in neonatal foals (Baker 1972, Raisis *et al.* 1996), also known as sleepy foal disease. Affected foals usually die within 24 hours. Sleepy foal disease is predominantly associated with nonhaemolytic strains of *A. equuli* (Kuhnert *et al.* 2003). Recently, *A. equuli* subsp. *haemolyticus* was associated with facial cellulitis in a 2-day-old filly (Castagnetti *et al.* 2008). In adult horses, *A. equuli* has been implicated as a cause of respiratory tract disease (Ward *et al.* 1998), abortion (Webb *et al.* 1976), haemorrhagic diathesis (Zakopal & Nesvadba 1968) due to subsp. *haemolyticus* (Pusterla *et al.* 2008), (epidemic) pericarditis (Dill *et al.* 1982, Bolin *et al.* 2005), endocarditis due to subsp. *equuli* (Aalbaek *et al.* 2007), periorchitis (Belknap *et al.* 1988), enteritis (Al-Mashat & Taylor 1986), and peritonitis (Gay & Lording 1980, Golland *et al.* 1994, Matthews *et al.* 2001). It should be realized that horses with *A. equuli* peritonitis present with similar clinical signs as horses with other causes of abdominal pain (Matthews *et al.* 2001).

Differential diagnosis

The differential diagnosis includes other causes of foal septicaemia (see p. 262).

Diagnosis

Actinobacillus spp. infections in foals were associated with leucopenia, neutropenia, lymphopenia and depression on hospital admission (Corley *et al.* 2007). A positive blood culture of *A. equuli* is diagnostic in foals. Abnormal colour with an elevated protein (25–84 g/l; normal <20 g/l) were features of an abdominal fluid sample in 98% of horses suffering from *A. equuli* peritonitis, and a marked elevation in nucleated cell count (46–810 × 10^9 cells/l; normal <10 × 10^9 cells/l) was present in all samples. Pleomorphic Gram-negative rods were seen on cytology in 53% of samples and a positive culture of *A. equuli* was returned in 72% of samples obtained from horses suffering from *A. equuli* peritonitis (Matthews *et al.* 2001).

Pathology

The presence of multifocal microabscesses in the renal and adrenal cortices is regarded as pathognomonic. Microscopically purulent exudates are centred on the bacteria and necrotic tissues. In fulminating bacteraemia other organs may be affected, resulting in embolic hepatitis (39–42) and polyarthritis.

Management/Treatment

Most isolates obtained from horses suffering from *A. equuli* peritonitis were sensitive to procaine penicillin, so treatment with procaine penicillin and gentamicin sulphate is recommended until antimicrobial sensitivity is known. In one study of 51 horses, all demonstrated a rapid response to treatment with procaine penicillin (20 mg/kg BW IM bid) alone, or a combination of procaine penicillin and gentamicin sulphate (6.6 mg/kg BW IV sid) and supportive therapy and were discharged from hospital (Matthews *et al.* 2001). In addition, cefquinome showed high activity against *A. equuli in vitro* (Thomas *et al.* 2006).

Public health significance

A. equuli is found in infected wounds of humans bitten by horses (Peel *et al.* 1991, Ashhurst-Smith *et al.* 1998, Kuhnert *et al.* 2003).

38 A positive blood culture of *Actinobacillus equuli* is diagnostic in foals with a tentative diagnosis of sleepy foal disease.

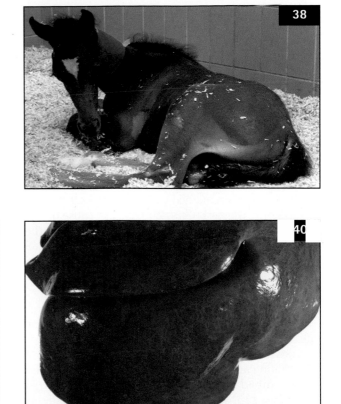

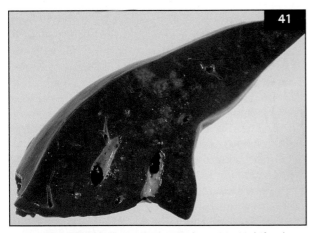

39, 40 Acute multifocal necrosuppurative hepatitis in a foal. Widespread miliary yellowish foci on the liver surface. *Actinobacillus equuli.*

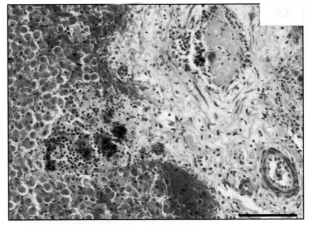

41 Acute multifocal necrosuppurative hepatitis. Multifocal to coalescing small yellowish areas of necrosis and suppuration on cut section of the liver. *Actinobacillus equuli.*

42 Acute multifocal necrosuppurative hepatitis. The hepatic parenchyma is affected by foci of hepatocellular necrosis with infiltrated neutrophils and surrounding haemorrhages. Note the intense basophilic bacterial colonies in the centre of such a focus (left middle). Near the top right corner a portal vein is obstructed by a thrombus also containing the causative bacteria (indicative of bacteraemia probably due to an umbilical infection). *Actinobacillus equuli.* (H&E stain. Bar 100 μm.)

Lawsonia intracellularis: EQUINE PROLIFERATIVE ENTEROPATHY

Phylum BXII Proteobacteria
Class IV Deltaproteobacteria/Family I
Desulfovibrionaceae/Genus III *Lawsonia*: Gram-negative nonspore-forming curved rods

Definition/Overview

Proliferative enteropathy caused by *Lawsonia intracellularis* is known as equine proliferative enteropathy (EPE) and is predominantly seen in older foals. Measurable colostral antibodies against *L. intracellularis* remained detectable in foals for 11–56 days only (Pusterla *et al.* 2009*c*). The cause of this proliferative enteropathy in pigs and horses is the same organism based on similarities between the 16S rRNA (Cooper & Gebhart 1998, McOrist & Gebhart 1999, Lavoie *et al.* 2000).

Aetiology

L. intracellularis is an obligate Gram-negative intracellular argyrophilic bacterium, which cannot be cultivated in cell-free media. These Gram-negative cells retain carbol–fuchsin when they are stained by the modified Ziehl–Nielsen method. Although *Rickettsia* spp. are the only obligate intracellular bacteria known to have a similar intracellular location, any relationship with these bacteria was clearly ruled out by the DNA sequence data. Cells characteristically replicate within the cytoplasm, are not enclosed by membrane-bound vacuoles, and occur in epithelial cells in the ilea of pigs. They are best revealed in histological sections by silver-staining techniques (McOrist *et al.* 1995).

Epidemiology

Mares residing on a farm known to be endemic for EPE are routinely exposed to *L. intracellularis,* and antibodies against *L. intracellularis* are passively transferred to foals (Pusterla *et al.* 2009*b*). The largest number of PCR-positive *L. intracellularis* faecal samples was observed in striped skunks, followed by Virginian opossums, jackrabbits, and coyotes. Because their faecal samples were collected at equine farms with confirmed cases of EPE, these animal species may act as potential sources of infection to susceptible weanlings (Pusterla *et al.* 2008).

Pathophysiology

Transmission generally occurs via the oral–faecal route. Infected crypt cells divide excessively, resulting in marked hyperplasia of the mucosa with poorly differentiated enterocytes and concurrent villous atrophy, leading to diarrhoea due to loss of intestinal absorptive capacity. The associated hypo-proteinaemia is due to malabsorption and protein loss into the intestinal lumen (Wuersch *et al.* 2006). Furthermore, impaired intestinal absorption of glucose has been reported (Wong *et al.* 2009).

Incubation period

A foal exposed via nasogastric intubation to 3×10^{10} *L. intracellularis* organisms developed fever (38.3°C) on days 19–20 post-inoculation and became mildly lethargic with partial anorexia on day 24 post-inoculation, which lasted for 4 days. Peripheral oedema in the distal extremities and throatlatch was first noticed on days 28 and 29 post-inoculation, respectively. The oedema lasted for 27 and 5 days in the distal extremities and throatlatch, respectively. Faecal shedding of *L. intracellularis* was detected starting between days 12 and 18 post-inoculation and lasted for 7–21 days after initial detection. Measurable antibodies (ranging from 240 to 3,840) against *L. intracellularis* were present 14–21 days post-inoculation with titres persisting up to the end of the study (90 days) (Pusterla *et al.* 2010*a*).

Clinical presentation

Clinical signs include weight loss, ventral oedema, lethargy, a prolonged period of decreased appetite or anorexia, fever (up to 41°C) or hypothermia, increased intestinal sounds, diarrhoea (**43**), and colic (Wuersch *et al.* 2006, Sampieri *et al.* 2006, Frazer 2008). Poor body condition with a rough coat and a pot-bellied appearance are common in affected foals (Lavoie *et al.* 2000, Wuersch *et al.* 2006). A sex predilection is not apparent (Frazer 2008), whereas an age predilection is obvious, with all horses being foals or weanlings between 3 and 13 months of age (Lavoie *et al.* 2000, Deprez *et al.* 2005, Wuersch *et al.* 2006, Frazer 2008). Clinical signs are usually seen after weaning (Lavoie *et al.* 2000, Wuersch *et al.* 2006). The disease is fatal in about 20% of cases (Sampieri *et al.* 2006).

Clinicopathological abnormalities include hypoproteinaemia, hypoalbuminaemia (range 9–33 g/l), hyperfibrinogenaemia, (transient) leukocytosis, azotaemia, and increased plasma activities of creatine kinase (CK; 388–13,300 IU/l), aspartate aminotransferase (AST) and lactate dehydrogenase (LDH) activity (associated with Zenker's degeneration of muscle), and sometimes anaemia (Lavoie *et al.* 2000, Sampieri *et al.* 2006, Wuersch *et al.* 2006, Frazer 2008).

Differential diagnosis

The combination of thickened intestinal (small bowel) wall (**44, 45**), as shown by means of abdominal ultrasound and hypoalbuminaemia in older foals, must be regarded as pathognomonic for

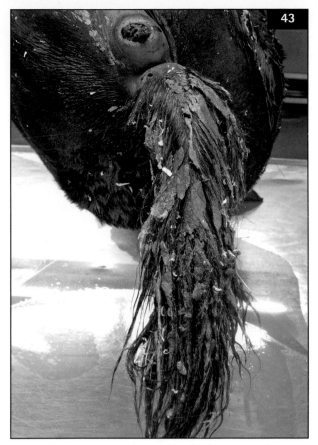

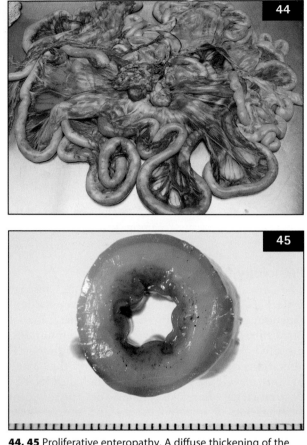

43 Proliferative enteropathy. Profuse diarrhoea as can be seen in *Lawsonia* enteritis-affected foal. Note also the rough haircoat.

44, 45 Proliferative enteropathy. A diffuse thickening of the small intestinal wall in a foal associated with a *Lawsonia intracellularis* infection. Note the swollen mesenteric lymph nodes in the centre of the small intestinal convolute. This particular case proved to be PCR-positive for the causative bacterium (**44**). Proliferative enteropathy. Transversely cut portion of the thickened small intestinal wall (ileum). *Lawsonia intracellularis*. (Scale in mm.) (**45**)

the disease. Weight loss and mild small bowel protein losing enteropathy might be associated with *Parascaris equorum* infection in older foals.

Diagnosis

Observation of older foals for typical clinical signs, abdominal ultrasound revealing thickened intestinal wall (range 4–8 mm, median 6 mm; normal range 3 mm at maximum [Reef 1998]), the presence of hypoalbuminaemia, and ruling out other differential diagnoses for enteric disease allow early initiation of treatment and aid in interpreting faecal PCR and serum immunoperoxidase monolayer assay (IPMA) results (Frazer 2008). An IPMA titre ≥60 is considered positive for *L. intracellularis* infection (Frazer 2008). Affected horses tested positive on faecal PCR and IPMA in 75% and 81% of cases, respectively. In comparison, age-matched, clinically normal herd mates also tested positive for *L. intracellularis* on faecal PCR (6%) and IPMA (33%) (Frazer 2008). In other studies, however, only 33–55% of horses with clinically suspected infection were found to be positive on faecal PCR analysis (Lavoie *et al.* 2000, Sampieri *et al.* 2006).

It should be realized that PCR testing does not differentiate between viable and nonviable DNA (Frazer 2008). Only 50% of horses with clinical signs of EPE tested positive on both faecal PCR and serum IPMA, which stresses the importance of running both of these diagnostic tests on all suspected horses (Frazer 2008). Rectal swabs should be considered as an alternative sample type for EPE-suspected patients with decreased or no faecal output. By analysing dual samples, the PCR detection rate for *L. intracellularis* increased from 76% and 79% for rectal swabs and faeces, respectively, to 90% (Pusterla *et al*. 2010*b*).

For diagnosis of EPE, hypoproteinaemia might be used as a screening test (Lavoie *et al*. 2000).

Pathology
The disease is characterized by the intense hyperplastic proliferation of crypt epithelium (adenomatosis) predominantly in the distal ileum, but can extend proximally into the jejunum and distally into the large intestine. Gross pathological alterations characterized by proliferative thickening of the ileal wall are pathognomonic in foals (**46, 47**). Post-mortem diagnosis relies on histological examination of infected tissues and use of silver stain, immunofluorescence, and PCR. Curved bacteria can be readily demonstrated by silver stain (Warthin–Starry) in the apical cytoplasm of the proliferating enterocytes. A more sensitive method is immunohistochemistry using a monoclonal antibody to *L. intracellularis*. PCR of intestinal lesions is the most sensitive and specific technique for diagnosis (Deprez *et al*. 2005, Wuersch *et al*. 2006). Histological examination reveals a necrotizing enteritis with focal adenomatosis and segmental mucosal ulceration (**48**). Haemorrhages and plasma cell infiltration are present in the lamina propria. Calcification of the lamina elastica interna of the small arteries might also be observed in the submucosa (Deprez *et al*. 2005, Frazer 2008). In addition, depletion of lymphoid nodules can be observed both on jejunum and colon samples (Sampieri *et al*. 2006).

Management/Treatment
Treatment with erythromycin estolate (25 mg/kg BW, PO, q8h) alone or combined with rifampicin (rifampin) (7 mg/kg BW, PO, q12h) for a minimum of 21 days is recommended, with additional symptomatic treatment including plasma transfusion, parenteral nutrition, and antiulcer medications when indicated (Lavoie *et al*. 2000, Deprez *et al*. 2005). Oxytetracycline (6.6 mg/kg BW bid IV) and doxycycline (10 mg/kg BW bid PO) are also effective treatments for EPE (Sampieri *et al*. 2006). Given the high prevalence of *L. intracellularis* in pigs, direct contact of foals with pigs should be prevented (Lavoie *et al*. 2000, Deprez *et al*. 2005). *L. intracellularis* is not able to survive outside the host for more than 2 weeks at room temperature (Collins *et al*. 2000).

Foals vaccinated intrarectally with a modified-live vaccine of *L. intracellularis* seroconverted after the first vaccine, compared to 50% and 0% of foals following oral drenching after pre-medication with a proton-pump inhibitor or orally without any pre-medication, respectively. Premedication with omeprazole prior to oral vaccination to increase stomach pH and decrease the effect of low pH on the viability of the challenged *L. intracellularis* led to an earlier and stronger detectable humoral response compared to non-premedicated foals (Pusterla *et al*. 2009*a*). Unfortunately, faecal shedding of *L. intracellularis* was detected in mares, immunized intrarectally with a modified-live *L. intracellularis* vaccine 3–5 weeks before the expected foaling dates, 12–15 days following administration, and lasted for 1–3 days (Pusterla *et al*. 2009*c*).

Public health significance
EPE is not currently reported to be a zoonosis (*Lavoie et al*. 2000).

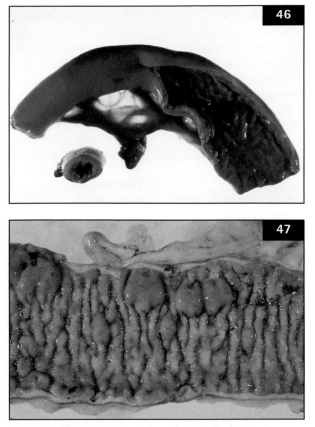

46, 47 Proliferative enteropathy. A longitudinal opened portion of the small intestine (ileum) gives a view of the raised corrugated mucosa as a result of the hyperplastic crypts and thickened submucosa. *Lawsonia intracellularis*.

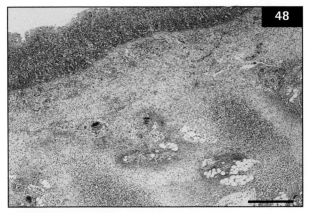

48 Proliferative enteropathy. Micrograph at small magnification of a portion of hyperplastic ileal mucosa with blunted villi (darker upper portion) and the underlying severely thickened oedematous and inflamed submucosa. *Lawsonia intracellularis*. (H&E stain. Bar 500 μm.)

Campylobacter spp.

Phylum BXII Proteobacteria
Class V Epsilonproteobacteria/Family 1
Campylobacteraceae/Genus I *Campylobacter*:
Aerobic/microaerophilic, motile, helical/vibrioid
Gram-negative bacteria

Definition/Overview

Campylobacter spp. are among putative pathogens
found at very low prevalence in foal diarrhoea.

Aetiology

Campylobacter spp. are thermophilic Gram-negative
rods.

Epidemiology

Birds are one of the most important reservoirs of
Campylobacter spp. With a relatively high internal
body temperature of around 42°C, they offer the
appropriate environment for these bacteria, which
show special thermal requirements (Wysok &
Uradziński 2009), whereas long-term survival of
Campylobacter jejuni at low temperature is
dependent on polynucleotide phosphorylase activity
(Haddad *et al.* 2009). Rats were found to be infected
with strains of *C. jejuni* with bacterial restriction
endonuclease DNA analysis patterns indistinguishable from those infecting humans, poultry, and a
horse (Kakoyiannis *et al.* 1988).

Pathophysiology

C. jejuni actively penetrates the intestinal mucus
layer, secretes proteins mainly via its flagellar
apparatus, is engulfed by intestinal cells, and can
disrupt the integrity of the epithelial lining.
Furthermore, *C. jejuni* stimulates the
proinflammatory pathway and the production of a
large repertoire of cytokines, chemokines, and innate
effector molecules (van Putten *et al.* 2009).

Incubation period

Not established in the equine species yet.

Clinical presentation

Campylobacter spp. were among putative pathogens
found at very low or zero prevalence in foal
diarrhoea (Al-Mashat & Taylor 1986, Browning *et
al.* 1991, Netherwood *et al.* 1996). In addition, *C.
fetus* subsp. *fetus* was cultured from jugular venous
blood in a 10-month-old Standardbred colt with
granulomatous enteritis. However, at necropsy the
bacterium could not be isolated from tissues
(Johnson & Goetz 1993). Furthermore, abortion
caused by *C. fetus* subsp. *fetus* was diagnosed in a
7-month-old equine fetus (Hong & Donahue 1989).

Differential diagnosis

The differential diagnosis includes various causes of
diarrhoea in foals (see p. 262).

Diagnosis

A fresh faecal sample and/or a rectal tissue biopsy
might reveal *Campylobacter* spp. with microaerobic
culture (Hurcombe *et al.* 2009). However, diagnosis
should depend on the detection of *Campylobacter*
spp. combined with clinical signs.

Pathology

Campylobacter spp. can incite a mild to moderate
enterocolitis possibly combined with epithelial
erosion.

Management/Treatment

Treatment of diseased animals is supportive,
especially with regard to diarrhoea. A 2-year-old
Quarter Horse evaluated for chronic diarrhoea and
weight loss of 5 weeks duration responded
transiently to fluoroquinolone administration,
forming discrete faecal balls after 72 hours of
treatment. However, at 5 months follow-up it
reverted back to having soft 'cow-pie' faeces
(Hurcombe *et al.* 2009).

Public health significance

Poultry appear to be a major source of infection for
C. jejuni in humans, with nearly half of the human
isolates giving patterns which are indistinguishable
from those isolated from poultry (Kakoyiannis *et al.*
1988).

Helicobacter equorum

Phylum BXII Proteobacteria
Class V Epsilonproteobacteria/Family II
Helicobacteraceae/Genus I *Helicobacter*: Aerobic/
microaerophilic, motile, helical/vibrioid Gram-
negative bacteria

Definition/Overview

To date, at least nine gastric and 20 enterohepatic
formally named *Helicobacter* spp. have been
identified in a large variety of animal species (Euzéby
2007). However, an association between
Helicobacter pylori and gastric ulceration (49, 50)
has not been established in the equine species yet.

Aetiology

Helicobacter equorum is an urease-negative
Helicobacter species (Moyaert *et al.* 2007*c*).

Incubation period

H. equorum DNA was detected in faecal samples
from 1–3 days following intragastric inoculation
(Moyaert *et al.* 2007*a*).

Clinical presentation

H. equorum has been isolated from faecal samples of
clinically healthy horses and sites of colonization are
caecum, colon, and rectum (Moyaert *et al.* 2007*c*)
indicating no appreciable clinical signs. The agent is
highly prevalent in <6-month-old foals. In adult
horses, the prevalence of *H. equorum* seems to be
rather low, but these animals may harbour low,
subdetectable numbers of this microorganism in their
intestines (Moyaert *et al.* 2009).

Differential diagnosis

Not appropriate as of yet.

Diagnosis

H. equorum DNA can be identified using PCR
amplifying a 1,074-bp fragment (Moyaert *et al.*
2007*b*).

Pathology

No apparent pathology.

Management/Treatment

Not considered necessary.

Public health significance

Not convincing yet. *H. equorum* DNA was not
detected in human faeces, indicating that this
microorganism does not commonly spread from
horses to humans (Moyaert *et al.* 2009).

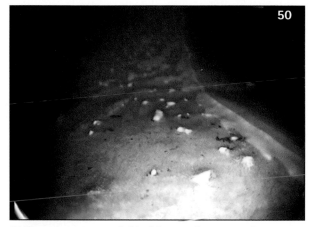

49 Erosions and ulceration of the squamous part (left) of the
gastric mucosa as visualized *in vivo* using an endoscope.

50 The squamous part (left) of the gastric mucosa almost
completely destroyed although the margo plicatus is still
distinguishable as visualized *in vivo* using an endoscope.

Clostridium botulinum: BOTULISM ('SHAKER FOAL DISEASE')

Phylum BXIII Firmicutes
Class I Clostridia/Order I Clostridiales/Family I Clostridiaceae/Genus I *Clostridium*: Endospore-forming Gram-positive rods and cocci

Definition/Overview

The botulinum neurotoxin, a marvel of protein design (Montal 2010), is the most potent toxin known, with as little as 30–100 ng potentially fatal, and is responsible for botulism, a severe neuroparalytic disease that affects humans, animals, and birds (Peck 2009). Botulism can arise from preformed toxin, wound infection, or intestinal toxico-infection. All three forms can occur in humans as well as in animals (Critchley 1991). Intoxication classically presents as an acute, symmetrical, descending flaccid paralysis (Dembek et al. 2007). Clinical suspicion of botulism remains the cornerstone of diagnosis (Sobel 2009) in the absence of electrophysiological testing. Early treatment with antitoxin generally results in a favourable outcome. Botulism can be prevented by vaccination (Whitlock & Buckley 1997).

Aetiology

The disease is caused by a neurotoxin released from *Clostridium botulinum*, a Gram-positive, obligate anaerobic rod-shaped bacterium transmitted as spores and present in soil throughout the world. Botulinum neurotoxins (BoNTs) are among the most potent naturally occurring toxins and are a category A biological threat agent. The seven toxin serotypes of BoNT (serotypes A–G) have different toxicities, act through three different intracellular protein targets, and exhibit different durations of effect (Dembek et al. 2007). The ability to form BoNT is restricted to six phylogenetically and physiologically distinct bacteria (*C. botulinum* groups I–IV and some strains of *C. baratii* and *C. butyricum*) (Peck 2009). It has also emerged that the BoNT-forming clostridia are not overtly pathogenic (unlike *C. difficile*), but saprophytic bacteria that use the neurotoxin to kill a host and create a source of nutrients. The neurotoxin gene is present within a cluster of associated genes, and can be located on the chromosome, a plasmid, or a bacteriophage (Peck 2009). Disease in horses has been attributed to serotypes A, B, C, and D (Kinde et al. 1991, Szabo et al. 1994, Gerber et al. 2006, Johnson et al. 2010). Horses appear to be more sensitive to botulinum toxin type B, compared with other species (Adam-Castrillo et al. 2004).

Epidemiology

Botulism may follow ingestion of food contaminated with BoNT, from toxin production of *C. botulinum* present in the intestine or wounds (e.g. open castration), or from inhalation of aerosolized toxin (Bernard et al. 1987, Dembek et al. 2007). Foals may especially suffer from toxico-infectious botulism, a condition where the *C. botulinum* might colonize and produce toxin within the GI tract (Galey 2001). One important feature that has contributed to the success of BoNT-forming clostridia is their ability to form highly resistant endospores. The spores, however, also present an opportunity to control these bacteria if escape from lag phase (and hence growth) can be prevented (Peck 2009).

Potential sources include carrion in hay, mouldy or otherwise rotted vegetation or forage, birds carrying material from animal burial or other similar sites, and contaminated carcasses on-site (Kinde et al. 1991, Galey 2001, Johnson et al. 2010). Equine fodder-borne botulism in Europe is most probably caused by BoNT/C and BoNT/D (Gerber et al. 2006). In addition, neurotoxin B genes were detected in 94% of soil samples. Fewer soil samples were positive for *C. botulinum* type B by the mouse bioassay (15%) than by any DNA-based detection system. Hybridization of a type B-specific probe to DNA dot blots (26% of the samples positive) and PCR-enzyme-linked assay (77% of the samples positive) were valid for rapid soil analysis, with conventional detection of PCR products by gel electrophoresis being the most sensitive method (300 cell limit) (Szabo et al. 1994). As a consequence, there is also the possibility that the development of pica through lack of essential nutrients could lead to the ingestion of contaminated substances facilitating botulinum intoxication (Critchley 1991).

A total of 31% horses were ELISA positive for anti-BoNT/C IgG antibodies in Israel. The farm and its geographical region were associated significantly with seropositivity; horse-level variables, such as gender and breed, were also associated with seropositivity. Quarter Horse and Warmblood mares placed in the southern region of Israel had the highest odds ratio to be tested positive for anti-BoNT/C IgG antibodies (Steinman et al. 2007). In Switzerland, the incidence of equine botulism had increased in the preceding 5 years (Gerber et al. 2006).

Shaker foal disease shows the highest incidence in Kentucky and the mid-Atlantic region of the USA (Wilkins & Palmer 2003a), whereas almost all type A cases and outbreaks occurred in the western USA, with Oregon and Idaho overrepresented (Johnson et al. 2010).

Pathophysiology

When *C. botulinum* spores were given orally to horses they were innocuous, and they produced toxicosis only when necrotic lesions were present (Swerczek 1980*a*). BoNT is a modular nanomachine: an N-terminal Zn^{2+}-metalloprotease, which cleaves the soluble N-ethylmaleimide-sensitive factor attachment protein receptor; a central helical protein-conducting channel, which chaperones the protease across endosomes; and a C-terminal receptor-binding module, consisting of two subdomains that determine target specificity by binding to a ganglioside and a protein receptor on the cell surface and triggering endocytosis. BoNT proteases disable synaptic vesicle exocytosis by cleaving their cytosolic soluble N-ethylmaleimide-sensitive factor attachment protein receptor substrates (Montal 2010). As a consequence, a presynaptic blockade of neuromuscular transmission with reduced release of acetylcholine occurs, associated with electrophysiological findings ranging from spontaneous activity and small motor unit potentials of short duration to complete electrical silence on needle EMG (Souayah *et al.* 2006). Protective antibodies when bound to the toxin at sites that coincide or overlap with synaptosomes-binding would prevent the toxin from binding to the nerve synapse and therefore block toxin entry into the neuron. Thus, analysis of the locations of the antibody-binding and the synaptosomes-binding regions provides a molecular rationale for the ability of protecting antibodies to block BoNT/A action *in vivo* (Atassi *et al.* 2007). On the other hand, the use of BoNT/A (Botox) is under study as a therapeutic option for stringhalt in horses (Wijnberg *et al.* 2009).

Incubation period

The incubation period is as short as 6 days following IM inoculation with BoNT/B and simultaneous induction of muscle necrosis and death 48–60 hours after the onset of clinical signs. However, yearling Thoroughbred colts died from respiratory arrest within 6 hours after IV inoculation with BoNT/B (Swerczek 1980*b*). In comparison, injection of 2,500 IU of BoNT/B toxin in the anal sphincter resulted in mild generalized weakness, low head carriage, diarrhoea, and dysphagia on day 10. Neuromuscular deficits had resolved by day 24 (Adam-Castrillo *et al.* 2004).

Clinical presentation

A tentative diagnosis is usually based on the presence of the following clinical findings: anxious attitude, delayed pupillary light response, mydriasis, ptosis, reduced tone of the tongue, throat, or lips, slow chewing, salivation, and difficulties swallowing (**51**),

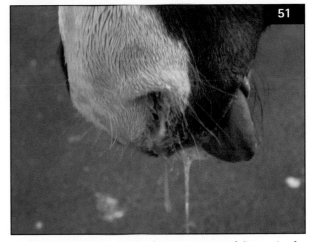

51 Clinical suspicion remains the cornerstone of diagnosis of botulism in the absence of electrophysiological testing, with clinical findings including reduced tone of the tongue, difficulties in swallowing, and salivation. However, dysphagia is not a consistent finding.

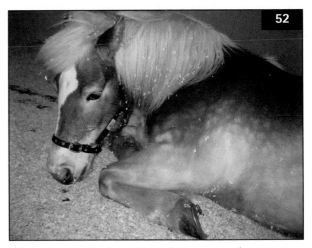

52 Generalized muscle weakness that progressed to recumbency in a 13-year-old Haflinger mare suffering from (fatal) botulism. Needle electromyography did not reveal the presence of motor unit action potentials in skeletal muscle.

generalized muscle weakness that progresses during a period of 1–4 days to lateral recumbency (**52**), decreased tail tone, small hard faecal balls, and slow prehension of feed. Botulism should also be considered in cases where intolerance to exercise might be seen in the horse. Dysphagia may also be present, although it is not a consistent finding (Kinde *et al.* 1991, Whitlock & Buckley 1997, Schoenbaum *et al.* 2000, Galey 2001, Gerber *et al.* 2006).

Affected animals might appear alert and interested in eating and drinking even while recumbent (Schoenbaum *et al.* 2000) or even show increased appetite (Kinde *et al.* 1991). Death occurs secondary to respiratory muscle paralysis (Swerczek 1980*b*, Wilkins & Palmer 2003*a*).

In 'Shaker foal' disease, the toxico-infectious botulism of foals, foals either were found dead without premonitory signs of illness or, most often, had signs of progressive and symmetric motor paralysis. Stilted gait, muscular tremors, and the inability to stand longer than 4–5 minutes were the salient clinical signs. Other clinical manifestations included dysphagia, constipation, mydriasis, and frequent urination. As the disease progressed, dyspnoea with extension of the head and neck, tachycardia, and respiratory arrest occurred. Death occurred most often 24–72 hours after the onset of clinical signs (Swerczek 1980*a*, Wilkins & Palmer 2003*a*). Approximately 50% of these cases required oxygen therapy, whereas 30% required mechanical ventilation. Mean duration of hospitalization was 14 days (Wilkins & Palmer 2003*a*). Mechanical ventilation of foals with botulism and respiratory failure appears to be an effective adjunct therapy, with survival in treated foals being 88–96% (Wilkins & Palmer 2003*b*). Lethality of type A and C botulism in horses was 91% (Johnson *et al.* 2010) and 82% (Kinde *et al.* 1991), respectively.

It has been suggested that *C. botulinum* types C and D are involved in the aetiology of equine grass sickness (EGS) (53–57) (Hunter *et al.* 1999, Nunn *et al.* 2007). However, it has been shown that with reference to synaptophysin, an integral membrane protein of synaptic vesicles regarded as an immunohistochemical marker for degenerating neurons, different mechanisms cause neuronal damage and/or dysfunction in EGS and botulism (Waggett *et al.* 2010). In addition, electro-myographic (EMG) findings seen in horses with grass sickness (Wijnberg *et al.* 2006) differ from the expected readings in botulism.

Differential diagnosis

Diagnosis of botulism is often a clinical diagnosis backed up by elimination of other possible infectious, injurious, or toxic causes of weakness of the horse. Definitive diagnosis and type identification in the laboratory are difficult and usually require a suitable sample of the source material (Galey 2001). The differential diagnosis predominantly includes various causes of acute neurological disease (see p. 262).

Diagnosis

Increased cerebrospinal fluid (CSF) creatine kinase (CK) activity was reported in CSF samples from horses with botulism (Furr & Tyler 1990). Definitive diagnosis requires detection of botulinum toxin in plasma, serum, GI contents, or body tissues like liver (Kinde *et al.* 1991, Szabo *et al.* 1994, Whitlock & Buckley 1997, Schoenbaum *et al.* 2000). Early diagnosis is important because antitoxin therapy is most effective when administered early in the course of the disease.. Confirmatory testing of botulism with BoNT assays or *C. botulinum* cultures is time consuming, and may be insensitive in the diagnosis of inhalational botulism and in as many as 32% of food-borne botulism cases (Dembek *et al.* 2007).

Sensitivity of an ELISA for detecting type C and D toxins compared with mouse inoculation was 70% and specificity 96% on samples from animals with botulism diagnosed on clinical signs and herd history. However, both mouse inoculation and the ELISA failed to detect toxin in many animals with a presumptive diagnosis of botulism. Some cross-reaction was seen with *C. novyi* type A, but not with other clostridial species. While the ELISA cannot replace mouse inoculation for the diagnosis of botulism, it is a useful additional test (Thomas 1991). In comparison, the mouse bioassay failed to detect botulinum toxin in the serum samples of nearly one-third of injection drug users with characteristic wound botulism (Wheeler *et al.* 2009). Single supramaximal stimulations is a simple and reliable electrodiagnostic test for botulism,

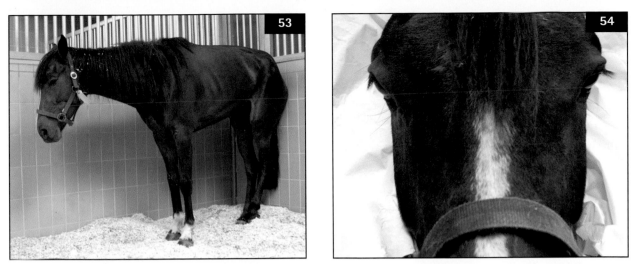

53, 54 Chronic grass sickness in a 3-year-old Warmblood mare (overview **53**) and photograph of the head *in vivo* (**54**) following administration of phenylephrine (α-1 adrenergic agonist) eyedrops (see Hahn & Mayhew 2000) in the left eye, resulting in a reduction in ptosis. In comparison, the right eye illustrates ptosis.

55 Left nostril of a 3-year-old Warmblood mare suffering from chronic grass sickness illustrating rhinitis sicca.

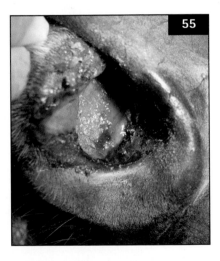

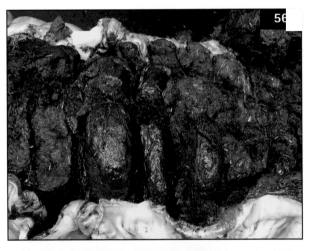

56 Grass sickness (dysautonomia). Colon ascendens containing dehydrated impacted ingesta/feed contents due to dysautonomic dysperistalsis as a sequel of autonomic ganglionic neuronal degeneration. *Clostridium botulinum* is associated as a probable aetiology. Possible additional lesions are gastric impaction and crusting of the nasal orifices.

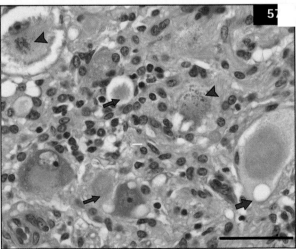

57 Grass sickness (dysautonomia). Neuronal chromatolysis in the coeliac autonomic ganglion. Close-up of several affected neurons displaying striking typical degenerative changes such as: severe chromatolysis with formation of a central eosinophilic core and cytoplasmic vacuolation (large arrow) and within the same neuron a flattened pyknotic marginated nucleus, cytoplasmic accumulation of light brown granular lipofuscin pigments (arrowheads), and interspersed shrunken eosinophilic necrotic perikarya with complete loss of their nucleus (small arrows). (H&E stain. Bar 50 μm.)

associated with a sensitivity of 95% and a specificity of 100% in humans (Witoonpanich *et al.* 2009). Single-fibre EMG (Wijnberg *et al.* 2010) allows rapid identification of botulism while bioassay studies are in progress, revealing an increase in jitter (**58**) (Padua *et al.* 1999).

Pathology

Pathology usually remains inconclusive; apart from the anaerobic entry wounds and predisposing sites for the development of toxico-infectious botulism like gastric ulcers, foci of necrosis in the liver, and abscesses in the navel and lungs, there are no characteristic gross and histopathological lesions in botulism (Swerczek 1980*a*).

Management/Treatment

Early treatment with antitoxin (Whitlock & Buckley 1997, Dembek *et al.* 2007) combined with intensive care (**59**) (Gerber *et al.* 2006) generally results in a favourable outcome. Seven of 10 horses treated with type C antitoxin and plasma obtained from horses hyperimmunized with *C. botulinum* type C toxoids survived (Kinde *et al.* 1991).

Aluminium hydroxide based mono- and bivalent recombinant HcBoNT/C and D vaccines were characterized by good compatibility and the ability to elicit protective antibody titres similar or superior to the commercially available toxoid vaccine (Stahl *et al.* 2009). The recombinant vaccine showed fewer adverse reactions compared to a commercially available vaccine, but induced similar concentrations of neutralizing antibodies (Frey *et al.* 2007).

Horse antiserum against BoNT/A or human and mouse (outbred) antisera against the toxoid recognized similar regions on BoNT/A, but exhibited some boundary frame shifts and differences in immunodominance of these regions among the antisera (Atassi *et al.* 1996).

Prevention (high standards of forage quality and vaccination) is of utmost importance (Whitlock & Buckley 1997, Gerber *et al.* 2006).

Public health significance

Botulism has public health significance since a case of a veterinarian, who was likely to be infected/intoxicated by *C. botulinum* during the handling of a diseased animal, has been reported. It should be realized that in horses with botulism, tonsils might contain both vegetative toxigenic bacteria and BoNT (Böhnel *et al.* 2008).

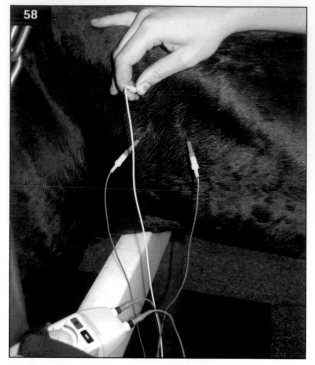

58 Single-fibre EMG is regarded as the gold standard diagnostic technique in botulism, allowing rapid identification while bioassay studies are in progress. This technique reveals an increase in jitter in botulism and is also available for use in horses.

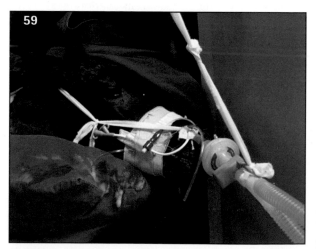

59 Botulism in an 8-day-old filly. Mechanical ventilation of foals with botulism and respiratory failure appears to be an effective adjunct therapy. (Courtesy of Dr M. Aleman, University of California, Davis, USA.)

Clostridium difficile

Phylum BXIII Firmicutes
Class I Clostridia/Order I Clostridiales/Family I
Clostridiaceae/Genus I *Clostridium*: Endospore-
forming Gram-positive rods and cocci

Definition/Overview

Acute enterocolitis (including duodenitis–
proximal jejunitis) (**60, 61**) eventually followed by
diarrhoea is caused by *Clostridium difficile* (formerly
Bacillus difficilis), in some cases preceded by
treatment with β–lactam antibiotics. It has been
suggested that *C. difficile* may also be a nosocomial
infection in horses (Båverud *et al.* 1997).

Aetiology

C. difficile is a Gram-positive or Gram-variable,
strictly anaerobic spore-forming bacterium that is an
important cause of diarrhoea in humans, and a
commonly identified nosocomial pathogen in human
hospitals (Norén 2005). In 1935, a new species of
bacterium was named *Bacillus difficilis*, the species
name given because of its difficult anaerobic
isolation from human faeces. Forty years later, it was
renamed *Clostridium difficile* and identified as the
cause of pseudomembranous colitis in man. This
organism is the most common cause of nosocomial
diarrhoea, and incidence has increased since the
appearance of a hypervirulent strain in 2000
(Kuipers & Surawicz 2008). Toxins A and B are
responsible for the pathological changes that result
in the clinical signs of disease (Weese *et al.* 1999).
Furthermore, metronidazole-resistant strains may be
associated with severe disease (Magdesian *et al.*
2006).

Epidemiology

A geographic association was found with areas in a
large animal clinic where nosocomial *C. difficile*
diarrhoea in horses had previously been diagnosed.
C. difficile was implicated in approximately 20–25%
of cases of enterocolitis in adult horses and foals at
the Ontario Veterinary College, Canada (Weese *et al.*
2000*a*).

Identical strains of *C. difficile* were present in
36% of mare–foal pairs indicating that mare–foal
pairs can harbour *C. difficile* subclinically and are
potential reservoirs for colonization of each other
(Magdesian & Leutenegger 2011).

Pathophysiology

The pathogenesis of the disease is attributable to a
number of virulence factors, including large
enterotoxins such as toxins A (enterotoxin)
and B (cytotoxin). Adenosine diphosphate
ribosyltransferase (binary toxin) has also been

detected in equine isolates of *C. difficile*. Its role in
the pathogenesis of disease has not yet been
established (Magdesian *et al.* 2006, Arroyo *et al.*
2006). Receptor-mediated endocytosis of the toxins
is followed by endosomal acidification, a necessary
step for conversion of the toxin to its active form in
the cytosol. Specific cell surface receptors have been

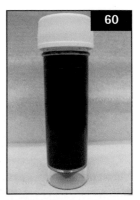

60 Haemorrhagic gastric reflux is associated with duodenitis–proximal jejunitis.

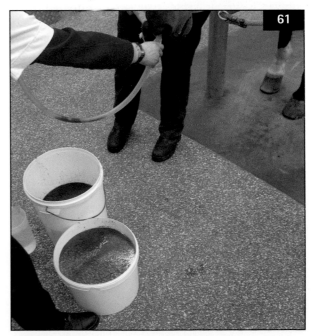

61 Large volumes of (haemorrhagic) gastric reflux are associated with duodenitis–proximal jejunitis. Additional clinical signs seen in duodenitis–proximal jejunitis are fever, sluggishness, and reactive hepatitis.

characterized for toxin A. Both toxins disrupt the actin cytoskeleton by disrupting Rho-subtype, intracellular signalling molecules. Disruption of the actin cytoskeleton is catastrophic for cellular function, but inflammation and neurogenic stimuli are also involved in the pathogenesis of the disease (Keel & Songer 2006).

Incubation period

C. difficile was isolated from faeces of foals between 24 and 72 hours after inoculation and toxins A or B or both were detected in the faeces of all foals by an enzyme-linked immunosorbent assay (Arroyo *et al.* 2004).

Clinical presentation

Clinical signs associated with *C. difficile* enterocolitis in horses can range from mild diarrhoea to severe haemorrhagic necrotizing enteritis (**62, 63**). In foals, the small intestine is more severely affected than the large intestine. Foals as young as 1 day old can have diarrhoea, probably because of the lack of a stable protective GI tract microflora (Weese *et al.* 1999). Clinical signs in foals after inoculation vary from mild abdominal discomfort and pasty faeces to colic and watery diarrhoea associated with haemorrhagic, necrotizing enterocolitis (Jones *et al.* 1988, Arroyo *et al.* 2004). Furthermore, lactose intolerance has been reported as a sequel to clostridial enterocolitis in a 12-hour-old Quarter Horse foal (Weese *et al.* 1999). *C. difficile* is also associated with acute colitis in mature horses treated with β-lactam antibiotics (Båverud *et al.* 1997). Duodenitis–proximal jejunitis has also been associated with toxigenic strains of *C. difficile* (Arroyo *et al.* 2006). Horses infected with strain B were 10 times as likely to have been treated with metronidazole prior to the onset of diarrhoea as horses infected with other strains. Duration from onset of diarrhoea to discharge (among survivors) was longer, systemic inflammatory response syndromes were more pronounced, and mortality rate was higher in horses infected with strain B than those infected with strains A and C combined (Magdesian *et al.* 2006). In contrast, it has been reported that horses with toxin A in their faeces had a significantly higher mortality rate than did horses negative for toxin A in their faeces (Ruby *et al.* 2009).

Differential diagnosis

The differential diagnosis includes various causes of acute diarrhoea (see p. 263).

Diagnosis

Diagnosis of *C. difficile* requires bacterial culture or demonstration of toxins in faeces. Culture does not differentiate carriers from those with disease nor does it confirm the presence of toxins (Kuipers & Surawicz 2008). Because nontoxigenic strains can be isolated, the association of *C. difficile* with enterocolitis is best made by culture of the organism and demonstration of cytotoxin in the faeces. An enzyme immunoassay to detect toxin production is a rapid, relatively inexpensive, and accurate test (Weese *et al.* 1999). Sensitivity and specificity of an ELISA for detection of *C. difficile* antigen were 93% and 88% when assay results were compared with results of microbial culture following direct plating, and 66% and 93% when assay results were compared with results of microbial culture following broth enrichment (Ruby *et al.* 2009). In addition, a commercially available *C. difficile* Tox A/B II ELISA was validated for detection of *C. difficile* toxins in horse faeces in comparison to a cell cytotoxicity assay (CTA), the accepted gold standard for *C. difficile* toxin detection (Medina-Torres *et al.* 2010).

A positive enzyme immunosorbent assay result was reported in 44% of diarrhoeic horses. Twenty-seven per cent of cases did not possess any toxin genes (A, B, or CDT [binary toxin]. There was no association between the presence of different ribotypes or strains and toxin gene profiles and the clinical outcome (Arroyo *et al.* 2007). Eighty per cent of isolates from horses with duodenitis–proximal jejunitis possessed genes encoding the production of both main toxins, A and B, while two were variant strains that produced toxin B but not toxin A. Additionally, genes encoding binary toxin (CDT) were present in one isolate that also carried the genes encoding toxins A and B. In one study, three of the 10 horses with duodenitis–proximal jejunitis developed diarrhoea during hospitalization and *C. difficile* was recovered from their faeces (Arroyo *et al.* 2006).

Pathology

Intestinal lesions due to *C. difficile* enterotoxaemia are typically comprised of a haemorrhagic necrotizing enterocolitis in foals and a necrotizing typhlocolitis in horses (McGavin & Zachary 2007).

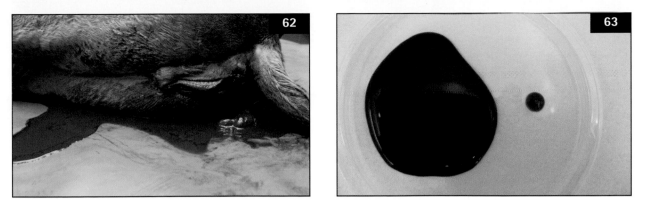

62, 63 Haemorrhagic necrotizing enterocolitis in foals is associated with *Clostridium difficile* infection.

Management/Treatment

Although the vegetative form of *C. difficile* does not survive for long periods of time in an aerobic environment, *C. difficile* organisms can survive for long periods of time in spore form. Whereas metronidazole has been suggested as the recommended treatment for horses with *C. difficile*-associated disease, antimicrobial susceptibility testing of isolates is warranted, as treatment with metronidazole predisposed horses to colonization with resistant strains (Magdesian *et al.* 2006). Several antimicrobials (like bacitracin zinc and metronidazole) have been advocated for the treatment of clostridial enterocolitis; however, substantial data regarding the efficacy of any of these are currently lacking (Weese *et al.* 1999). Interestingly, *Lactobacillus pentosus* WE7 isolated from the faeces of healthy horses was inhibitory against *C. difficile*, making it potentially useful as a therapeutic probiotic (Weese *et al.* 2004). In contrast to *C. difficile* organisms stored aerobically at 4°C, *C. difficile* toxins were considerably more stable and could be detected in faecal samples for at least 30 days at 4°C (Weese *et al.* 2000*b*). However, the spores persist in the environment and are difficult to eradicate (Kuipers & Surawicz 2008).

Public health significance

Since 1978, *C. difficile* has been clearly connected to human antibiotic-associated diarrhoea. For decades, standard treatment has been vancomycin or metronidazole with equal efficacy in man. Drawbacks such as the rise of vancomycin-resistant enterococci have limited the use of vancomycin in human cases (Norén 2005).

Horse and human isolates are usually positive for both toxins A and B, but human isolates produced greater amounts of toxin B. Furthermore, there is host–species dependency on the ability to attach to intestinal epithelial cells (Taha *et al.* 2007). However, colitis associated with infection by *C. difficile* NAP1/027 comprising the current human 'epidemic strain', which is associated with human *C. difficile*-associated disease was reported in a 14-year-old Quarter Horse with a 48-hour history of colic euthanized after failure to respond to treatment (Songer *et al.* 2009).

Clostridium perfringens

Phylum BXIII Firmicutes
Class I Clostridia/Order I Clostridiales/Family I
Clostridiaceae/Genus I *Clostridium*: Endospore-
forming Gram-positive rods and cocci

Definition/Overview

Acute typhlocolitis (including antibiotic-associated
or nosocomial typhlocolitis) eventually followed by
diarrhoea in horses of all ages is caused by the
ubiquitous enterotoxigenic bacterium *Clostridium
perfringens* (Jones 2000, Weese *et al.* 2001).
Clostridia produce the highest number of toxins of
any type of bacteria and are involved in severe
diseases in humans and other animals (Popoff &
Bouvet 2009). Equine clostridial enterotyphlocolitis
is being recognized with increasing frequency.
Perhaps it is time to consider clostridial enterocolitis
as yet another consequence of the use of
antimicrobials analogous to the selective pressures
that result in the emergence of multiple drug-
resistant pathogens (Jones 2000).

Aetiology

C. perfringens is a Gram-positive, strictly anaerobic
spore-forming rod-shaped bacterium that is an
important cause of diarrhoea, occurring worldwide
as constituents of soil and in the GI tracts of animals.
C. perfringens type A was the most common
genotype identified (85%) with the enterotoxin gene
identified in 2.1% of samples, and *C. perfringens*
type C was identified in < 1% of samples from
broodmares and foals (Tillotson *et al.* 2002).

Sequence comparison of the *cpb2* gene of beta2-
toxigenic *C. perfringens* revealed two genetically
different populations with most of the isolates from
horses carrying the *cpb2* gene (Johansson *et al.*
2006) prone to antibiotic-induced ribosomal
frameshifting by aminoglycosides (Vilei *et al.* 2005).

C. perfringens type A with the beta2-toxin gene
was identified in 12% of samples from broodmares
and foals (Tillotson *et al.* 2002). The *cpb2* gene of
equine and other nonporcine isolates differed from
that of porcine isolates by the absence of an adenine
in a poly A tract immediately downstream of the
start codon in all nonporcine *C. perfringens* strains.
Expression of the beta2 toxin was absent in equine
and the other nonporcine strains under standard
culture conditions (Vilei *et al.* 2005). The high
incidence of beta2-toxigenic *C. perfringens* in
samples of ingesta, biopsy specimens of the
intestinal wall, and faeces from horses suffering or
dying from typhlocolitis, together with the absence
of this organism in healthy horses provides strong
evidence that beta2-toxigenic *C. perfringens* plays
an important role in the pathogenesis of

typhlocolitis (Herholz *et al.* 1999); however,
decreased transcription and/or message instability
may be involved, at least in part, in the low cpb2
production noted for horse GI disease isolates in
comparison to that noted for pig GI disease isolates
(Waters *et al.* 2005).

Epidemiology

The prevalence of equine clostridial typhlocolitis in
horses with diarrhoea was 25%. *C. perfringens*
enterotoxin was detected in 16%, the cpa-encoded
alpha-toxin in 14%, and both toxins in 5% of faecal
samples collected from horses with diarrhoea.
However, a significant association was not found
between detection of enterotoxins in faeces and
development of diarrhoea as a complication of colic
(Donaldson & Palmer 1999). In comparison, *C.
perfringens* enterotoxin was detected in diarrhoeic
adults (19%) and diarrhoeic foals (29%), but was
not detected in adult horses or foals with normal
faeces. The positive predictive value of isolation of
C. perfringens with respect to the presence of
enterotoxin in faeces was 60% in adult horses and
64% in foals. There was no association between
total faecal *C. perfringens* spore count (versus the
vegetative form) and enterotoxin in faeces (Weese *et
al.* 2001).

Rotavirus was most frequently detected (20%)
followed by *C. perfringens* (18%), *Salmonella* spp.
(12%), and *C. difficile* (5%) in hospitalized foals
with diarrhoea. Foals below 1 month of age were
significantly more likely to be positive for *C.
perfringens* (OR = 15) or to have negative faecal
diagnostic results (OR = 3) than older foals.
However, the type of infectious agent identified in
the faeces or bacteraemia was not significantly
associated with survival (Frederick *et al.* 2009).
Enterocolitis associated with *C. perfringens*
infection in neonatal foals is often severe and has
been associated with a high case-mortality risk.
Multivariable logistic regression revealed that foals
of the stock horse type, housing in a stall or drylot
in the first 3 days of life, other livestock present on
the premises in the past, foal born on soil, sand, or
gravel surface, and low amounts of grass hay and
grain fed post-partum were significantly associated
with an increased risk of equine clostridial
enterocolitis. Low grain amounts fed prepartum
represented a decreased risk (East *et al.* 2000).

The prevalence of *C. perfringens* in ileal contents
from horses suffering from EGS was not
significantly greater than that for matched-control
horses with non-GI disease (Waggett *et al.* 2010).

64 Clostridial enterotoxaemia. Acute haemorrhagic typhlocolitis. The voluminous haemorrhagic content spills from the incised colon and caecum. Clostridial exotoxins cause severe necrosis of the mucosa and blood vessels resulting in diffuse intraluminal haemorrhage.

65 Clostridial enterotoxaemia. Acute haemorrhagic enterocolitis in a foal. Both small and large intestines are diffusely hyperaemic and include profuse thin haemorrhagic contents. *Clostridium perfringens*.

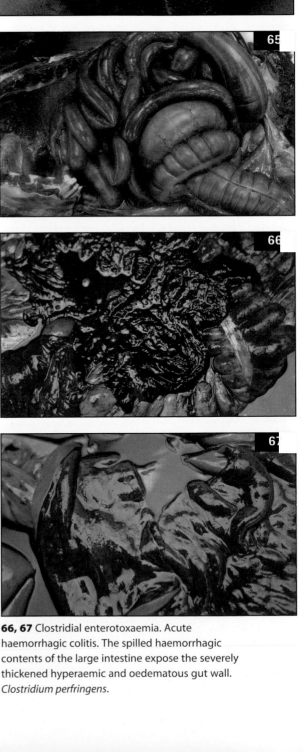

Pathophysiology

Most of the clostridial toxins are responsible for gangrenes and GI diseases. Three groups of clostridial toxins have the ability to enter cells: large clostridial glucosylating toxins, binary toxins, and neurotoxins. The binary and large clostridial glucosylating toxins alter the actin cytoskeleton by enzymatically modifying the actin monomers and the regulatory proteins from the Rho family, respectively. Clostridial neurotoxins proteolyse key components of neuroexocytosis (Popoff & Bouvet 2009). *C. perfringens* alpha-toxin is able to induce haemolysis due to Ca^{2+} uptake through T-type Ca^{2+} channels activated by the toxin (Ochi *et al.* 2003). Furthermore, marked fatal hyperammonaemia has been attributed to *C. perfringens* via increased intestinal bacterial production of ammonia that was readily absorbed through the inflamed bowel wall, exceeding the hepatic capacity for deamination (Stickle *et al.* 2006).

Incubation period

Not established in the equine species yet due to the variety of types of clostridia involved and the difficulty of experimentally reproducing the disease (Jones 2000), but may be as short as 12 hours. It should be realized that oral administration of oxytetracycline to horses was rapidly followed by the appearance of *C. perfringens* type A in large numbers and the accumulation of watery fluid in the rectal contents, whereas these changes were not seen following administration of trimethoprim–sulphadiazine (White & Prior 1982).

Clinical presentation

The clinical course usually involves acute typhlocolitis (including antibiotic-associated or nosocomial typhlocolitis) eventually followed by diarrhoea ranging from mild diarrhoea to severe haemorrhagic necrotizing enteritis in horses of all ages (**64–67**).

66, 67 Clostridial enterotoxaemia. Acute haemorrhagic colitis. The spilled haemorrhagic contents of the large intestine expose the severely thickened hyperaemic and oedematous gut wall. *Clostridium perfringens*.

In foals, the small intestine might be more severely affected than the large intestine. Foals less than 7 days old that have enterocolitis associated with *C. perfringens* infections, especially type C, have a guarded prognosis (East *et al.* 1998) although enterotoxigenic *C. perfringens* type A may also cause fatal enteric disease in horses (Bueschel *et al.* 1998). Other clinical signs include cellulitis and associated gas gangrene (Reef 1983), myonecrosis (Peek *et al.* 2003, Choi *et al.* 2003), urachitis and uroperitoneum in neonatal foals (Hyman *et al.* 2002), corneal infections (Rebhun *et al.* 1999), and purulent pericarditis as a sequela to clostridial myositis (May *et al.* 2002). Clostridial myonecrosis can occur following the IM or inadvertent perivascular administration of a wide variety of commonly administered drugs. It is most common in the neck musculature. The most common antecedent condition prior to referral was colic. Aggressive treatment can be associated with survival rates of up to 81% for cases due to *C. perfringens* alone. Survival rates for other *Clostridia* spp. tend to be lower (Peek *et al.* 2003).

Furthermore, severe fatal neurological abnormalities, including depression, repetitive muscle fasciculations, muscle stiffening, and collapse associated with severe hyperammonaemia (1,369.0 µmol/l compared with 15.3 µmol/l in controls) due to intestinal *C. perfringens* as a source of hyperammonaemia in the absence of hepatic disease has been reported in a 2-year-old Quarter Horse filly (Stickle *et al.* 2006).

Differential diagnosis

The differential diagnosis includes various causes of acute diarrhoea (see p. 263).

Diagnosis

Diagnosis of *C. perfringens* enterocolitis requires bacterial culture and/or demonstration of toxins in faeces combined with clinical signs. As *C. perfringens* type C is not frequently isolated from the faeces of healthy horses, high counts or monoculture of *C. perfringens* type C suggests its predominance in the flora of the large bowel, and might support the tentative clinical diagnosis of equine clostridial typhlocolitis. *C. perfringens* is probably part of the normal microflora of neonatal foals.

Most isolates from broodmares and foals are *C. perfringens* type A; thus, the clinical relevance of culture results alone is questionable for type A (Tillotson *et al.* 2002). Agreement between culture and enterotoxin ELISA for the detection of *C. perfringens* in the faeces was poor (κ = 0.085) in hospitalized foals with diarrhoea (Frederick *et al.* 2009). The *C. perfringens* alpha-toxin and the gene encoding beta2-toxin are frequently detected by means of phenotypical and PCR examination of bacterial isolates originating from field samples (Sting 2009). The presence of type III echinocytes or spheroechinocytes may be helpful in diagnosing immune-mediated haemolytic anaemia associated with clostridial infections in horses. In addition, automated reticulocyte counts may detect very low levels of reticulocytosis (Weiss & Moritz 2003).

Pathology

Pathology might reveal a haemorrhagic necrotizing typhlocolitis with degeneration of parenchymatous organs (68–72). The beta2 toxin might be demonstrated in sections of stomach, small intestine, and large intestine by immunohistochemical methods (Bacciarini *et al.* 2003).

Management/Treatment

Treatment of diseased horses is supportive (including transfaunation) especially with regard to diarrhoea. Of importance, *Clostridia* in general show a very good susceptibility to penicillins. Metronidazole appears to be an effective adjunctive treatment (McGorum *et al.* 1998). It should be realized that aminoglycosides are not effective against anaerobic bacteria. In addition, treatment of *C. perfringens* with the aminoglycosides gentamicin and streptomycin induced expression of the *cpb2* gene, presumably by frameshifting. This result may explain the finding that treatment with aminoglycosides of horses affected by beta2-toxigenic *C. perfringens* leads to a more accentuated and fatal progression of equine typhlocolitis (Vilei *et al.* 2005). A combination of high-dose IV antibiotic therapy and surgical fenestration/debridement is the best approach to cases of clostridial myonecrosis (Peek *et al.* 2003).

Di-tri-octahedral smectite effectively adsorbed *C. perfringens* exotoxins *in vitro* and had a dose-dependent effect on the availability of equine colostral antibodies, suggesting that it may be an appropriate adjunctive treatment in the management of neonatal clostridiosis in horses (Lawler *et al.* 2008).

Probiotics have not been demonstrated to provide any beneficial health effects in horses so far. However, *Lactobacillus pentosus* WE7 possesses *in vitro* and *in vivo* properties that may be useful for the prevention and treatment of equine clostridial typhlocolitis due to *C. perfringens* (Weese *et al.* 2004). Furthermore, to combat diseases caused by

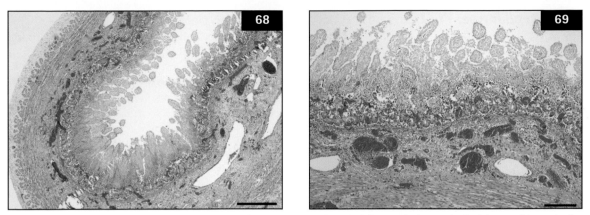

68, 69 Clostridial enterotoxaemia. Acute necrohaemorrhagic enteritis. Sharply delineated, the top half of the small intestinal mucosa including villi (jejunum) is diffusely pale eosinophilic with loss of cellular detail (necrosis). *Clostridium perfringens.* (H&E stain. Bars 500/200 μm, respectively.)

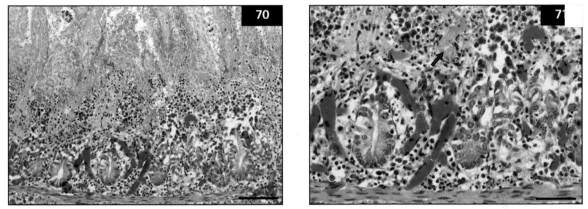

70, 71 Clostridial enterotoxaemia. Close-up micrograph of the affected mucosa on the junction of several intact crypts and overlying necrosis where an intravascular eosinophilic fibrinous thrombo-embolus is present (arrow). *Clostridium perfringens.* (H&E stain. Bars 100/50 μm, respectively.)

72 Clostridial enterotoxaemia. Close-up micrograph of pale eosinophilic villi that lack any cellular detail, i.e. necrotic villi, which are lined by numerous large basophilic bacterial rods. *Clostridium perfringens.* (H&E stain. Bar 50 μm.)

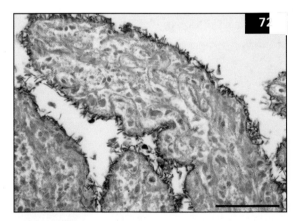

toxin-producing *C. perfringens* successfully, the implementation of consistent vaccination regimens in combination with controlled feeding is recommended (Timoney *et al.* 2005, Sting 2009).

Public health significance
Clostridia are not normally considered to be zoonotic pathogens, although many species affect both humans and domestic animals. Strains of *C. perfringens* that produce enterotoxin are typically transmitted to humans in contaminated, improperly handled foods (Songer 2010).

Clostridium piliforme: TYZZER'S DISEASE

Phylum BXIII Firmicutes
Class I Clostridia/Order I Clostridiales/Family I
Clostridiaceae/Genus I *Clostridium*: Endospore-
forming Gram-positive rods and cocci

Definition/Overview

Tyzzer's disease, an acute sporadically occurring
highly fatal hepatitis followed by sepsis of foals is
caused by *Clostridium piliforme* (formerly named
Bacillus piliformis).

Aetiology

C. piliforme is a spore-forming soil and manure-
borne, Gram-variable obligate intracellular
bacterium. A monoclonal antibody inhibition assay
detected large amounts of antibody to the flagellar
antigens of *C. piliforme* type E (horse origin), type
R1 (rat origin), or both in horse sera, indicating that
horses are susceptible to infection with at least two
distinct strains and that there is no apparent cross-
reacting immunity (Hook *et al.* 1995).

Epidemiology

In one study, foals born between March 13 and April
13 in California had a 7.2 times higher risk of
developing *C. piliforme* infection than those born at
any other time of the foaling season. Foals of
nonresident mares were 3.4 times more likely to
develop disease than were foals born to resident
mares, suggesting that passive transfer of *C.
piliforme*-specific antibodies through colostrum may
play a role in protection (Fosgate *et al.* 2002).

Pathophysiology

Oral exposure by ingestion of spore-containing
faeces from carrier horses with subsequent infection
of the liver via the portal circulation is presumed
(Swerczek 1976).

Incubation period

Not established in the equine species yet, but may be
as short as several hours.

Clinical presentation

Common clinical signs include fever, icterus (73, 74),
lethargy, recumbency, and seizures, with a poor
prognosis illustrated by a median survival time from
onset of disease in nonsurviving foals of 30 hours
(mean 34.5 ± 20.1; range 16–62 hours) (Borchers *et
al.* 2006).

Differential diagnosis

EHV1-infection is the most important differential
diagnosis with reference to clinical signs and the
concurrent multifocal hepatic coagulative necrosis in
neonatal foals.

Diagnosis

Tyzzer's disease is usually diagnosed by post-mortem
examination disclosing multifocal hepatic
coagulative necrosis given its nonspecific and
peracute course. Furthermore, a real-time TaqMan
assay has been developed to detect *C. piliforme* gene
sequences in liver tissue from affected foals (Borchers
et al. 2006).

Pathology

Post-mortem examination usually discloses
hepatomegaly with multifocal coagulative necrosis
(75–79) and hepatitis with intracytoplasmic
filamentous bacilli consistent with *C. piliforme*
(Borchers *et al.* 2006).

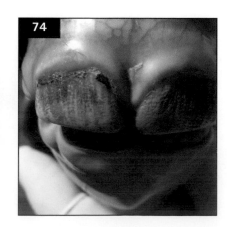

73 Icterus is a predominant clinical
sign in Tyzzer's disease in foals as
illustrated in the mucous
membranes of the oral cavity.

74 Bilirubin accumulation as
a sequela of icterus in a foal seen
in the dorsal parts of the
upper teeth.

Management/Treatment

Survival is rare and successful outcome is possible if the disease is identified early in its course and aggressive treatment (ampicillin and gentamicin, as well as partial parenteral nutrition) is instituted promptly (Borchers *et al.* 2006).

Public health significance

Spontaneous Tyzzer's disease has been reported in multiple species of laboratory, domestic, and wild animals but it is extremely rare in humans and nonhuman primates, e.g. cotton-top tamarins (*Saguinus oedipus*) (Sasseville *et al.* 2007).

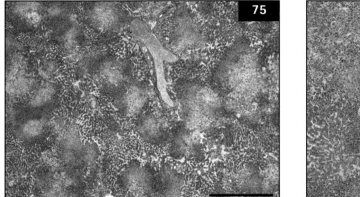

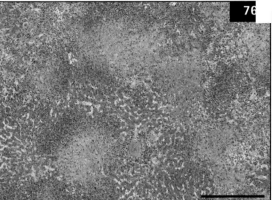

75, 76 Tyzzer's disease. Multifocal hepatic necrosis. Liver of a foal with randomly scattered pale foci of hepatocellular necrosis. *Clostridium piliforme*. (**75**: Giemsa stain. Bar 1 mm; **76**: H&E stain. Bar 500 μm.)

77 Tyzzer's disease. Hepatic necrosis. Close-up of a necrotic focus surrounded by an inflammatory infiltrate comprised of neutrophils and mononuclear cells. *Clostridium piliforme*. (H&E stain. Bar 200 μm.)

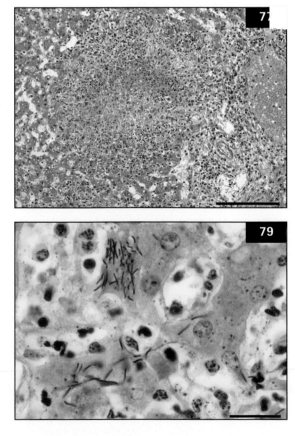

78, 79 Tyzzer's disease. At the margin of a necrotic focus viable hepatocytes contain numerous stacked intracytoplasmic large filamentous black-stained bacilli. *Clostridium piliforme*. (Warthin–Starry stain. Bars 50/20 μm, respectively.)

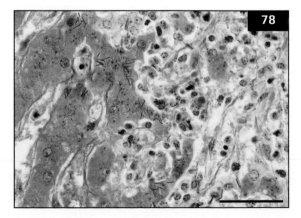

Clostridium tetani: TETANUS

Phylum BXIII Firmicutes
Class I Clostridia/Order I Clostridiales/Family I
Clostridiaceae/Genus I *Clostridium*: Endospore-
forming Gram-positive rods and cocci

Definition/Overview

Tetanus is caused by a neurotoxin released from
wounds infected with *Clostridium tetani*, a Gram-
positive bacterium present in soil throughout the
world.

Aetiology

Clostridium tetani, a Gram-positive, obligate
anaerobic rod-shaped bacterium, is transmitted as
spores.

Epidemiology

C. tetani spores occur worldwide as constituents of
soil and in the GI tracts of animals (including
humans) (Roper *et al.* 2007). The bacterium is
present in the GI tract in 5–9% of healthy horses
(Wilkins *et al.* 1988). Tetanus affects mammals
worldwide, but the horse seems to be one of the most
susceptible domestic animals (Ansari & Matros
1982, Green *et al.* 1994). In horses, the umbilical
cord in neonates, retained placenta, puncture
wounds of the foot, and surgical wounds are known
to be frequent sites of *C. tetani* infection (Ansari &
Matros 1982, Kay & Knottenbelt 2007).

Pathophysiology

Tetanus toxin is one of the most potent toxins ever
identified, with a minimum lethal dose of less than
2.5 ng/kg BW in humans. At autolysis, after death of
the bacterium, the toxin molecule is released and
transformed by bacterial or tissue proteases into its
active form. By cleaving synaptobrevin proteins in
synaptic vesicle membranes, the action of inhibitory
neurons is thereby impeded, leaving α-motor neuron
excitation unopposed, resulting in the muscle rigidity
and long-lasting painful spasms that are
characteristic of tetanus. In addition to its action on
the motor system, tetanus toxin can have profound
and life-threatening effects on the autonomic
nervous system by interrupting spinal inhibitory
sympathetic reflexes, resulting in a hyperadrenergic
state. The action of tetanus toxin within neurons
persists for several weeks; the mechanism of
functional recovery remains unclear (Wassilak *et al.*
2004, Roper *et al.* 2007).

Incubation period

The time from inoculation of tetanus spores
into damaged tissue to the appearance of
the first symptom, or incubation period, is usually
3–21 days in man, although cases have been
reported with incubation periods as short as 1 day,
or longer than 1 month (Roper *et al.* 2007). The
incubation period ranged from 2 days to 2 months in
horses (Green *et al.* 1994, Galen *et al.* 2008) and was
not significantly different between survivors and
nonsurvivors (Galen *et al.* 2008).

Clinical presentation

As consciousness is preserved, tetanus presents a
truly dreadful disease (Roper *et al.* 2007). The
neurotoxin blocks neurotransmitter release from the
inhibitory pathways of the motor and autonomic
nervous systems, resulting in unrestrained neuronal
activity of both pathways (Humeau *et al.* 2000). As
a consequence, tetanus is a painful and protracted
disease characterized by increased muscle tone,
muscle spasm (**80–82**), and, in severe cases,
autonomic dysfunction (Thwaites *et al.* 2006).
Autonomic dysfunction leading to severe sustained
or labile hypertension, hypotension, tachycardia,
bradycardia, and arrhythmias can also result in life-
threatening haemodynamic instability and cardiac
arrest (Roper *et al.* 2007). The spontaneous
protrusion of the third eyelid (nictitating membrane)
is regarded as almost pathognomonic for the
disease (**83**).

Affected horses were reported to have a mean
heart rate of 61±17 bpm, respiratory rate of 42±27
rpm, and age of 4.3±4.0 years (Galen *et al.* 2008).
Most of the equine patients (84%) were 5 years old
or younger; young horses are particularly
vulnerable to tetanus and their prognosis is poorer
than that of older horses (Galen *et al.* 2008).
Survivors left the hospital between 16 and 32 days
after observation of the first signs (mean±SD:
25.8±5.6 days) (Galen *et al.* 2008). This is in
agreement with a hospitalization period ranging
from 14 days (Green *et al.* 1994) to 3–4 weeks
(Ansari & Matros 1982) in other studies in horses.

Differential diagnosis

The differential diagnosis includes meningitis, brain
trauma, tetany (hypocalcaemia), myopathy,
laminitis, and severe lameness. Especially with
reference to the protrusion of the nictitating
membrane hyperkalaemic periodic paralysis (HYPP)
and other channelopathies should be considered.

Diagnosis

The diagnosis of tetanus is made strictly on clinical
grounds (predominantly protrusion of the nictitating
membrane in horses eventually following lifting of
the head), as cultures of human tetanus patients'
wounds frequently fail to detect growth of *C. tetani*;
moreover, the organism occasionally grows in

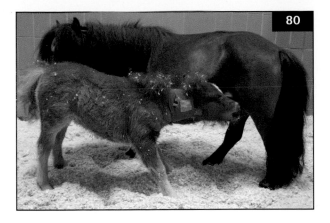

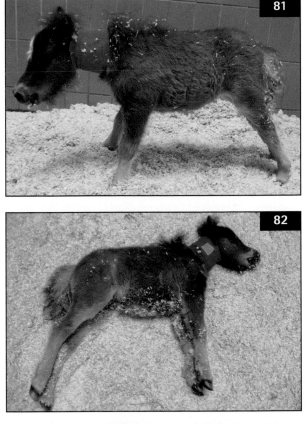

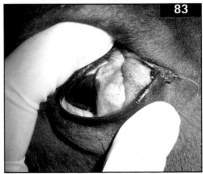

80 Neck stiffness in a 4-week-old Shetland pony mare with tetanus.

81 Extensor rigidity in a 4-week-old Shetland pony mare with tetanus.

82 Tonic muscle spasms in a 4-week-old Shetland pony mare with tetanus.

cultures from patients without tetanus. Furthermore, negligible serum tetanus antibody concentrations can support but cannot prove the diagnosis (Roper *et al*. 2007).

Pathology

Pathology usually remains inconclusive; apart from the anaerobic entry wound there are no characteristic gross and histopathological lesions in tetanus.

Management/Treatment

The specific objectives of tetanus treatment are to stop the production of toxin at the site of infection, with appropriate wound care and antibiotic use (preferably metronidazole); to neutralize circulating toxin with antitetanus immunoglobulin; and to provide effective management of muscle spasm (preferably using acepromazine), respiratory failure, autonomic dysfunction, and complications that arise during the course of the illness (Roper *et al*. 2007).

Equine patients should be placed in a padded, dark, quiet stable, treated with tetanus antitoxin (IV, IM, or SC), sedatives, muscle relaxants, and antibiotics. Any wound or foot abscess should be thoroughly cleaned and treated appropriately. If needed, patients are fed by stomach tube and intravenous infusion implemented to maintain fluid balance. Intrathecal treatment with

83 Protrusion of third (nictitating) eyelid is pathognomonic for tetanus.

tetanus antitoxin increased survival rate from 50 to 75% as compared with IV or IM treatment (Muylle *et al*. 1975).

Magnesium sulphate has several attractive therapeutic properties in tetanus including muscle relaxation and cardiovascular effects, which might ameliorate the effects of autonomic dysfunction (Altura & Altura 1981). However, magnesium sulphate heptahydrate infusion did not reduce the need for mechanical ventilation in human adults with severe tetanus, but did reduce the requirement for other drugs to control muscle spasms and cardiovascular instability (Thwaites *et al*. 2006). To the authors' knowledge no information regarding potential beneficial effects of magnesium sulphate in equine tetanus is available.

Equine survival rates ranged from 25% to 75% (Muylle *et al.* 1975, Green *et al.* 1994) and the case fatality rate was 68% (Galen *et al.* 2008). Of the nonsurvivors, 66% were reported to present with pulmonary lesions (Green *et al.* 1994). The development of dyspnoea, recumbency, and the combination of dysphagia, dyspnoea, and recumbency was observed significantly more in the nonsurvivors (Galen *et al.* 2008). All nonsurvivors died within 8 days of the first signs (Galen *et al.* 2008). The timing of tetanus antitoxin administration (either immediately after the onset of suggestive signs or after a delay) was not different between the two groups (Galen *et al.* 2008).

In comparison, the prognosis of generalized human tetanus is strongly predicted by the incubation and onset periods. Short incubation and onset periods correlate with increased disease severity and higher mortality. Autonomic dysfunction also predicts high mortality, especially if it manifests early in the disease course (Brauner *et al.* 2002, Roper *et al.* 2007).

The only reliable immunity against tetanus is that induced by vaccination with tetanus toxoid (Roper *et al.* 2007), with carbopol-based adjuvants showing greatest efficacy (Holmes *et al.* 2006). Horses that are incompletely vaccinated against tetanus are not protected against the disease (Galen *et al.* 2008), whereas annual revaccination might generate 24 months duration of immunity against tetanus (Heldens *et al.* 2010).

The spores are extremely hardy; destruction requires autoclaving or prolonged exposure to iodine, hydrogen peroxide, formalin, or glutaraldehyde (Wassilak *et al.* 2004).

Public health significance

Maternal and neonatal tetanus are important causes of maternal and neonatal mortality, claiming about 180,000 lives worldwide every year, almost exclusively in developing countries (Roper *et al.* 2007).

Mycoplasma spp.

Phylum BXIII Firmicutes
Class II Mollicutes/Order I Mycoplasmatales/
Family I Mycoplasmataceae/Genus I *Mycoplasma*

Definition/Overview

Mycoplasma are putative pathogens and it is generally thought that most species are very host specific, but there are many reports of *Mycoplasma* spp. in hosts that are not perceived as their normal habitat (Pitcher & Nicholas 2005). *M. equigenitalium* and *M. subdolum* have been associated with infertility, endometritis, vulvitis, and abortions in mares, and with reduced fertility and balanoposthitis in stallions (Tortschanoff *et al.* 2005).

Aetiology

Prokaryotic organisms of the genus *Mycoplasma* are characterized by their small body and genome size – 0.6–1.35 Mbp. The *Mycoplasma* genus stems from the class Mollicutes (for soft skin), which lacks the cell walls and external motility appendages often present in other bacteria. To date, there are more than 200 known species of *Mycoplasma* (Fadiel *et al.* 2007, Waites *et al.* 2008). Mycoplasmas are generally likely to survive for a long period (a maximum of 8 days) in horse serum, although the survival period depends on the species, strain, and temperature (Nagatomo *et al.* 1997).

Epidemiology

Clinically healthy stallions may present a permanent reservoir for infection of mares via venereal transmission (Spergser *et al.* 2002).

Pathophysiology

Clinical manifestations of respiratory tract disease occur as a result of cytadherence of the organism to the host's respiratory epithelium, followed by the production of a variety of substances that induce local damage and stimulate release of inflammatory mediators by the host. Severity of disease appears to be related to the degree to which the host immune response reacts to the infection (Waites *et al.* 2008). Despite their role in equine genital disorders, determinants of virulence and pathogenesis as well as factors provoking specific host immune responses have not been identified to date (Tortschanoff *et al.* 2005). It has been shown that impaired bactericidal activity of equine neutrophils did not predispose equids to bacterial *M. felis* pleuritis (Rosendal *et al.* 1987).

Incubation period

Not established in the equine species yet.

Clinical presentation

Inflammatory airway disease was associated with tracheal infection with *M. equirhinis* (Shams Eldin & Kirchhoff 1994, Wood *et al.* 2005, Waites *et al.* 2008) and *M. felis* (Wood *et al.* 1997, Newton *et al.* 2003). *M. felis* was also identified as the cause of acute pleuritis with the pleural exudate being proteinaceous (84), containing large numbers of neutrophils, and having a markedly increased lactate concentration (Hoffman *et al.* 1992). Haemotrophic mycoplasmas are parasites on the surface of red blood cells and species closely related to *M. haemofelis* and 'Candidatus Mycoplasma haemobos' were found in horses suffering from poor performance, apathy, weight loss, and anaemia (Dieckmann *et al.* 2010).

However, *Mycoplasma* were rarely isolated and were not associated with disease in the equine species in other studies (Christley *et al.* 2001, Szeredi *et al.* 2003, Baczynska *et al.* 2007).

Diagnosis

Although serology is a useful epidemiological tool for investigating and characterizing outbreaks in circumstances where the likelihood of mycoplasmal disease is high, it is less suited for assessment of individual patients. The fastidious growth requirements and length of time necessary to culture *M. pneumoniae* (as much as 6 weeks) make growing the organism impractical for patient management. Serological assays used to detect acute *M. pneumoniae* infection include immunofluorescent antibody assays, direct and indirect haemagglutination using IgM capture, particle agglutination antibody assays, and enzyme immunoassays (EIAs). The PCR assay is valuable in identifying a mycoplasmal aetiology in patients with a variety of extrapulmonary syndromes in which an obvious contribution of respiratory infection may not be readily apparent. Detection of the organism by PCR is possible in blood and CSF, where culture has rarely been successful. Use of the PCR assay combined with serology in symptomatic persons may be the optimum approach for the diagnosis of *M. pneumoniae* respiratory infection (Waites *et al.* 2008).

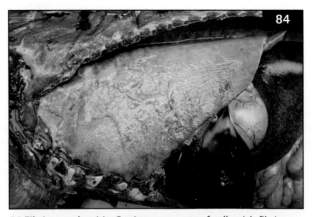

84 Fibrinous pleuritis. Copious amounts of yellowish fibrin cover the visceral pleura. Implicated aetiologies in the horse are: *Streptococcus* spp., *Nocardia* spp., and *Mycoplasma felis*.

A fast and simple method to detect mycoplasmal contamination in simulated samples of animal sera by using a PCR has been developed (Dussurget & Roulland-Dussoix 1994). Of swabs from the genital tract, pre-ejaculatory fluid and semen samples, 80% of samples were positive by PCR and 29% were positive by culture. Mycoplasmas were isolated predominantly from the fossa glandis and urethra and less frequently from the penis shaft and from semen. *M. equigenitalium* (25%) and *M. subdolum* (20%) were the predominant species identified and *M. equirhinis* and *M. felis* were detected in 8% and 2% of samples, respectively (Spergser *et al.* 2002). The growth of *M. equigenitalium* and *M. subdolum* from specimens collected from the clitoral fossa of Standardbred mares was not diminished by freezing of the specimens in liquid nitrogen (−196°C) for up to 30 days when compared to samples cultured immediately (Bermudez *et al.* 1988).

Rising serum antibody titres to *M. felis* were demonstrated in horses suffering from acute pleuritis, with *M. felis* isolated in pure culture from pleural fluid (Hoffman *et al.* 1992).

Pathology
M. felis has been associated with a fibrinopurulent pleuritis (Hoffman *et al.* 1992, Jubb *et al.* 2007).

Management/Treatment
Treatment of diseased horses is supportive.

Public health significance
The most common atypical pneumonias are caused by three zoonotic pathogens, *Chlamydophila psittaci* (psittacosis), *Francisella tularensis* (tularemia), and *Coxiella burnetii* (Q fever), and three nonzoonotic pathogens, *Chlamydophila pneumoniae*, *Mycoplasma pneumoniae*, and *Legionella* (Cunha 2006). Although more than 200 species in the genus *Mycoplasma* are now recognized, relatively few are pathogenic in humans. The best known and most intensely studied of these species is *M. pneumoniae*. *M. pneumoniae* is a common cause of upper and lower respiratory tract infections in persons of all ages and may be responsible for up to 40% of community-acquired pneumonias (Waites *et al.* 2008). Effective management of *M. pneumoniae* infections can usually be achieved with macrolides, tetracyclines, or fluoroquinolones, but the recent emergence of macrolide resistance in Japan is of concern (Waites *et al.* 2008).

Erysipelothrix rhusiopathiae
Phylum BXIII Firmicutes
Class II Mollicutes/Order V Incertae sedis/Family I Erysipelotrichaceae/Genus I *Erysipelothrix*: Regular, nonsporing Gram-positive rods

Definition/Overview
Endocarditis caused by *Erysipelothrix rhusiopathiae* is uncommon and only a few sporadic cases have been reported in horses.

Aetiology
E. rhusiopathiae is a facultative, nonspore-forming, nonacid-fast, small, Gram-positive bacillus. Protective antisera from swine, horses, and mice recognized prominent bands of molecular mass of 66–64 and 40–39 kDa. Mice immunized with preparations of the 66–64 kDa band purified by preparative electrophoresis were protected. Both antigens were trypsin sensitive, contained no detectable polysaccharide, and showed a marked tendency to aggregate in the absence of sodium dodecyl sulphate (Groschup *et al.* 1991).

Epidemiology
The organism is ubiquitous and able to persist for a long period of time in the environment, including marine locations. It is a pathogen or a commensal in a wide variety of wild and domestic animals, birds, and fish. Swine erysipelas caused by *E. rhusiopathiae* is the disease of greatest prevalence and economic importance. Diseases in other animals include erysipelas of farmed turkeys, chickens, ducks, and emus, and polyarthritis in sheep and lambs (Wang *et al.* 2010).

Pathophysiology
Neuraminidase plays a significant role in bacterial attachment and subsequent invasion into host cells. The role of hyaluronidase in the disease process is controversial. The presence of a heat labile capsule has also been reported as important in virulence (Wang *et al.* 2010). *E. rhusiopathiae* can cause endocarditis, which may be acute or subacute and has a male predilection in man. It usually occurs in previously damaged valves, predominantly the aortic valve. Endocarditis does not occur in patients with valvular prostheses and is not associated with intravenous drug misuse (Veraldi *et al.* 2009).

Incubation period
Not established in the equine species yet.

Clinical presentation
Clinical signs are predominantly associated with endocarditis and/or disseminated infection

(McCormick *et al.* 1985, Seahorn *et al.* 1989). *E. rhusiopathiae* serotype 5 was isolated from blood obtained antemortem from a horse with presenting problems of laminitis, uveitis, acute blindness, localized ventral oedema, and depression. The patient failed to respond to therapy and died 96 hours after the onset of clinical signs. Cultures of the lung post-mortem yielded *E. rhusiopathiae* serotype 5, beta-haemolytic *Streptococcus* sp., *Escherichia coli*, *Proteus* sp., and *Klebsiella* sp. (Seahorn *et al.* 1989).

Diagnosis

Diagnosis should depend on the detection of the bacteria combined with (most obviously) an endocarditis.

Pathology

Pathological examination might reveal an endocarditis.

Management/Treatment

Control of animal disease by sound husbandry, herd management, good sanitation, and immunization procedures is recommended (Wang *et al.* 2010). In individual cases, a course of oral antimicrobial therapy for several weeks preferably based on antibiotic sensitivity testing might be indicated.

Public health significance

Three forms of human disease have been recognized. These comprise a localized cutaneous lesion form, so-called erysipeloid, a generalized cutaneous form, and a septicaemic form often associated with endocarditis. Infection due to *E. rhusiopathiae* in humans is occupationally related, principally occurring as a result of contact with contaminated animals, their products or wastes, or soil. Erysipeloid is the most common form of infection in humans (Veraldi *et al.* 2009, Wang *et al.* 2010). Erysipeloid is an infection of the skin caused by traumatic penetration of *E. rhusiopathiae*. The disease is characterized clinically by an erythematous oedema, with well-defined and raised borders, usually localized to the back of one hand and/or fingers. Vesicular, bullous, and erosive lesions may also be present. The lesions may be asymptomatic or accompanied by mild pruritus, pain, and fever. Diagnosis of localized erysipeloid is based on the patient's history (occupation, previous traumatic contact with infected animals or their meat) and clinical picture (typical skin lesions, lack of severe systemic features, slight laboratory abnormalities, and rapid remission after treatment with penicillin or cephalosporin) (Veraldi *et al.* 2009). Endocarditis induced by *E. rhusiopathiae* is an uncommon disease. Most of the infected persons (90%) work in environments with frequent exposure to *E. rhusiopathiae* (butchers, fishermen). Although the clinical picture of endocarditis induced by *E. rhusiopathiae* is indistinguishable from other forms of subacute endocarditis, this infection has a mortality rate of 40% and a high morbidity. Microbiological diagnosis should consider the possibility of making a mistake, considering that isolation of a Gram-positive bacillus may represent contamination by an agent without clinical relevance. Treatment with penicillin G for 4 weeks is commonly sufficient to cure the disease (Azofra *et al.* 1991).

Bacillus anthracis: ANTHRAX

Phylum BXIII Firmicutes
Class III Bacilli/Order I Bacillales/Family I
Bacillaceae/Genus I *Bacillus*: Endospore-forming
Gram-positive rods and cocci

Definition/Overview

Anthrax is a dramatic, rapidly fatal infectious disease that affects many animal species and humans, particularly herbivores, whereas the horse seems to be less susceptible to anthrax than ruminants. The disease is caused by *Bacillus anthracis* characterized by septicaemia with the exudation of tarry blood from the orifices of the body (Parkinson *et al.* 2003, Fasanella *et al.* 2010*b*).

Aetiology

B. anthracis belongs to the family Bacillaceae. It is a Gram-positive bacterium, rod-shaped, aerobic, immobile, capsulated and spore forming. The bacterium is 1–1.5 μm wide by 5–6 μm in length. In tissue or culture smears, other pathological bacteria are found singly, as clusters, or as short chains, with rounded ends, while *B. anthracis* cells with square ends are arranged in long chains that gives them a particular look similar to bamboo canes. Outside the body and at temperatures between 14°C and 42°C (optimum 21–37°C) *B. anthracis* will sporulate. The spores are oval, and are released after lysis of the bacterium. Sporulation is completed within 48 hours, but it does not happen in the presence of high concentrations of carbon dioxide, a condition that occurs in infected putrefying carcasses (Fasanella *et al.* 2010*b*). The long lasting and highly resistant spores when exposed to the air can, under favourable conditions, persist for decades in the environment before infecting a new host (Parkinson *et al.* 2003). *B. anthracis* grows well in ordinary medium under aerobic or microaerophilic conditions, at temperatures between 12°C and 44°C, but optimal growth occurs around 37°C and at a pH of 7.0–7.4. On nutrient agar it forms white colonies 3–4 mm in diameter with a rough surface, called 'glass beads', and with irregular margins that, if observed at a small magnification, have the appearance of a 'Medusa's head' (Fasanella *et al.* 2010*b*). Analysis showed that *B. anthacis* strains in Italy predominantly belong to a single clonal lineage, the subgenotype sgt - eB (Fasanella *et al.* 2010*a*), whereas most isolates in Kazakhstan belonged to the A1.a, the A3.b, and the A4 genetic cluster (Aikembayev *et al.* 2010).

Epidemiology

Anthrax is distributed worldwide although the incidence varies geographically. Outbreaks originating from a soil-borne infection usually occur following weather changes: anthrax incidents have been reported after long periods of unusually warm and dry spring weather followed by heavy rainfall (Parkinson *et al.* 2003, Constable *et al.* 2007, Fasanella *et al.* 2010*b*).

Pathophysiology

Infections develop after inhalation of the spores into the respiratory system or ingestion into the GI tract. Furthermore, spores can enter the body following penetration of the skin via biting insects. Following ingestion, the spores lodge in the mucosa, germinate, and encapsulate. The vegetative cells start to produce toxin causing oedema and tissue necrosis. The production of toxin usually precedes septicaemia by several hours (Constable *et al.* 2007, Himsworth & Argue 2009). *B. anthracis* survives within alveolar macrophages, after germination within the phagolysosome, then enters the external medium where it proliferates. Oedema toxin and lethal toxin are the major genetic determinants mediating the survival of germinated spores within macrophages (Guidi-Rontani 2002).

Incubation period

Not established in the equine species yet but probably a few days.

Clinical presentation

Clinical disease is almost invariably fatal in horses without treatment and most will die within 2–4 days of the clinical onset. Horses either die suddenly or develop the acute form of anthrax with clinical signs including fever, cyanosis, tachypnoea, tachycardia, muscle tremors, severe depression, colic, dyspnoea, haemorrhagic diarrhoea, and generalized subcutaneous oedema, with tarry blood oozing from the orifices of the body (Constable *et al.* 2007, Himsworth & Argue 2009, Fasanella *et al.* 2010*a*). It has been stated that subcutaneous oedema (particularly in the inguinal, preputial, and ventral thoracic and abdominal areas) is a predominant clinical sign of anthrax in live horses (85) (Himsworth & Argue 2009). Subcutaneous oedema suggests a cutaneous reaction to bites from contaminated horseflies. When there is an infection of the pharynx or intestine from contaminated feed or forage there is often diffuse haemorrhagic ulcerative enteritis. The regional lymph nodes are red and swollen, with yellowish areas of necrosis (Fasanella *et al.* 2010*a*).

Differential diagnosis
The differential diagnosis includes various causes of blood-clotting disorders and various causes of sudden death (86, 87) (see p. 262).

Diagnosis
When taking a sample from an animal suspected of anthrax, one needs to take precautions to prevent human infection, bacterial sporulation, and a resulting environmental contamination. From live animals, blood can be collected in a vacutainer. From dead animals, traditionally ears are collected as they are convenient and far from the intestinal tract, but a better sample would be nasal turbinates, which are well vasculated and therefore should have plenty of spores but with minimal tissue that is only little affected by putrefaction. The sample should be taken as soon as possible since decomposition leads to rapid disintegration of the bacilli (Fasanella *et al.* 2010*b*). Diagnosis is usually based either on the

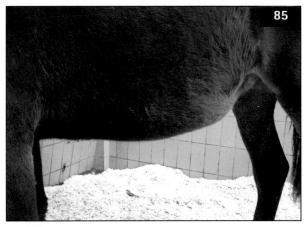

85 Subcutaneous oedema (particularly in the inguinal, preputial, and ventral thoracic and abdominal areas) is a predominant clinical sign of anthrax in horses.

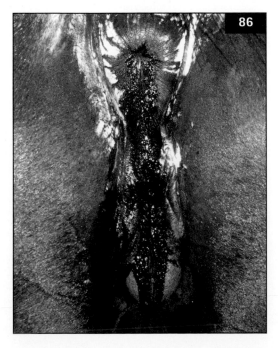

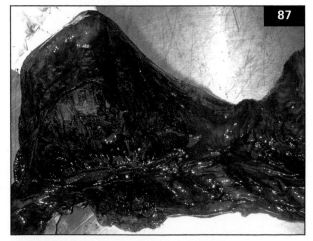

86, 87 Fresh blood oozing from the anus (**86**) in a 14-year-old Warmblood mare due to a grade IV rectal tear (**87**) following rectal exploration indicated by the gel around the anus. In case of anthrax tarry blood usually oozes from multiple orifices of the body.

detection of rod-like forms or typical bamboo canes in a fresh blood smear stained with Gram stain, which stains the bacilli violet, or preferably Giemsa stain, which stains the bacilli purple and the capsule a characteristic red-mauve, or a culture test (Fasanella *et al.* 2010*b*). PCR is the method of choice as a parallel diagnostic test, whether performed directly on clinical samples after nonselective enrichment of mixed cultures or as a confirmation test for suspect colonies (Constable *et al.* 2007, Himsworth & Argue 2009, Fasanella *et al.* 2010*b*). In addition, a sensitive enzymatic assay able to detect functional oedema factor, a calmodulin-activated adenylyl cyclase toxin which contributes to cutaneous and systemic anthrax, has been developed for use in human and animal plasma. Oedema factor can be detected at concentrations of 1 pg/ml in plasma from humans or at 10 pg/ml in the plasma of various animal species using only a blood volume of 5 μl (Duriez *et al.* 2009).

Pathology

The presence of incomplete or absent rigor mortis with unclotted, tarry blood oozing from the orifices of the body is indicative of the disease. Pathological examination reveals systemic haemorrhagic oedema, subcutaneous swellings containing gelatinous material, the presence of haemorrhagic fluid in the body cavities, and enlargement of lymphoid tissue including splenomegaly (Constable *et al.* 2007, Himsworth & Argue 2009). Failure of blood to clot was the most reliable indicator of anthrax in carcasses (Himsworth & Argue 2009). Splenic lesions will be absent if the animal dies as a result of local reaction (e.g. pharynx or intestines), without septicaemia (Fasanella *et al.* 2010*b*).

Management/Treatment

Anthrax is a reportable disease. *B. anthracis* is very sensitive to various antibiotics like penicillin combined with streptomycin. This combination is curative if administered in an early stage of the disease and it also prevents spread of the disease to other animals and man (Constable *et al.* 2007). Results from testing some 1,200 isolates showed that 3–6% were resistant to penicillin, depending also on the region in the world the isolate came from (Fasanella *et al.* 2010*b*). Furthermore, vaccination is used successfully to control anthrax (Constable *et al.* 2007, Fasanella *et al.* 2010*b*). Horses and other equids can respond poorly and need two doses 4–8 weeks apart (live attenuated noncapsulated Sterne vaccine) (Fasanella *et al.* 2010*b*).

Public health significance

Anthrax has important public health significance. Man is usually resistant to acquiring infection, but when infected may show three different clinical forms: the cutaneous, like eyelid anthrax and cicatricial ectropion (Devrim *et al.* 2009), intestinal, and respiratory forms (including a rare, but catastrophic cause of meningoencephalitis [Narayan *et al.* 2009]) (Fasanella *et al.* 2010*b*). The current human standard for anthrax inhalation post-exposure therapy is ciprofloxacin twice a day for 60 days (IV treatment initially (400 mg bid) and switch to oral therapy when clinically appropriate). (Friedlander *et al.* 1993, Fasanella *et al.* 2010*b*).

Listeria monocytogenes: LISTERIOSIS

Phylum BXIII Firmicutes
Class III Bacilli/Order I Bacillales/Family IV
Listeriaceae/Genus I *Listeria*: Regular, nonsporing
Gram-positive rods

Definition/Overview

A rare bacterial disease in horses caused by *Listeria monocytogenes* is associated with encephalitis, abortion, eye infections, and diarrhoea.

Aetiology

L. monocytogenes is an ubiquitous Gram-positive, facultative anaerobic, intracellular, rod-shaped bacterial pathogen in the environment and in the digestive tract (Evans *et al.* 2004) with forms without cell walls (so called L-forms of a protoplastic type) (Edman *et al.* 1968). Disease in horses is predominantly associated with serovars 1/2a and 4b (Gudmundsdottir *et al.* 2004).

Epidemiology

Although silage has been well established as a common source of systemic listeriosis infection in farm ruminants, it has also been hypothesized that *Listeria*-contaminated silage may be a source of listerial eye infections. For example, some reports noted that silage on farms with cases of listerial ocular infections was fed at or above the height of the animal's head (Evans *et al.* 2004). It has been stated that ocular listeriosis is not caused by specific strains with an ocular tissue tropism (Evans *et al.* 2004). Molecular subtyping allows specific determination of the sources of listeriosis outbreaks (Gudmundsdottir *et al.* 2004). Single-strand conformation polymorphism PCR (SSCP-PCR) is a promising method with sensitive detection limits and moderate sample variances and can be applied to epidemiological studies using environmental dust (Korthals *et al.* 2008). *L. monocytogenes*, containing 30% spores, showed visible bands at 7×10^2 cfu/g.

Free-living amoebae feed on bacteria, fungi, and algae. However, some microorganisms have evolved to become resistant to these protists. These amoeba-resistant microorganisms include established pathogens, such as *L. monocytogenes*. Free-living amoebae represent an important reservoir of amoeba-resistant bacteria and may, while encysted, protect the internalized bacteria from chlorine and other biocides (Greub & Raoult 2004).

Pathophysiology

This intracellular pathogen has evolved multiple strategies to face extracellular innate defence mechanisms of the host and to invade and multiply intracellularly within macrophages and nonphagocytic cells (Dussurget 2008).

Incubation period

Not established in the equine species yet.

Clinical presentation

Although regarded as a rare cause of disease in horses, *L. monocytogenes* can induce encephalitis, uterine infections resulting in abortion, eye infections, diarrhoea, and septicaemia (Evans *et al.* 2004, Gudmundsdottir *et al.* 2004). *L. monocytogenes* septicaemia has been associated with diarrhoea or signs of neurological disease in foals. Initial complaints and clinical signs in these animals were depression, weakness, fever, diarrhoea, abdominal pain, and seizures in foals aged 2 days to 3 weeks (Jose-Cunilleras & Hinchcliff 2001). Equine cerebral listeriosis in a Freiberger gelding showed sudden onset and the animal collapsed within 24 hours and was humanely killed (Rütten *et al.* 2006). Typical signs associated with listerial eye infections include swollen, hyperaemic conjunctivae, epiphora, photophobia, corneal clouding, miosis, and scattered white corneal foci with uptake of fluorescein dye (Sanchez *et al.* 2001, Evans *et al.* 2004).

Diagnosis

Isolation of the organism is possible on blood culture (Jose-Cunilleras & Hinchcliff 2001), preferably preceded by cold-enrichment. *L. monocytogenes* can be cultured from a conjunctival swab or corneal scraping obtained from an animal with an eye infection (Evans *et al.* 2004). The detection of *L. monocytogenes* in the faeces of a horse does not necessarily indicate listeriosis. Faeces from horses with no other clinical signs than a slightly increased temperature contained $1–10^3$ cfu/g. On the other hand, large numbers of *L. monocytogenes* ($>10^6$ cfu/g) were often found in the faeces of horses with severe signs of listeriosis (Gudmundsdottir *et al.* 2004). However, *L. monocytogenes* was not isolated from the faeces of foals affected with diarrhoea. In addition, CSF culture in a case also failed to yield any growth (Jose-Cunilleras & Hinchcliff 2001), demonstrating the difficulties in diagnosing the disease.

Differential diagnosis

The differential diagnosis predominantly includes various causes of acute neurological disease (see p. 262).

Pathology

Three archetypal separate disease forms are acknowledged in listeriosis: infection of the gravid uterus and abortion, septicaemia with generalized microabscess formation in foals, and encephalitis in adults. Histologically encephalitis is characterized by multifocal small aggregates of neutrophils and/or microglial nodules, white matter oedema, and lymphohistiocytic perivascular cuffing (Jubb *et al.* 2007). Necropsy in a Freiberger gelding with cerebral listeriosis revealed multiple small brown to reddish foci within the brain stem and pons. Histopathology demonstrated multifocal suppurative meningoencephalitis with microabscesses (Rütten *et al.* 2006).

Management/Treatment

Most of the antibiotics used routinely in horses, with the exception of ceftiofur, should be effective against *L. monocytogenes*. In foals there was a favourable clinical response to potassium penicillin G and amikacin sulphate administered IV for 7–11 days (Jose-Cunilleras & Hinchcliff 2001). Treatment with ciprofloxacin ophthalmic preparation and topical ticarcillin/clavulanic acid resulted in resolution of ocular listeriosis (Evans *et al.* 2004). Treatment options of ocular listeriosis also include ofloxacin (2 drops 5 times daily), phenylbutazone (1 g orally bid for 3 days, then decreasing to 500 mg orally every 12 h), topical itraconazole/DMSO 2% ointment every 4–6 h as prophylactic antifungal treatment, and 1% atropine ointment topically every 12 h for mydriasis and cycloplegia (Sanchez *et al.* 2001).

Public health significance

L. monocytogenes is the causative agent of human listeriosis, a potentially fatal foodborne infection. Clinical manifestations range from febrile gastroenteritis to more severe invasive forms including meningitis, encephalitis, abortions, and perinatal infections (Dussurget 2008). As a consequence, its zoonotic risk should be minimized.

Methicillin-resistant Staphylococcus aureus

Phylum BXIII Firmicutes
Class III Bacilli/Order I Bacillales/Family VIII
Staphylococcaceae/Genus I *Staphylococcus*: Gram-positive cocci

Definition/Overview

Staphylococcus aureus colonizes the skin and is present in the anterior nares in about 25–30% of healthy people (Casewell & Hill 1986). Methicillin-resistant *S. aureus* (MRSA) appears to be an emerging pathogen in horses (Baptiste *et al.* 2005, Weese & Lefebvre 2007, Duijkeren van *et al.* 2010).

Aetiology

S. aureus is a coagulase-positive and Gram-positive bacterium. Of all the resistant traits *S. aureus* has acquired since the introduction of antimicrobial chemotherapy in the 1930s, methicillin resistance is clinically the most important, since a single genetic element confers resistance to the most commonly prescribed class of antimicrobials, namely the β-lactam antibiotics, which include penicillins, cephalosporins, and carbapenems. It should be realized that methicillin resistance is also possible in coagulase-negative species (Grundmann *et al.* 2006). Genotypic analysis includes PCR, pulsed-field gel electrophoresis (PFGE), the staphylococcal cassette chromosome element carrying the *mecA* gene (SCCmec), the encoding gene of protein A (*spa*), and multilocus sequence typing (MLST) (Eede Van den *et al.* 2009). Virulence genes were detected in 92% of the equine strains, with a majority of *seh* or *sei* enterotoxin genes (Haenni *et al.* 2010). Whereas strains of community-associated (CA)-MRSA, the majority of which carry genes encoding Panton–Valentine leukocidin, are spreading rapidly in human populations, only sporadic cases have been reported in animals to date (Morgan 2008) including horses (Weese & Lefebvre 2007). However, whereas the clonal relationship between MRSA strains of CC398 is straightforward in livestock this is less obvious in horses (Catry *et al.* 2010).

Epidemiology

Previous colonization of the horse, previous identification of colonized horses on the farm, antimicrobial (predominantly penicillin and trimethoprim-potentiated sulphonamide [TMP/S]) administration within 30 days, admission to the neonatal intensive care unit, and admission to a service other than the surgical service were risk factors for CA colonization (Weese & Lefebvre 2007). In contrast, none of 13 putative risk factors (other than that animals presenting for veterinary treatment more frequently carried MRSA than healthy animals) were found to be significant in selected companion animal populations (including horses). It has been suggested that the absence of these typical risk factors indicates that companion animals act as contaminated vectors rather than as true reservoirs (Loeffler *et al.* 2010).

Nosocomial transmission has been suggested in equine clinics (Duijkeren van *et al.* 2010). CA-MRSA colonization was identified in 2.0% of horses in Canada from which a nasal swab was collected at admission (Weese & Lefebvre 2007, Tokateloff *et al.* 2009) similar to that found in the Greater London area (Loeffler *et al.* 2011) and Ireland (Abbott *et al.* 2010). Colonization tended to be transient and seemed unrelated to stress or administration of antimicrobials (Tokateloff *et al.* 2009). One study of horses on farms in Ontario and in New York State, USA, reported a prevalence of colonization of 4.7% (Weese *et al.* 2005b), and colonization of horses at the time of admission to veterinary hospitals ranged from 2.7 to 10.9% (Weese *et al.* 2006b, Duijkeren van *et al.* 2010, Eede Van den *et al.* 2009). In the Netherlands, the percentage of MRSA isolates found in equine clinical samples increased from 0% in 2002 to 37% in 2008 (Busscher *et al.* 2005, Duijkeren van *et al.* 2010). In comparison, colonization by methicillin-resistant (predominantly coagulase-negative) staphylococci was identified in 36% of healthy horses in Italy, and 4% of the humans in close contact with these horses were found to be carriers of methicillin-resistant staphylococci (De Martino *et al.* 2010). In Ireland, the isolation rate of MRSA was 5.2% for horses based on clinical samples and the isolation rate for healthy horses was 1.7% (Abbott *et al.* 2010).

Pathophysiology

The bacterium readily acquires resistance against all classes of antibiotics by one of two distinct mechanisms: mutation of an existing bacterial gene or horizontal transfer of a resistance gene from another bacterium (Grundmann *et al.* 2006). Adaptation of certain MRSA genotypes to more than one mammalian species has been shown, reflecting their extended host spectra (Walther *et al.* 2009).

Incubation period

Not established in the equine species yet.

Clinical presentation

Clinical signs involve opportunistic infections of various wounds (**88, 89**) or puncture sites (like thrombophlebitis [90] and arthritis), with sepsis seen as a sequela. Colonization of up to 5 months duration has been reported (Weese & Rousseau 2005). Previous hospitalization and treatment with gentamicin were associated significantly with CA-MRSA, whereas infected incision sites were associated significantly with hospital-associated (HA)-MRSA. Factors significantly associated with nonsurvival included IV catheterization, CA-MRSA infection, and dissemination of infection to other body sites, although the overall prognosis for survival to discharge (84%) is good (Anderson *et al.* 2009).

Morbidity associated with coagulase-positive staphylococci was 1.7% in horses, with isolates identified almost exclusively as *S. aureus* and rarely as *S. pseudintermedius* (1.7%). Coagulase-positive staphylococci (alone or in association with another bacterial species) were associated with the death or euthanasia of 90% of the cases. Proportions of antibiotic resistance to penicillin G and tetracycline reached 63% and 24%, respectively (Haenni *et al.* 2010).

Differential diagnosis

The differential diagnosis predominantly includes other opportunistic infections of various wounds or puncture sites.

Diagnosis

Diagnosis is usually established by culturing the bacterium from exudate followed by assessment of methicillin resistance. Compared with culture screening, the use of rapid screening tests was not associated with a significant decrease in MRSA acquisition rate (risk ratio 0.87, 95% CI 0.61–1.24) (Tacconelli *et al.* 2009). However, it should be realized that *S. aureus* infection usually does not result in the development of clinical signs. Nasal swabs are helpful in the identification of carriers. Bilateral collection of nasal swabs revealed the presence of different or identical methicillin-resistant staphylococci strains in both nostrils in 8% of cases, and 27% of the cohort were colonized by methicillin-resistant staphylococci strains in one nostril only (De Martino *et al.* 2010).

Pathology

Aspecific inflammatory lesions may be present such as thrombophlebitis, arthritis, dermatitis, and sepsis.

Management/Treatment

Horses with a tentative diagnosis of MRSA infection should be isolated to prevent possible human exposure, regarding it as a zoonosis or humanosis (Morgan 2008). Treatment should be based on *in vitro* antimicrobial susceptibility testing.

Public health significance

Colonized horses may transmit MRSA to other horses and humans, and zoonotic MRSA infections from horses have occurred (Weese *et al.* 2005*a*, Weese *et al.* 2006*a*, De Martino *et al.* 2010).

Colonization with MRSA was found in 10% of participants (being predominantly primary care veterinary personnel) at the 2006 convention of the American Association of Equine Practitioners. However, a significant association between practice type and MRSA colonization was not found. An increased risk of MRSA colonization was associated with having been diagnosed with, or having treated a patient diagnosed with, MRSA colonization or infection in the previous year, whereas hand washing between infectious cases and hand washing between farms were protective. Equine veterinary personnel need to be aware of the potential risk of MRSA colonization, and practise appropriate hand hygiene to help limit transmission (Anderson *et al.* 2008).

The vast majority of MRSA isolates from horses identified in North America have been classified by PFGE as subtypes of Canadian MRSA-5. This clone is relatively uncommon in humans (Christianson *et al.* 2007) but is the predominant clone found in equine personnel and veterinarians, suggesting that it may be somewhat adapted to survival in horses (Weese *et al.* 2005*a*, Weese *et al.* 2005*b*). Surveillance is warranted because of the potential for MRSA to cause disease in horses and humans (Tokateloff *et al.* 2009).

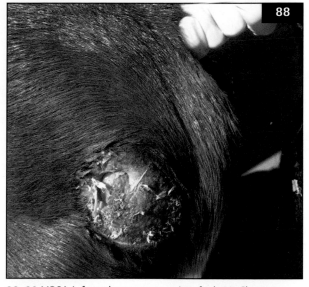

88, 89 MRSA-infected pressure sore in a foal; **89**: Close-up.

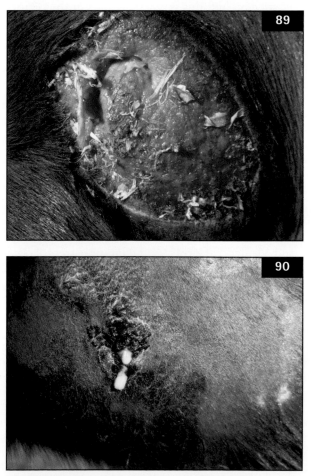

90 Clinical signs associated with methicillin-resistant *Staphylococcus aureus* infection involve thrombophlebitis (left jugular vein shown) following IV catheterization, with sepsis seen as a sequela.

Streptococcus equi subsp. *equi*: 'STRANGLES'

Phylum BXIII Firmicutes
Class III Bacilli/Order II Lactobacillales/Family VI
Streptococcaceae/Genus I *Streptococcus*: Gram-positive cocci

Definition/Overview

Acute onset of fever is caused by *Streptococcus equi* subsp. *equi* infection, commonly referred to as 'strangles' (Sweeney *et al.* 2005). Strangles is characterized by abrupt onset of fever followed by upper respiratory tract catarrh, as evidenced by mucopurulent nasal discharge and acute swelling with subsequent abscess formation in submandibular and retropharyngeal lymph nodes. The name strangles was coined because affected horses were sometimes suffocated by enlarged lymph nodes that obstructed the airway (Sweeney *et al.* 2005). The guttural pouch is regarded as the predominant site in healthy carriers of *S. equi* subsp. *equi* and this is usually associated with varying degrees of pathology commonly evident endoscopically as visible empyema or chondroids (Newton *et al.* 1997). Chondroids formed after strangles can harbour *S. equi* subsp. *equi* (**91**) (Sweeney *et al.* 2005).

Aetiology

S. equi subsp. *equi* is a beta-haemolytic, Gram-positive, facultative anaerobic, coccoid bacterium belonging to Lancefield group C (Facklam 2002, Timoney 2004). There is compelling evidence that it is derived from an ancestral *S. equi* subsp. *zooepidemicus* as a genovar or biovar of the latter (Sweeney *et al.* 2005), with which it shares greater than 98% DNA homology and therefore expresses many of the same proteins and virulence factors (Timoney 2004). An important virulence factor and vaccine component, the antiphagocytic fibrinogen binding SeM of *S. equi* subsp. *equi,* is a surface anchored fibrillar protein, and N-terminal variation of SeM alters a conformational epitope of significance in mucosal IgA and systemic T cell responses, but does not affect antibody-mediated phagocytosis and killing (Timoney *et al.* 2010).

Epidemiology

Transmission of infection occurs when there is either direct or indirect transfer of *S. equi* subsp. *equi* within purulent discharge (Sweeney *et al.* 2005). Nasal shedding of *S. equi* subsp. *equi* usually begins 2–3 days after onset of the fever. Some animals never shed. In others, persistent guttural pouch infection may result in intermittent shedding for years (Newton *et al.* 1997, Chanter *et al.* 1998, Sweeney *et al.* 2005). Of infected horses, 9–44% were identified as carrying *S. equi* subsp. *equi* after clinical signs had disappeared and the predominant site of carriage was the guttural pouch. Prolonged carriage of *S. equi* subsp. *equi*, which lasted up to 8 months, did not cease spontaneously before treatment was initiated to eliminate the infection (Newton *et al.* 2000, Sweeney *et al.* 2005).

When PCR and culture methods were compared, many more nasopharyngeal swabs were found to be positive using PCR (56% *vs.* 30%) from established guttural pouch carriers of *S. equi* subsp. *equi*. Similar results were obtained for guttural pouch samples from these established carriers (76% *vs.* 59%). However, it should be realized that PCR also detects dead organisms and is, therefore, liable to yield false-positive results (Newton *et al.* 2000).

S. equi subsp. *equi* may be cultured from lavages collected by direct percutaneous sampling of the pouch, although this is not recommended because of the high risk of injury to important anatomical structures in the region (Sweeney *et al.* 2005).

A multiphasic approach can be used to answer specific diagnostic questions pertaining to the source of infection and/or outbreak, or to address quarantine concerns (Ivens *et al.* 2009, Lanka *et al.* 2010), eventually expanded to serology (Knowles *et al.* 2010).

Pathophysiology

S. equi subsp. *equi* enters via the mouth or nose and spread may be haematogenous or via lymphatic channels, which results in abscesses in lymph nodes and other organs. This form of the disease has been known as 'bastard strangles' (Sweeney *et al.* 2005). Hyaluronate lyases, which degrade connective tissue hyaluronan and chondroitins, are thought to facilitate streptococcal invasion of the host. Prophage-encoded hyaluronan-specific hyaluronate lyases play a direct role in *S. equi* subsp. *equi* disease pathogenesis (Lindsay *et al.* 2009).

Incubation period

In a recent study, although very small numbers of *S. equi* subsp. *equi* entered the lingual and nasopharyngeal tonsils, carriage to regional lymph nodes occurred within hours of inoculation (Timoney & Kumar 2008). Bacteraemia occurs on days 6–12 in horses inoculated intranasally with virulent *S. equi* subsp. *equi* (Evers 1968), whereas fever as the first clinical sign of infection occurs between 3 and 14 days after exposure (Sweeney *et al.* 2005). The submandibular and retropharyngeal lymph nodes are about equally involved in *S. equi* subsp. *equi* infections and become swollen and painful about 1 week after infection (Sweeney *et al.* 2005).

Clinical presentation

Lymphadenopathy is a major clinical sign (92, 93). Older horses often exhibit a mild form of the disease characterized by nasal discharge (94), small abscesses, and rapid resolution of disease, whereas younger horses are more likely to develop severe lymph node abscessation that subsequently opens and drains. Pharyngitis, laryngitis, and rhinitis may occur and contribute to bilateral nasal discharge.

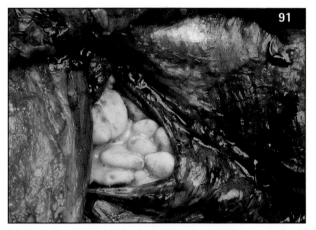

91 Strangles. Guttural pouch pyoliths. Pyoliths (i.e. pus stones) or chondroids can develop from chronic guttural pouch empyema during constant inspissation. *Streptococcus equi* subsp. *equi*.

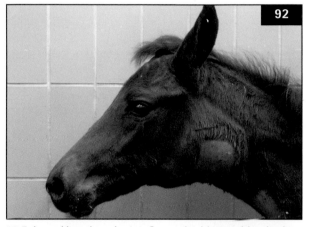

92 Enlarged lymph nodes in a 2-month-old Warmblood colt suffering from strangles.

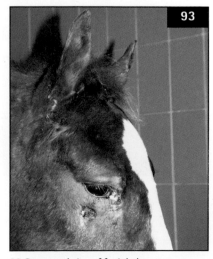

93 Ruptured site of facial abscess associated with strangles.

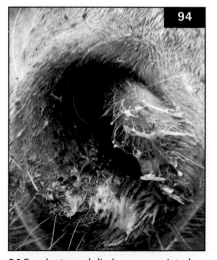

94 Purulent nasal discharge associated with strangles in a 7-year-old Draft horse gelding.

Retropharyngeal lymph nodes may drain into and cause empyema of the guttural pouch (**95, 96**) (Sweeney *et al.* 2005).

Sequelae include compression of the pharynx, larynx, or trachea due to enlarged lymph nodes, necessitating a tracheostomy in severe cases (**97**) (Sweeney *et al.* 2005). Other complications of *S. equi* subsp. *equi* infection include dysphagia resulting from lymph node enlargement, neuritis of adjacent nerves leading to laryngeal hemiplegia, retroversion of the epiglottis, pharyngeal collapse or DDSP, guttural pouch empyema, purpura haemorrhagica (**98–100**), myositis/rhabdomyolysis, agalactia, periorbital abscessation, panophthalmitis, arthritis, necrotic bronchopneumonia, endocarditis, myocarditis, vaginitis (**101**), and metastatic abscesses in the mesentery and various organs such as liver, spleen, kidneys, and brain (Sweeney *et al.* 1987*a*, Sweeney 1996, Chiesa *et al.* 2000, Spoormakers *et al.* 2003, Sweeney *et al.* 2005).

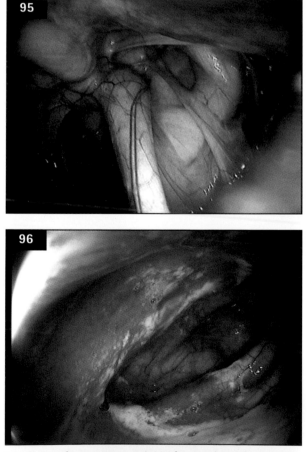

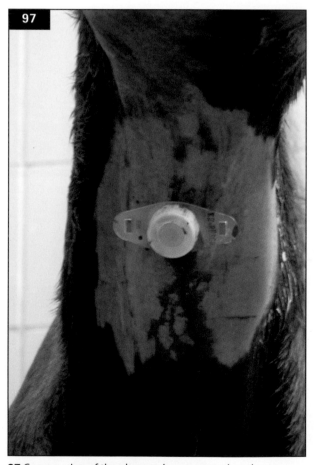

95, 96 Specific treatment options of guttural pouch empyema (**95**) due to *S. equi* subsp. *equi* include topical installation of 20% (w/v) acetylcysteine solution via a specially designed catheter (**96**).

97 Compression of the pharynx, larynx, or trachea due to enlarged lymph nodes necessitating a tracheostomy in severe cases as in this 2-month-old Warmblood colt.

The overall complication rate associated with *S. equi* subsp. *equi* infection is approximately 20% (Ford & Lokai 1980 1987*b*), Sweeney *et al.*, including metastatic abscessation to various organs. A recovered horse may be a potential source of infection for at least 6 weeks after its clinical signs of strangles have resolved (Sweeney *et al.* 2005). Approximately 75% of horses develop a solid, enduring immunity to strangles which persists for 5 years or longer after recovery from the disease (Todd 1910, Hamlen *et al.* 1994). Older horses with residual immunity have limited susceptibility and develop a mild form of strangles, often termed 'catarrhal strangles'. These animals shed virulent *S. equi* subsp. *equi* that will produce severe disease in more susceptible, often younger horses (Sweeney *et al.* 2005). Foals that suckle immune mares are usually resistant to *S. equi* subsp. *equi* infection until weaning owing to the presence of protective antibodies in milk (Sweeney *et al.* 2005).

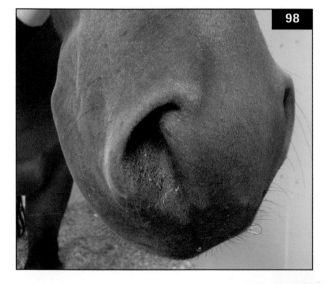
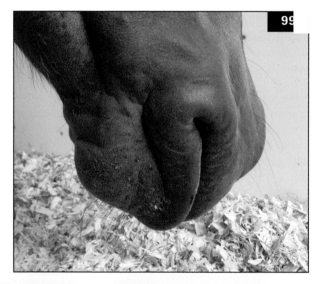
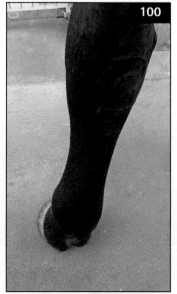
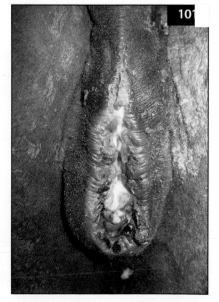

98, 99 Purpura haemorrhagica (morbus maculosis, immune complex deposition-mediated leucocytoclastic vasculitis) may develop as a sequela in a few cases of strangles, and results in generalized petechiae and oedema of the head.

100 Purpura haemorrhagica (morbus maculosis, immune complex deposition-mediated leucocytoclastic vasculitis) may develop as a sequela in a few cases of strangles, and results in oedema of the limbs.

101 Purulent discharge from the vagina due to *S. equi* subsp. *equi*.

Differential diagnosis

This includes various causes of unilateral (rhinitis, sinusitis, and other causes of guttural pouch empyema) or bilateral nasal discharge (chronic bronchitis [102]). Mandibular lymphadenopathy caused by *Actinomyces denticolens* might mimic strangles (Albini *et al.* 2008). The differential diagnosis with reference to various causes of internal abscessation includes *S. equi* subsp. *zooepidemicus*, *Corynebacterium pseudotuberculosis*, *Burkholderia pseudomallei*, and *Rhodococcus equi* (see p. 262).

Diagnosis

Culture of nasal swabs, nasal washes, or pus aspirated from abscesses remains the gold standard for the detection of *S. equi* subsp. *equi*. A PCR based on SeM, the gene for the antiphagocytic M protein of *S. equi* subsp. *equi*, offers an adjunct to culture for detection of *S. equi* subsp. *equi*. PCR is approximately three times more sensitive than culture. However, PCR does not distinguish between dead and live organisms and so a positive test result must be confirmed by culture (Timoney & Eggers 1985, Timoney *et al.* 1997, Newton *et al.* 2000, Sweeney *et al.* 2005). The presence of other beta-haemolytic streptococci, especially *S. equi* subsp. *zooepidemicus*, may complicate interpretation of cultures (Sweeney *et al.* 2005). In addition, radiography and/or ultrasonography revealing abscesses support(s) the tentative diagnosis of strangles as well as increased total protein and gamma-globulin content of blood.

Pathology

The affected lymph nodes (submandibular and retropharyngeal) and guttural pouches are swollen, firm to fluctuant and contain copious amounts of pus (103). Infection may spread and induce abscessation of mediastinal and mesenteric lymph nodes and other organs such as lungs, spleen, and liver (104–109). Purpura haemorrhagica (morbus maculosis, immune complex deposition-mediated leucocytoclastic vasculitis) may develop in a few cases and results in generalized petechiae and oedema of head and limbs (Jubb *et al.* 2007).

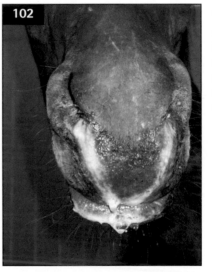

102 For comparison, bilateral nasal discharge (saliva) associated with oesophageal obstruction.

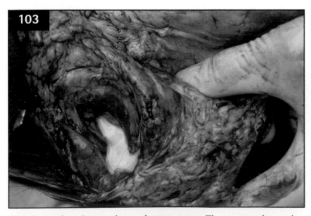

103 Strangles. Guttural pouch empyema. The guttural pouch contains creamy liquefied pus. *Streptococcus equi* subsp. *equi*.

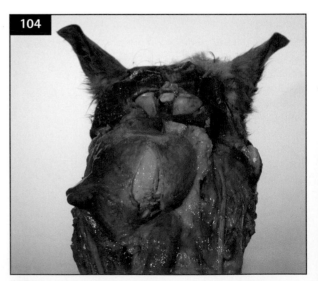

104 Strangles. Unilateral guttural pouch empyema. In posterior view exposed is the left guttural pouch gravely distended with inspissated pus. *Streptococcus equi* subsp. *equi*.

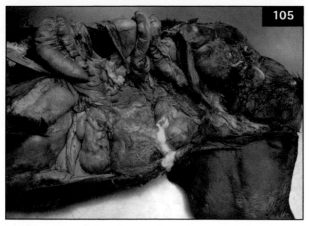

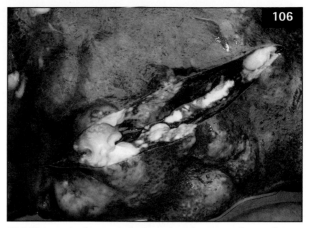

105 Bastard strangles. Abscessation of mesenteric lymph nodes. A large confluent intra-abdominal swelling reveals copious amounts of pus when incised. *Streptococcus equi* subsp. *equi*.

106 Metastatic abscesses in the spleen known as bastard strangles. (Courtesy of Dr E. Gruys.)

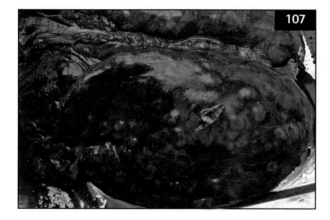

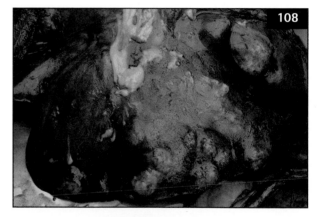

107 Bastard strangles. Extensive multifocal pulmonary abscessation. The lung abscesses contain copious amounts of thick liquid pus. *Streptococcus equi* subsp. *equi*.

108 Bastard strangles. Multifocal hepatic abscessation. The liver abscesses contain copious amounts of creamy pus. *Streptococcus equi* subsp. *equi*.

109 Strangles. Micrograph at high magnification of an abscess harbouring a bacterial colony of numerous streptococci bordered by degenerated neutrophils. *Streptococcus equi* subsp. *equi*. (H&E stain. Bar 20 μm.)

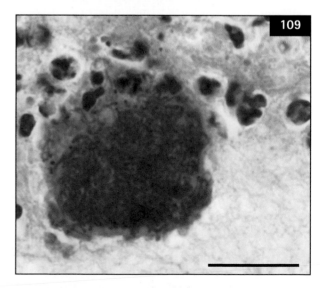

Management/Treatment

Veterinary opinion as to whether or not to use antibiotic treatment remains markedly divided. However, the majority of strangles cases require no treatment other than proper rest and adequate feeding (Sweeney *et al.* 2005). Immediate treatment of horses that show the earliest clinical sign of fever could be an effective way of controlling strangles outbreaks. Once an external lymphadenopathy is detected in an otherwise alert and healthy horse, antibiotic therapy is probably contraindicated (Sweeney *et al.* 2005). Therapy should be directed toward enhancing maturation and drainage of the abscesses. Daily flushing of the open abscess with a 3–5% povidone iodine solution should be continued until the discharge ceases (Sweeney *et al.* 2005). Penicillin is considered the antibiotic of choice for *S. equi* subsp. *equi* (Sweeney *et al.* 2005). A percutaneous ultrasound-guided technique for draining abscesses of the retropharyngeal lymph nodes has been described in horses suffering from a deep lymph node infection that has persisted following antibiotic treatment (De Clercq *et al.* 2003). Once again, high risk of injury to important anatomical structures in the region should be a consideration.

Carriers can be successfully treated by endoscopic removal of inflammatory material via flushing of the guttural pouches with large volumes (up to 3 l) of saline (**110**) and antibiotic treatment without surgical intervention. Furthermore, solid chondroids can either be macerated and subsequently removed using saline irrigation and aspiration, or (preferably) be removed entire with endoscopically guided grabbing forceps, a basket snare, or a memory-helical polyp retrieval basket. Topical as well as systemic antimicrobial therapy consists primarily of TMP/S. Systemic therapy consists initially of one or two 21-day courses of oral TMP/S at 30 mg/kg BW. Thirty percent of carriers originally given potentiated sulphonamide required further therapy with procaine penicillin IM at 10 mg/kg BW or ceftiofur at 2 mg/kg BW administered for 7–10 days both systemically and topically, before *S. equi* subsp. *equi* infection and associated inflammation of the guttural pouches were eliminated (Verheyen *et al.* 2000). It has been shown that a gelatin–penicillin mix (containing 10,000,000 IU sodium benzylpenicillin G) is more effective at remaining in the pouches than a straight aqueous solution (Verheyen *et al.* 2000). In addition, topical installation of 20% (w/v) acetylcysteine solution has also been used to aid the treatment of guttural pouch empyema (Sweeney *et al.* 2005). Treatment was generally regarded as successful when the guttural pouches appeared normal and *S. equi* subsp. *equi* was not detected in nasopharyngeal swabs and pouch lavages on three consecutive occasions (Verheyen *et al.* 2000).

Horses with strangles and their contacts should be maintained in well-demarcated quarantine areas and *S. equi* subsp. *equi* should be eliminated from guttural pouches (Sweeney *et al.* 2005). In addition, pastures used to hold infectious animals should be rested for 4 weeks, as it has been suggested that *S. equi* subsp. *equi* does not readily survive in the presence of other soil-borne flora (Sweeney *et al.* 2005).

An effective recombinant multicomponent subunit vaccine (comprising five surface localized proteins and two IgG endopeptidases) has been developed (Guss *et al.* 2009).

Public health significance

S. equi subsp. *equi* infection is possible in humans and may cause meningitis (Elsayed *et al.* 2003, Popescu *et al.* 2006) or cellulitis (Breiman & Silverblatt 1986).

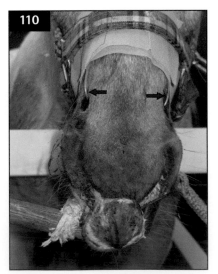

110 Bilateral guttural pouch catheters (arrows) in a pony.

Streptococcus equi subsp. *zooepidemicus*

Phylum BXIII Firmicutes
Class III Bacilli/Order II Lactobacillales/Family VI
Streptococcaceae/Genus I *Streptococcus*: Gram-positive cocci

Definition/Overview

Streptococci pathogenic for the horse include *Streptococcus equi* subsp. *equi*, *S. equi* subsp. *zooepidemicus* (formerly *S. zooepidemicus*), *S. dysgalactiae* subsp. *equisimilis*, and *S. pneumoniae* capsule type III. *S. equi* subsp. *zooepidemicus* is the most frequently isolated opportunist pyogen of the horse (Timoney 2004). This zoonotic pathogen is commonly found harmlessly colonizing the equine nasopharynx. Occasionally, strains can invade host tissues or cross species barriers, and *S. equi* subsp. *zooepidemicus* is associated with numerous different diseases in a variety of hosts, including inflammatory airway disease and abortion in horses, pneumonia in dogs, and meningitis in humans (Webb *et al.* 2008). *S. dysgalactiae* subsp. *equisimilis* is predominantly seen in uterine pathology.

Aetiology

The determination of haemolysis is one of the most useful characteristics for the identification of streptococci. Nonhaemolytic variants of *S. pyogenes, S. agalactiae*, and members of the *S. anginosus* group are well documented. *S. equi* subsp. *zooepidemicus* is identified by beta-haemolysis and Lancefield's group C antigen presence (Facklam 2002). The Gram-positive bacterium *S. equi* subsp. *zooepidemicus* is a commensal of horses, an opportunistic pathogen in many animals and humans, and a well-known cause of pyogenic disease. *S. equi* subsp. *equi* is widely believed to be a clonal descendant or biovar of an ancestral *S. equi* subsp. *zooepidemicus* strain with which it shares greater than 98% DNA homology and therefore expresses many of the same proteins and virulence factors (Timoney 2004, Webb *et al.* 2008, Tiwari & Timoney 2009). A striking difference is the fact that *S. equi* subsp. *equi* bacteriophage SeP9 binds to group C carbohydrate but is not infective for *S. equi* subsp. *zooepidemicus* in contrast to *S. equi* subsp. *equi* (Tiwari & Timoney 2009). In equids, the bacterium is not a homogeneous, clonal population but instead represents a wide diversity of strain types. *S. equi* subsp. *zooepidemicus* isolated from 23% of study samples comprised 24 different types of varying prevalence. The four most common types, A1HV4, A1HV2, C1HVu, and D1HV1, accounted for 45% of all the typed isolates (Barquero *et al.* 2009). In comparison, using multilocus sequence typing (MLST) for *S. equi* subsp. *zooepidemicus* a total of 130 unique sequence types were identified from isolates of diverse geographical and temporal origin (Webb *et al.* 2008). Variation in the protectively immunogenic surface-exposed proteins (SzP) has been well characterized (Timoney 2004). About 50% of *S. equi* subsp. *zooepidemicus* strains contained the superantigen-encoding genes szeN, szeF, or szeP and horizontal transfer of these novel superantigens from and within the diverse *S. equi* subsp. *zooepidemicus* population is likely to have implications for veterinary and human disease (Paillot *et al.* 2010).

Epidemiology

S. equi subsp. *zooepidemicus* was isolated from 9% of horses suffering from infectious upper respiratory disease at the Seoul race park in the spring, 22% in the summer, and 17% in winter. The bacterium was also identified in 5% of isolates from clinically normal horses (Ryu *et al.* 2009). *S. equi* subsp. *zooepidemicus* infection was highly prevalent based on isolates collected sequentially from recently weaned, pasture maintained Welsh mountain ponies, with bacteria causing naturally occurring respiratory disease being isolated from 94% of tracheal washes and 88% of nasopharyngeal swabs. Among different *S. equi* subsp. *zooepidemicus* types isolated, more were isolated from the trachea than the nasopharynx (Newton *et al.* 2008). It should also be realized that the stallion and use of semen for artificial insemination represent major risk factors for the transmission of bacterial contaminants of the penis, including *S. equi* subsp. *zooepidemicus*, *Pseudomonas aeruginosa*, and *Klebsiella pneumoniae*, known to cause endometritis and infertility in the mare (Samper & Tibary 2006).

Pathophysiology

Little is known about the virulence factors or protective antigens of *S. equi* subsp. *zooepidemicus* (Hong 2006), although it has been shown that immune responses to the bacterium during uterine infection is partly strain-specific (Causey *et al.* 2006). Streptokinases secreted by nonhuman isolates of group C streptococci (*S. equi* subsp. *equi*, *S. dysgalactiae* subsp. *equisimilis*, and *S. equi* subsp. *zooepidemicus*) have been shown to bind to different mammalian plasminogens but exhibit preferential plasminogen activity (Caballero *et al.* 1999).

Incubation period

In one study, at 17–20 hours following endobronchial inoculation, transient increases in rectal temperature to between 38.6°C and 39.2°C, inappetence, and lethargy were observed. Clinical

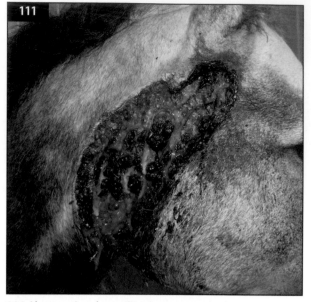

111 Abscessation due to *Streptococcus equi* subsp. *zooepidemicus*.

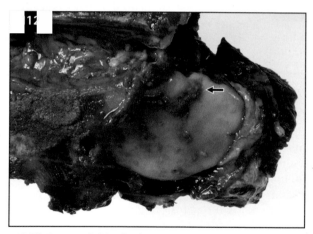

112 Fibrinous arthritis of a thoracic intervertebral joint. Note the fibrinopurulent flecks on the articular surface (arrow). *Streptococcus equi* subsp. *zooepidemicus*.

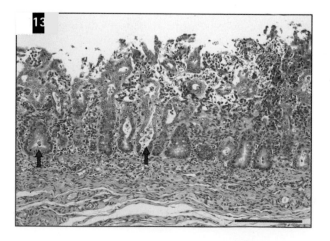

signs of respiratory disease developed within 48 hours after inoculation and continued until 12 days later just before euthanasia (Yoshikawa *et al.* 2003).

Clinical presentation

Infection is best characterized as opportunistic pyogenic disease involving various organ systems (**111–113**) with *S. equi* subsp. *zooepidemicus* also associated with strangles-like disease, pharyngeal lymphoid hyperplasia, and abnormal endoscopic appearance of guttural pouches (Laus *et al.* 2007). Tracheal infection (**114**) with *S. equi* subsp. *zooepidemicus* was associated with both clinical respiratory disease and subclinical inflammatory airway disease (IAD) when compared with controls with no evidence of IAD (Newton *et al.* 2003). On the other hand, *S. equi* subsp. *zooepidemicus* and *S. pneumoniae* play an important aetiological role in the pathogenesis of IAD in young horses. *S. equi* subsp. *zooepidemicus* and *S. pneumoniae* decreased in parallel with age, consistent with increased disease resistance, perhaps by the acquisition of immunity (Wood *et al.* 2005). In addition, *S. equi* subsp. *zooepidemicus* was the most frequently isolated (33%) bacterial organism in equine ulcerative keratitis (Keller & Hendrix 2005). Co-infection by *S. equi* subsp. *zooepidemicus* with *Chlamydophila caviae* has been reported in horses with rhinitis and conjunctivitis, implying that primary lesions were set by *C. caviae* and subsequently aggravated by *S. equi* subsp. *zooepidemicus* (Gaede *et al.* 2010). Furthermore, *S. equi* subsp. *zooepidemicus* was associated with more positive endometrial cytology results than coliforms (**115**) (Riddle *et al.* 2007).

Differential diagnosis

The differential diagnosis includes various causes of internal abscessation (see p. 262). Of importance, the absence of *S. equi* subsp. *equi* and the frequent detection of *S. dysgalactiae* subsp. *equisimilis* (**116, 117**) and *S. equi* subsp. *zooepidemicus* suggest that beta-haemolytic streptococci other than *S. equi* subsp. *equi* could be the causative agent of strangles-like disease (Laus *et al.* 2007).

113 Necrotizing colitis in a donkey. The mucosa is eroded with necrosis and loss of superficial epithelial cells. Note the scant amounts of inflammatory cells within crypt lumina, i.e. crypt abscesses (arrows). *Streptococcus equi* subsp. *zooepidemicus*. (H&E stain. Bar 200 μm.)

114 Haemopurulent transtracheal aspirate recovered from a necrohaemorrhagic and suppurative bronchopneumonia.

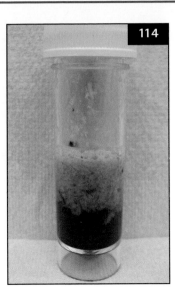

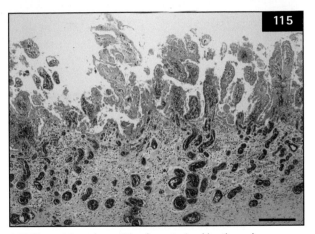

115 Necrotizing placentitis, characterized by the pale eosinophilic necrotic maternal endometrial villi. *Streptococcus equi* subsp. *zooepidemicus*. (H&E stain. Bar 200 μm.)

116 Necrohaemorrhagic and suppurative bronchopneumonia. Widespread pulmonary alveolar haemorrhage and extensive neutrophilic infiltrates. Note the broadened interlobular septa due to interstitial oedema (arrow). *Streptococcus dysgalactiae* subsp. *equisimilis*. (H&E stain. Bar 500 μm.)

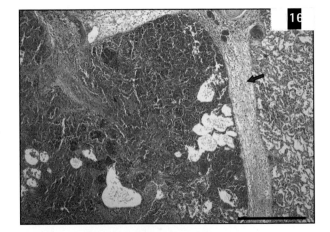

117 Necrohaemorrhagic and suppurative bronchopneumonia. Close-up micrograph displaying numerous intra-alveolar bluish cocci, degenerated neutrophils, erythrocytes, and protein-rich oedema. *Streptococcus dysgalactiae* subsp. *equisimilis*. (H&E stain. Bar 20 μm.)

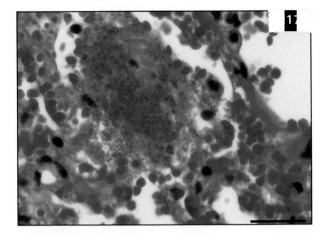

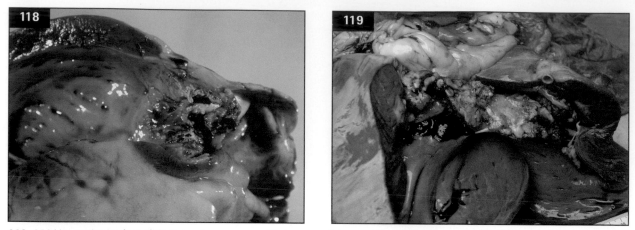

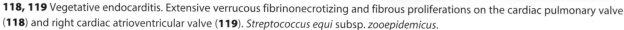

118, 119 Vegetative endocarditis. Extensive verrucous fibrinonecrotizing and fibrous proliferations on the cardiac pulmonary valve (**118**) and right cardiac atrioventricular valve (**119**). *Streptococcus equi* subsp. *zooepidemicus*.

Diagnosis

Ultrasonographic examination can be helpful for detecting internal abscesses. Clinical signs combined with culture of transtracheal or uterine aspirates, or pus aspirated from abscesses, remain the gold standard for the detection of *S. equi* subsp. *zooepidemicus*. However, a developed real-time PCR, based on the sodA and seeI genes was found to be more sensitive than conventional cultivation, although some strains biochemically identified as *S. equi* subsp. *zooepidemicus* were found by sequencing of the 16S rRNA gene to have a sequence homologous with *S. equi* subsp. *ruminatorum* (Båverud *et al.* 2007). The latter is seen in spotted hyenas (*Crocuta crocuta*) and plains zebras (*Equus quagga*, formerly *Equus burchelli*) (Speck *et al.* 2008).

Pathology

S. equi subsp. *zooepidemicus* is commonly involved in cases of equine endocarditis (**118–122**) and it can be a complication of septic jugular thrombophlebitis (**123**) (Jubb *et al.* 2007). Opportunistic (respiratory tract) infections with pyogenic *S. equi* subsp. *zooepidemicus* or *S. dysgalactiae* subsp. *equisimilis* typically induce exudation of plasma proteins, fibrin, infiltrating neutrophils and macrophages. In later stages organization of necrotic debris with fibrosis may be more evident.

Management/Treatment

Treatment should be based on *in vitro* antimicrobial susceptibility testing. It should be realized that prophylactic administration of SC trimethoprim/sulphadiazine (TMP/SDZ) was unable to eliminate *S. equi* subsp. *zooepidemicus* from tissue chambers (Ensink *et al.* 2005). In addition, resistance of *S. equi* subsp. *zooepidemicus* to trimethoprim–sulfamethoxazole differed between Kirby–Bauer agar disc diffusion and quantitative microbroth dilution methods (Feary *et al.* 2005).

Public health significance

Zoonotic transmission cannot be excluded although *Streptococcus equi* subsp. *zooepidemicus* infections are infrequent in humans; they have been associated with meningitis (Downar *et al.* 2001, Ural *et al.* 2003, Lee & Dyer 2004, Bordes-Benítez *et al.* 2006, Jovanović *et al.* 2008, Eyre *et al.* 2010), septicaemia, arthritis (Kuusi *et al.* 2006, Friederichs *et al.* 2010), and glomerulonephritis (Thorley *et al.* 2007).

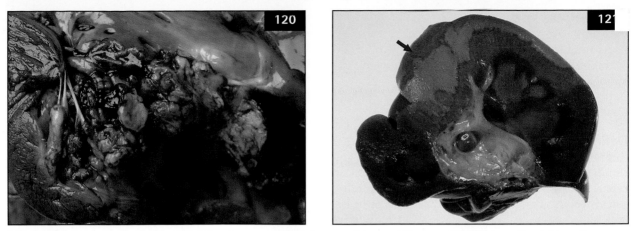

120, 121 Vegetative endocarditis. **120**: Extensive verrucous fibrinonecrotizing and fibrous proliferations on the right cardiac atrioventricular valve; **121**: cut surface of kidney showing renal infarction; well-delineated, wedge-shaped, pale necrotic cortical areas (arrow) resulting from dislodged thromboemboli in endocarditis. *Streptococcus equi* subsp. *zooepidemicus*.

122 Pulmonic valvular necrosuppurative endocarditis with fibrosis and extensive basophilic dystrophic mineralizations (arrow). *Streptococcus equi* subsp. *zooepidemicus*. (H&E stain. Bar 500 μm.)

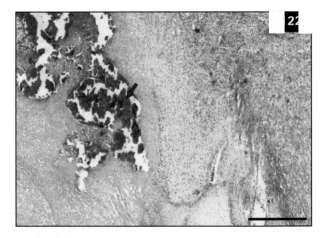

123 Septic thrombophlebitis of the jugular vein. The incised jugular vein reveals a hyperaemic thrombotic plaque that may spread and incite endocarditis.

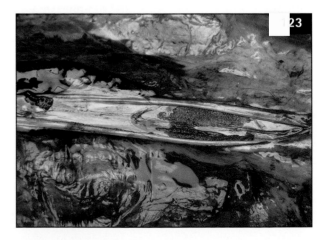

Actinomyces spp.

Phylum BXIV Actinobacteria
Class I Actinobacteria/Subclass V
Actinobacteridae/Order I Actinomycetales/
Suborder VIII Actinomycinae/Family I
Actinomycetaceae/Genus I *Actinomyces*: Irregular,
nonsporing Gram-positive rods

Definition/Overview

Actinomyces infections are reported in humans and
ruminants and only a few sporadic cases have been
reported in horses. In the equine species,
osteomyelitis, abscesses, skin nodules and pustules,
and septicaemia in colostrum-deprived foals were
associated with *Actinomyces* infections. Once
recognized, treatment of these infections requires
long courses of parenteral and oral therapy (Sullivan
& Chapman 2010) besides surgical debridement.

Aetiology

The order Actinomycetales includes phylogenetically
diverse but morphologically similar aerobic and
anaerobic bacteria that exhibit filamentous
branching structures which fragment into bacillary
or coccoid forms. The aerobic members are a large,
diverse group of Gram-positive bacteria including
*Nocardia, Gordona, Tsukamurella, Streptomyces,
Rhodococcus, Streptomycetes, Mycobacteria*, and
Corynebacteria spp. The anaerobic genera of
medical importance include *Actinomyces, Arachnia,
Rothia*, and *Bifidobacterium*. Both *Actinomyces* and
Nocardia cause similar clinical syndromes involving
the lung, bone and joint, soft tissue, and the central
nervous system (CNS) in man. The medically
important *Actinomyces* organisms cause infections
characterized by chronic progression and abscess
formation, with fistulous tracts and draining sinuses
(Sullivan & Chapman 2010).

Epidemiology

Among the isolated obligate anaerobic bacteria from
ulcerative keratitis in horses, 9% were *Actinomyces*
spp. compared to 73% *Clostridium* spp. (Ledbetter
& Scarlett 2008).

Pathophysiology

Modes of infection and transmission are as yet
unknown.

Incubation period

Not established in the equine species yet.

Clinical presentation

Horses with abscesses caused by *Actinomyces* spp.
(including *A. denticolens*) (**124, 125**) ranged in age
from 1 to 11 years, and the abscesses were most
commonly located in the submandibular and
retropharyngeal regions. The bacterium was usually
cultured as the sole isolate and the horses were most
often affected in the autumn. Most of the abscesses
were treated with antimicrobials and drainage, but
some of them recurred. The horses with
submandibular abscesses had residual scar tissue that
in some cases did not resolve (Fielding *et al.* 2008).
Actinomyces sp. was cultured from a meningeal
abscess surrounding the pituitary gland and from
resolving lung abscesses in a 3-year-old female
Morgan horse with anorexia and nasal discharge
(Rumbaugh 1977). Skin nodules and pustules in a
12-year-old Arabian stallion were associated with *A.
viscosus* (Specht *et al.* 1991). Osteomyelitis of the
mandible with *Actinomyces* spp. (both *A. viscosus*
and *A. odontolyticus*) was diagnosed in a 4-year-old
male sports horse (Vos 2007). *A. pyogenes* was
cultured during septicaemia in colostrum-deprived
foals (Robinson *et al.* 1993).

Differential diagnosis

The differential diagnosis includes various causes of
internal abscessation (see p. 262). Mandibular
lymphadenopathy caused by *A. denticolens* might
mimick strangles (Albini *et al.* 2008).

Diagnosis

Diagnosis of actinomycosis and nocardiosis
sometimes called 'great masqueraders', is often
delayed (Sullivan & Chapman 2010). Diagnosis
should depend on the detection of the bacteria
combined with appropriate clinical signs. Ultrasound
might be used to evaluate the abscesses and
ultrasonographic guidance might be used to drain
them (Fielding *et al.* 2008).

Pathology

Histological examination of biopsy specimens
revealed globular eosinophilic structures in
A. viscosus dermatitis in a 12-year-old Arabian
stallion (Specht *et al.* 1991). Of interest,
immunostaining with polyclonal anti-bacillus
Calmette–Guérin is a suitable screening technique
for the rapid identification of most common
bacterial and fungal organisms in paraffin-embedded
specimens (Bonenberger *et al.* 2001).

Management/Treatment

Once recognized, treatment of these infections requires long courses of parenteral and oral therapy (Sullivan & Chapman 2010). For instance, concomitant treatment with isoniazid (8 mg/kg BW, q 24h for 8 weeks), trimethoprim–sulfadiazine (30 mg/kg BW, q 24h for 8 weeks), and sodium iodide solution (66 mg/kg BW, every 1, 2, or 4 weeks, for 32 weeks) resolved *A. viscosus* dermatitis in a 12-year-old Arabian stallion (Specht *et al.* 1991). Surgical debridement with intravenous and local iodine solution treatment were administered to a 4-year-old male sports horse suffering from osteomyelitis of the mandible with *Actinomyces* spp. The horse was discharged after 7 days treatment with TMP/S at 30 mg/kg BW, PO, sid for 2 weeks, and a sodium iodide solution (Lugol), 60 mg/kg BW, diluted in 40 ml of 0.9% NaCl, slowly every 2 weeks for 2 months (Vos 2007). In horses with abscesses caused by *Actinomyces* spp., the submandibular abscesses were treated by lavage and drainage. Some of the horses were also treated with systemic antimicrobials, including doxycycline (10 mg/kg BW orally bid) and/or trimethoprim/sulfamethoxazole (30 mg/kg BW orally bid). All the abscesses eventually stopped draining and sealed over, after periods ranging from 2 weeks to 6 months. Some of the horses were left with excessive, firm, but nonpainful fibrous scar tissue in the affected areas.

Public health significance

Actinomyces spp. are not normally considered to be zoonotic pathogens, although a case of septic arthritis and osteomyelitis of the left ankle due to *A. pyogenes* has been reported in a diabetic farmer (Lynch *et al.* 1998).

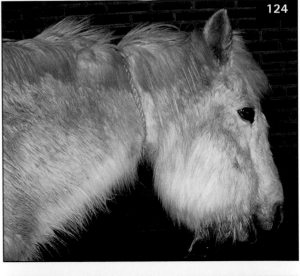

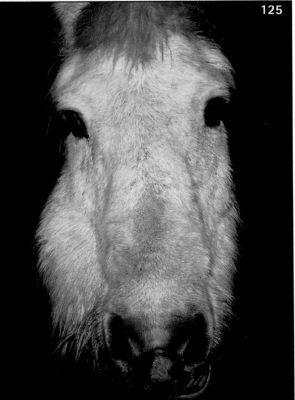

124, 125 Actinomycosis. Extensive unilateral swelling of the mandible due to a severe chronic osteomyelitis in a pony. *Actinomyces* spp. was isolated from the lesion. (Courtesy of Dr V.M. van der Veen.)

Dermatophilus congolensis: 'RAIN SCALD' or STREPTOTRICHOSIS

Phylum BXIV Actinobacteria
Class I Actinobacteria/Subclass V
Actinobacteridae/Order I Actinomycetales/
Suborder IX Micrococcineae/Family VIII
Dermatophilaceae/Genus I *Dermatophilus*:
Nocardioform actinomycetes

Definition/Overview

Dermatophilus congolensis is the pathogenic actinomycete that causes dermatophilosis (also known as streptotrichosis) in cattle, lumpy wool in sheep, and rain scald in horses and has public health significance (Larrasa *et al.* 2002).

Aetiology

D. congolensis is a filamentous branching Gram-positive actinomycete (Ambrose *et al.* 1998). The protein patterns observed in all isolates of *D. congolensis* reveal global antigenic similarities and distinct differences among isolates which could not be associated with either geographic, climatic or host factors when examined by sodium dodecyl sulphate polyacrylamide gel electrophoresis (SDS-PAGE) and by Western blotting (Makinde & Gyles 1999). However, DNA extraction and random amplified polymorphic DNA methods correlated with host species but not with geographical location (Larrasa *et al.* 2002).

Epidemiology

The disease has global distribution and is most prevalent following periods of prolonged rainfall. Transmission of *D. congolensis* by stable fly (*Stomoxys calcitrans*) and house fly (*Musca domestica*) has been reported (Richard & Pier 1966). The organism could not be isolated from soil samples collected from the immediate environment of the diseased animals (Pal 1995).

Pathophysiology

The pathogenesis of this disease is poorly understood and virulence factors of *D. congolensis* have not yet been characterized (Ambrose *et al.* 1998).

Incubation period

The *in vitro* incubation period is 12 days at 37°C (Hänel *et al.* 1991).

Clinical presentation

Clinical presentation includes a highly exudative dermatitis with crusts and 'paint-brush' formation localized predominantly at the dorsal midline, flanks, and distal limbs, usually without pruritis (**126–128**). In progressive disease, poor appetite, depression, fever, lymphadenopathy, and weight loss can be seen. Occasionally abortion might occur as a sequela (Sebastian *et al.* 2008).

Differential diagnosis

Although the multiple papules and crusts with 'paint-brush' formation are regarded as pathognomonic, *Staphylococcus hyicus* (subsp. *hyicus*) mono-infection or co-infection should be considered (DeVriese *et al.* 1983). However, *D. congolensis* should be considered as a possible aetiological agent associated with (mandibular) lymphadenopathy and granulomatous inflammation in the horse (Byrne *et al.* 2010).

Diagnosis

Diagnosis is usually based either on the detection of the typical 'railroad tracks' appearance of *D. congolensis* in a fresh impression smear stained with Gram or Giemsa stain or a culture test (**129**). A monoclonal antibody was used to demonstrate *D. congolensis* in clinical material from confirmed bovine and ovine cases and presumptive equine cases of dermatophilosis by indirect immunofluorescent staining (How *et al.* 1988).

Pathology

Dermatophilosis lesions are mostly situated on the dorsal areas with downward expansions resembling rain drops (hence the disease nomenclature rain scald). Affected distal extremities only (grease heal) may be apparent in horses kept in wet and muddy conditions (Stannard 2000, Jubb *et al.* 2007). Macroscopically the integument shows oedema, erythema, and a crusting exudative serous to suppurative dermatitis. Histological features include oedema of the congested dermis and epidermal neutrophilic exocytosis, with pustule formation and eventually formation of thick alternating orthokeratotic and parakeratotic serocellular crusts embedded within which are the causative large filamentous bacteria (**130, 131**).

126, 127 *Dermatophilus congolensis* is the pathogenic actinomycete that causes dermatophilosis or rain scald in horses (**126**) and has public health significance. Note the crusts with 'paint-brush' formation (**127**) regarded as pathognomonic for *D. congolensis*.

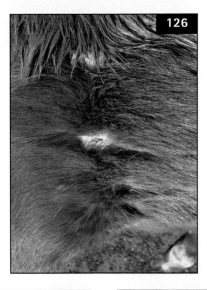

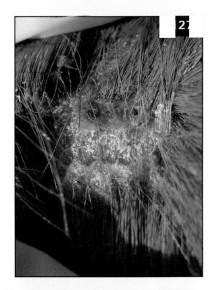

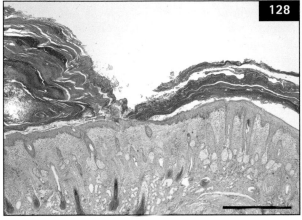

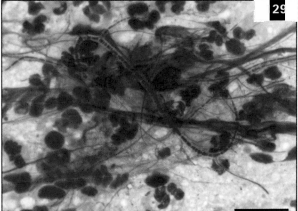

128 Dermatophilosis (streptotrichosis) or rain scald. Haired skin covered with typical extensive multilayered serocellular crusts containing the causative bacteria. Note the moderately thickened hyperplastic epidermis. *Dermatophilus congolensis*. (H&E stain. Bar 1 mm.)

129 Dermatophilosis (streptotrichosis) or rain scald. Superficial cytological smear of a crusting skin lesion. Note the typical longitudinal subdivisions of the serpentine branching bacteria known as 'railroad tracks' appearance. *Dermatophilus congolensis*. (May–Grünwald–Giemsa stain. Bar 20 μm.)

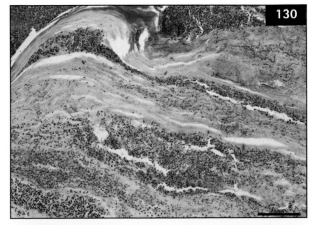

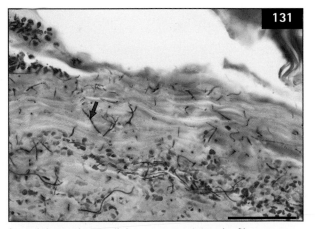

130, 131 Dermatophilosis (streptotrichosis) or rain scald. Close-up of a multilayered serocellular crust containing the filamentous Gram-positive bacteria. Several bacteria display longitudinal subdivisions (arrow). *Dermatophilus congolensis*. (Gram stain. Bars 100/50 μm, respectively.)

Management/Treatment

Frequent topical application of a 3–5% povidone iodine solution following clipping will usually cure the dermatitis. The horse's riding equipment should be desinfected as well. Although isolates were sensitive to penicillin G, ampicillin, streptomycin, gentamicin, lincomycin, erythromycin, tetracycline, oxytetracycline, bacitracin, and ceftiofur (Krüger *et al.* 1998), systemic antimicrobial treatment is usually not necessary. A dry coat will prevent future disease. There is no vaccine available yet for horses.

Public health significance

D. congolensis has public health significance as it might cause chronic dermatitis (Albrecht *et al.* 1974, Burd *et al.* 2007).

Corynebacterium pseudotuberculosis: 'PIGEON FEVER'

Phylum BXIV Actinobacteria
Class I Actinobacteria/Subclass V
Actinobacteridae/Order I Actinomycetales/
Suborder X Corynebacterineae/Family I
Corynebacteriaceae/Genus I *Corynebacterium*:
Irregular, nonsporing Gram-positive rods

Definition/Overview

Corynebacterium pseudotuberculosis causes disease in horses, sheep, and goats, and sporadically affects other species, such as cattle and man (Costa *et al.* 1998). It is also called 'pigeon fever' due to the swelling of the horse's pectoral region resembling a pigeon's breast (Spier 2008).

Aetiology

C. pseudotuberculosis is a Gram-positive, facultative, intracellular, pleomorphic bacterium. On the basis of ribotyping, sheep and goat isolates throughout the world appear to be distinct from equine isolates (Costa *et al.* 1998). Only *C. diphtheriae*, *C. ulcerans*, and *C. pseudotuberculosis* are known to harbour the phage-borne gene for production of toxin. *C. diphteriae* has been associated with wound infection in a 16-year-old Thoroughbred mare (Henricson *et al.* 2000).

Epidemiology

Disease incidence is seasonal with the highest number of cases occurring during the dry months of the year. As a consequence, high environmental temperatures and drought conditions usually precede outbreaks (Spier 2008). Many insects, particularly flies (house fly, *Musca domestica*; stable fly, *Stomoxys calcitrans*; and horn fly, *Haematobia irritans*) can all act as vectors of the disease (Spier *et al.* 2004).

Pathophysiology

The portal of entry for this soil-borne organism is thought to be through abrasions or wounds in the skin and mucous membranes (Aleman *et al.* 1996). Furthermore, the disease could be transmitted through horse-to-horse contact or from infected to susceptible horses via insects, other vectors, or contaminated soil (Doherr *et al.* 1999).

Incubation period

The incubation period is 3–4 weeks (Doherr *et al.* 1999).

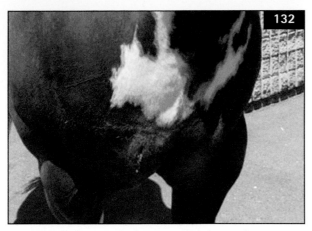

132 External abscesses in the pectoral abdomen due to *Corynebacterium pseudotuberculosis* infection. (Courtesy of Dr M. Aleman, University of California, Davis, USA.)

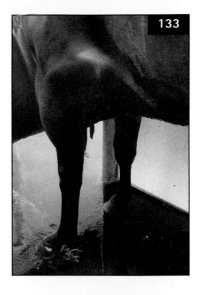

133 External abscess in the axillary region due to *Corynebacterium pseudotuberculosis*. (Courtesy of Dr M. Aleman, University of California, Davis, USA.)

134 Internal organ abscessation of the right kidney due to *Corynebacterium pseudotuberculosis*. (Courtesy of Dr M. Aleman, University of California, Davis, USA.)

135 Ulcerative lymphangitis of the left hind limb due to *Corynebacterium pseudotuberculosis*. (Courtesy of Dr M. Aleman, University of California, Davis, USA.)

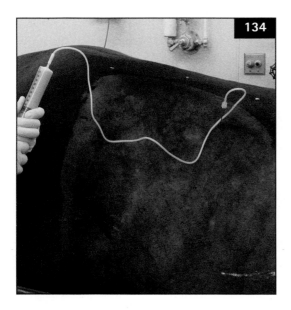

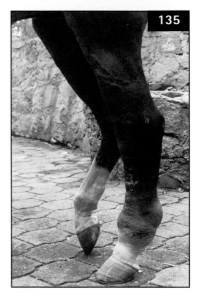

Clinical presentation

Three clinical forms of the disease occur: external abscesses in the pectoral or ventral abdomen (**132, 133**); internal organ abscesses including involvement of liver, lungs, kidneys, and spleen (**134**); and ulcerative lymphangitis of the limbs (**135**), with the first form being most common. Residual lameness or limb swelling is seen as a sequela of ulcerative lymphangitis/cellulitis (Pratt *et al*. 2005, Spier 2008). About 9% of horses with *C. pseudotuberculosis* infection have recurrent infections in subsequent years (Aleman *et al*. 1996). *C. pseudotuberculosis* has also been associated with epididymitis–orchitis in an 11-year-old Tennessee Walking horse stallion (Gonzalez *et al*. 2008). The mortality rate for horses with internal abscessation has been reported to vary from 28% to 40% (Aleman *et al*. 1996, Vaughan *et al*. 2004, Pratt *et al*. 2005). Interestingly, of 53 horses with purpura haemorrhagica 17 had been exposed to or infected with *Streptococcus equi* subsp. *equi*, whereas nine had been infected with *C. pseudotuberculosis* (Pusterla *et al*. 2003).

Differential diagnosis

The differential diagnosis includes various causes of internal abscessation (see p. 262).

Diagnosis

Ultrasonography examinations can be helpful for detecting internal abscesses (**136, 137**) (Aleman *et al.* 1996, Vaughan *et al.* 2004). The ultrasonographic appearance of these abscesses is characterized by focal or multifocal hypoechoic areas or cavities without an identifiable capsule or accumulation of hyperechoic material (Vaughan *et al.* 2004). The synergistic (with the exotoxins of *R. equi*) haemolysis inhibition (SHI) test is currently regarded as the most useful serological test available to detect IgG antibody to *C. pseudotuberculosis* in horses with internal infections. Dilution titres ≥512 are suggestive of the presence of internal abscessation (Knight 1978, Aleman *et al.* 1996, Vaughan *et al.* 2004, Spier 2008).

Pathology

Ulcerative lymphangitis typically affects initially the fetlocks of the hindlimbs, where diffuse swellings develop into dermal abscesses that may rupture and produce haemorrhagic purulent exudate. Various stages in the development and healing of ulcerated abscesses and lymphangitis may be present. Inflammation can advance and spread to pectoral and cervical regions. Furthermore, *C. pseudotuberculosis* infection can cause folliculitis (contagious acne) (Aleman *et al.* 1996, Jubb *et al.* 2007).

Management/Treatment

The use of antimicrobials for external abscesses is not necessary in most horses and may prolong the time to resolution (Aleman *et al.* 1996). However, antimicrobials are clearly indicated for horses with ulcerative lymphangitis or internal abscesses. Rifampicin (2.5–5.0 mg/kg BW bid orally) combined with ceftiofur (2.5–5.0 mg/kg BW bid IV or IM) appears highly effective for the treatment of internal abscesses. In addition, internal abscesses have reportedly responded to procaine penicillin (20,000 IU/kg BW bid IM), TMP/S (5.0 mg/kg BW bid orally) and potassium penicillin (20,000–40,000 IU/kg BW qid IV) (Pratt *et al.* 2005, Spier 2008).

In cases of ulcerative lymphangitis/cellulitis physical therapy, including hydrotherapy, hand walking, and wraps, as well as nonsteroidal anti-inflammatory drugs (NSAIDs) for pain management are recommended as additional therapy. For prevention of disease, good sanitation and fly control are suggested (Spier 2008).

Public health significance

C. pseudotuberculosis is also associated with lymphadenitis in humans (Peel *et al.* 1997).

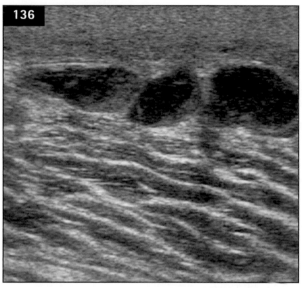

136 Ultrasonographic appearance of limb abscesses in *Corynebacterium pseudotuberculosis* infection. (Courtesy of Dr M. Aleman, University of California, Davis, USA.)

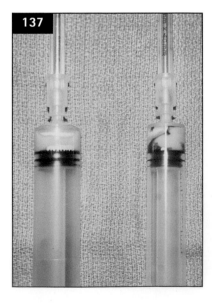

137 Purulent exudate associated with *Corynebacterium pseudotuberculosis* infection. (Courtesy of Dr M. Aleman, University of California, Davis, USA.)

Mycobacterium spp.: TUBERCULOSIS

Phylum BXIV Actinobacteria
Class I Actinobacteria/Subclass V
Actinobacteridae/Order I Actinomycetales/
Suborder X Corynebacterineae/Family IV
Mycobacteriaceae/Genus I *Mycobacterium*:
mycobacteria

Definition/Overview

Tuberculosis (TB) is a chronic, granulomatous disease caused by mycobacteria. Mycobacterial disease is considered to be uncommon in horses (Tasler & Hartley 1981, Cline *et al.* 1991, Gunnes *et al.* 1995, Keck *et al.* 2010, Monreal *et al.* 2001).

Aetiology

Mycobacteria are characterized as aerobic, acid-fast, nonspore-forming, slow-growing bacterial rods. As horses are considered to have a high innate resistance to *Mycobacterium bovis*, most reported equine cases of mycobacteriosis are caused by *M. avium complex* (Monreal *et al.* 2001) including subsp. *hominissuis* (Kriz *et al.* 2010).

Epidemiology

Historically most of the reported equine TB cases were caused by *M. bovis*, but with the implementation of eradication programmes for bovine TB the preponderance has shifted towards *M. avium* (Mair *et al.* 1986, Monreal *et al.* 2001).

Pathophysiology

Although the alimentary infection route appears to be the most common in the horse with primary involvement of the mesenteric lymph nodes (Gunnes *et al.* 1995, Jubb *et al.* 2007), airborne infection cannot be excluded (Gunnes *et al.* 1995). In comparison, transmission of TB occurs with the highest frequency from human patients with extensive, cavitary, pulmonary disease and positive sputum smear microscopy (Helke *et al.* 2006).

Incubation period

Not established in the equine species yet.

Clinical presentation

Clinical signs of TB in horses are extremely variable including fever, anorexia, weight loss (**138**), (intermittent) diarrhoea (Lofstedt & Jakowski 1989, Flores *et al.* 1991, Gunnes *et al.* 1995, Monreal *et al.* 2001, Kriz *et al.* 2010), poor racing performance (Sills *et al.* 1990), subcutaneous oedema in the ventral abdominal and scrotal regions (Lofstedt & Jakowski 1989, Gunnes *et al.* 1995), diffuse granulomatous dermatitis (Mair *et al.* 1986, Flores *et al.* 1991), neck stiffness (Binkhorst *et al.* 1972), and

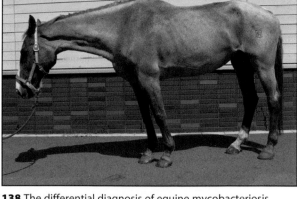

138 The differential diagnosis of equine mycobacteriosis includes (intermittent) fever and chronic weight loss.

spread to the vertebrae (Mair *et al.* 1986, Flores *et al.* 1991). Secondary lesions consisting of miliary or nodular tubercles have been reported in the lungs, liver, spleen, pancreas, myocardium, kidneys, serous membranes, and vertebrae, and less frequently in the skin, eyes, and other lymph nodes (Mair *et al.* 1986, Lofstedt & Jakowski 1989, Flores *et al.* 1991, Leifsson *et al.* 1997, Monreal *et al.* 2001). Abortion due to *M. avium complex* has been described in a 6-year-old Standardbred at approximately 300 days of gestation (Hélie & Higgins 1996) as well as in a 17-year-old Standardbred at 160 days of gestation due to *M. avium* (Cline *et al.* 1991).

Differential diagnosis

The differential diagnosis includes various causes of chronic weight loss and (intermittent) fever (see p. 263).

Diagnosis

Although abdominal palpation per rectum revealed mild thickening of the wall of the large colon (Lofstedt & Jakowski 1989), taut bands and small nodules on the small and large intestines (Gunnes *et al.* 1995), and an enlarged spleen with a very stiff consistency and big nodules in a generalized distribution (Monreal *et al.* 2001) antemortem diagnosis of equine mycobacteriosis remains a challenge, as failure to demonstrate acid-fast rods in direct smears and tissue sections using Ziehl–Nielsen staining does not exclude TB (Mair *et al.* 1986, Gunnes *et al.* 1995). Furthermore, an antemortem diagnosis is very difficult to achieve in horses, as intradermal skin testing (Cline *et al.* 1991) is unreliable in horses because up to 70% of clinically normal horses may have positive test results (Konyha & Kreier 1971). However, histological evaluation of liver biopsy tissue revealed granulomatous hepatitis associated with acid-fast Gram-positive bacilli characterized as *M. avium* serotypes 1 and 8 in a 15-month-old Appaloosa colt (Lofstedt & Jakowski 1989). When the spleen is affected as shown by multiple hypoechoic nodules ranging from 1 to 5 cm in diameter ultrasonographically, the diagnosis can also be confirmed by biopsy (Monreal *et al.* 2001). On the other hand, a biopsy of a chronic lingual ulcer in a 17-year-old Standardbred mare did not reveal the causative *M. avium* by acid-fast staining in contrast with post-mortem examination (Cline *et al.* 1991). It can be difficult to diagnose TB with culture. A rough colony variant of *M. avium complex* was cultured from a mare's faeces and ileocaecal lymph node after 4 weeks of incubation at 37°C (Cline *et al.* 1991).

Microscopy and culture still comprise the major backbone of laboratory diagnosis of TB (Chang *et al.* 2010). A PCR assay may be used to diagnose TB in horses and to identify the mycobacteria much faster than traditional methods (Monreal *et al.* 2001). Furthermore, the *M. tuberculosis complex* detection rate was 63% by PCR restriction fragment length polymorphism (PCR-RFLP) analysis, 79% by acid-fast stain, and 85% by a gene chip membrane array method in culture-positive human sputum specimens (Chang *et al.* 2010).

Histopathology – the results of which are available within days – is important in diagnosing difficult cases and should be requested early on (Malipeddi *et al.* 2007). However, whereas samples of lung, liver, spleen, and mesenteric lymph nodes taken at post-mortem examination yielded growth of *M. avium* serotype 4 from all organs, no acid-fast bacteria were seen in direct smears or tissue sections (Gunnes *et al.* 1995).

Abnormal laboratory findings included anaemia, hypoalbuminaemia, hyperglobulinaemia (Lofstedt & Jakowski 1989), mild leucocytosis, and neutrophilia (Monreal *et al.* 2001).

Pathology

According to Luke (1958), the pathological lesions in equine mycobacteriosis do not resemble those seen in mycobacteriosis in other animals. As caseation and necrosis are usually absent, the lesions are reported to take on a neoplastic appearance. This observation agrees with the findings in another report (Gunnes *et al.* 1995). However, horses also develop cavitary lesions with *M. bovis* (Francis 1958). Other animals that develop cavitary lesions with *M. bovis* include elephants, goats, sheep, and dogs. Interestingly, cattle rarely, if ever, develop cavitary lesions (Helke *et al.* 2006).

Myriads of intracytoplasmic acid-fast (Ziehl–Nielsen) bacilli are commonly observed in multinucleated giant cells, Langhans giant cells, and macrophages, with other findings including diffuse chronic granulomatous inflammation in various organs and tissues usually containing acid-fast bacilli (Sills *et al.* 1990, Flores *et al.* 1991, Malipeddi *et al.* 2007). Granulomatous enterocolitis generally represents the primary complex with involvement of the mesenteric lymph nodes (Lofstedt & Jakowski 1989, Gunnes *et al.* 1995, Jubb *et al.* 2007).

Management/Treatment

Usually not appropriate, as TB due to *M. bovis* is a reportable disease.

Public health significance

M. bovis (as well as *M. tuberculosis*) has important public health significance and is a reportable disease. *M. bovis* affects 17% of registered cattle farms in Devon, UK, and unpasteurized milk is consumed by an estimated 22% of Devon families with *M. bovis* reactor herds (Collinson *et al.* 2007). Most cases of human TB are caused by *M. tuberculosis*, and reliable information is not generally available on the incidence of *M. bovis* TB in humans. *M. bovis* is now estimated to account for less than 1% of human TB in most industrialized countries (Thoen & LoBue 2007).

Nocardia spp.

Phylum BXIV Actinobacteria
Class I Actinobacteria/Subclass V
Actinobacteridae/Order I Actinomycetales/
Suborder X Corynebacterineae/Family V
Nocardiaceae/Genus I *Nocardia*: Nocardioform
actinomycetes

Definition/Overview

Abortion and opportunistic (fatal) pneumonia or disseminated infection can be caused by *Nocardia* spp., but are uncommon and only a few sporadic cases have been reported in horses.

Aetiology

The genus *Nocardia* contains Gram-positive, catalase-positive, rod-shaped bacteria including *N. asteroides*.

Pathophysiology

Modes of infection and transmission are as yet unknown (Volkmann *et al.* 2001).

Incubation period

Not established in the equine species yet.

Clinical presentation

Clinical signs include abortion associated with placentitis and as a consequence foal losses from late abortions, stillbirths, prematurity, or early neonatal deaths. The foals are usually not infected, but may be small or emaciated. Furthermore, infertility and endometritis are mentioned as sequelae (Volkmann *et al.* 2001).

In addition, in immunocompromised horses (e.g. those suffering from severe combined immuno-deficiency disease, pituitary pars intermedia dysfunction, or lymphosarcoma), *N. asteroides* infection was associated with fatal pulmonary or disseminated infections (Biberstein *et al.* 1985).

Diagnosis

Diagnosis should depend on detection of the bacteria combined with appropriate clinical signs. A murine model has been used to develop a sensitive and specific serological test for clinical and subclinical infections caused by *Nocardia* spp. The following tests were able to differentiate between mice infected with and without nocardiae: (a) ELISAs with culture filtrate and cytoplasmic extract antigens from *N. asteroides*; (b) ELISA with *N. asteroides* trehalose dimycolate (cord factor); (c) indirect immuno-fluorescent antibody assay with whole cells of *N. asteroides*; and (d) Western-blot analysis for the 54–55 kDa, 36 kDa, and 62 kDa proteins of *N. asteroides* (Kjelstrom & Beaman 1993).

Pathology

Pathological examination might reveal an exudative placentitis.

Management/Treatment

In one study after a 2-week course of oral trimethoprim and sulphamethoxazole, based on antibiotic sensitivity testing, a uterine flush yielded no further growth (Volkmann *et al.* 2001). In two equine cases, *N. asteroides* infection was traumatic in origin and local in extent and the horses recovered without relevant antimicrobial therapy (Biberstein *et al.* 1985).

Public health significance

Zoonotic transmission cannot be excluded as a 75-year-old man who worked at a horse racing track developed pulmonary disease associated with *N. asteroides*. Occupational inhalation of soil has been suggested to have caused his disease (Nakagawa *et al.* 1996).

Rhodococcus equi: 'RATTLES'

Phylum BXIV Actinobacteria
Class I Actinobacteria/Subclass V
Actinobacteridae/Order I Actinomycetales/
Suborder X Corynebacterineae/Family V
Nocardiaceae/Genus II *Rhodococcus*:
Nocardioform actinomycetes

Definition/Overview

Pyogranulomatous lesions caused by the soil actinomycete *Rhodococcus* (formerly *Corynebacterium*) *equi* are seen most commonly in foals aged 30–60 days (Bain 1963, Higuchi *et al.* 1997). The pyogranulomatous lung lesions characteristic of *R. equi* infections reflect its ability to survive in macrophages, a characteristic also of *M. tuberculosis*, to which it is closely related (Meijer & Prescott 2004).

Aetiology

R. equi is a Gram-positive facultative intracellular pathogen that replicates in macrophages, and is one of the most important causes of pneumonia in foals between 3 weeks and 5 months of age (Giguère & Prescott 1997). *R. equi* belongs to the Mycolata, a phylogenetically distinct group of high G+C Gram-positive bacteria that contains a number of pathogens, including species of the genera *Mycobacterium*, *Nocardia* and *Corynebacterium* (Goodfellow & Alderson 1977). The possession of a large virulence plasmid containing a 27 kb pathogenicity island that encodes seven related virulence-associated proteins (Vaps) is crucial for virulence in foals (Meijer & Prescott 2004). Serotype 1 was the type most commonly isolated (72%) from clinical samples of foals or from the soil of horse facilities in Hungary. Six out of eight *R. equi* strains from humans belonged to serotype 2, and two human strains were untypable (Makrai *et al.* 2008). However, it has been shown that individual foals can be infected with multiple strains of virulent *R. equi* (Bolton *et al.* 2010).

Epidemiology

The majority of cases of *R. equi* infection are diagnosed during dry, warm summers; not only are these conditions optimal for bacterial multiplication but also they give rise to a dusty environment causing foals to inhale contaminated dust particles (Meijer & Prescott 2004).

Pathophysiology

The basis of pathogenicity of *R. equi* is its ability to multiply in and eventually to destroy alveolar macrophages. Immunity to *R. equi* pneumonia in foals is likely to depend on both the antibody- and cell-mediated components of the immune system (Meijer & Prescott 2004).

Both the oral and pulmonary routes of infection are possible (Smith & Robinson 1981). The distinct peribronchiolar distribution of the lesions observed in foals after multiple challenges with aerosols containing *R. equi* is precisely the type of distribution to be expected in a bacterial infection spread by aerosol (Martens *et al.* 1982). In addition, the intrabronchial instillation of *R. equi* also resulted in pulmonary lesions that were histologically representative of the natural disease (Magnusson 1938, Johnson *et al.* 1983a). On the other hand, the intragastric inoculation of *R. equi* induced lesions typical of the intestinal form of the naturally occurring disease, but failed to cause pneumonia (Johnson *et al.* 1983b). Furthermore, *R. equi* can produce subcutaneous abscesses when it is injected experimentally by the subcutaneous route (Magnusson 1938), suggesting migrating helminth larvae, such as *S. westerii*, as a source of infection.

Incubation period

The incubation period is about 18 days (Barton & Embury 1987).

Clinical presentation

The clinical signs of the disease are variable, but include increased respiratory rate, fever, cough, nasal discharge, harsh airway sounds, and wheezing. The respirations can have a characteristic rattle, which gave rise to the local appellation of 'rattles' for the disease (Bain 1963). Two clinical forms of *R. equi* pneumonia have been distinguished in foals. In the subacute form, apparently normal foals suddenly develop respiratory distress and severe pneumonia, and die within a few days. This form of the disease is characterized by a diffuse miliary pyogranulomatous pneumonia. In the chronic form, foals have a history of chronic unresponsive pneumonia and/or systemic disease (**139**). This chronic form is characterized by a chronic pyogranulomatous pneumonia with focal abscessation of the lung and pulmonary lymph nodes (Martens *et al.* 1982). Abscesses associated with *R. equi* can be found in organs other than the lungs, for example in the liver, kidneys, spleen, or the cervical lymph nodes. Cases also occur with intestinal ulcers and large abscesses in the mesenteric lymph nodes associated with diarrhoea (Magnusson 1938, Bain 1963, Higuchi *et* *al.* 1997). Kidney abscesses have been described in an 8-day-old foal (Bain 1963). Other less common clinical manifestations of infection with *R. equi* in foals include ulcerative enterocolitis, colonic or mesenteric lymphadenopathy, ulcerative lymphangitis, immune-mediated synovitis and uveitis, osteomyelitis, and septic arthritis (Giguère & Prescott 1997, Meijer & Prescott 2004). A chronic active, nonseptic synovitis (**140**) was found in 36% of cases. These foals were either apparently sound or were only mildly lame. The swelling of the joints usually disappears with no permanent effects as the pneumonia resolves (Sweeney *et al.* 1987).

At least one of 39 extrapulmonary disorders was found in 74% of foals infected with *R. equi.* Survival was significantly higher among foals without extrapulmonary disorders (82%) than among foals with extrapulmonary disorders (43%), but many extrapulmonary disorders were only recognized after death (Reuss *et al.* 2009). Furthermore, *R. equi* pneumonia is rarely seen in adult horses (Morresey & Waldridge 2010).

Differential diagnosis
The differential diagnosis includes various causes of internal abscessation (see p. 262).

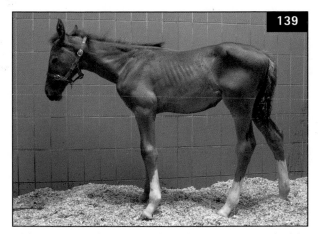

139 Depression, dyspnoea, and weight loss in a 2-month-old Warmblood filly suffering from *Rhodococcus equi* pneumonia.

140 Chronic active, nonseptic synovitis in a 2-month-old Warmblood filly. The swelling of the joints usually disappears with no permanent effects as the *Rhodococcus equi* pneumonia resolves.

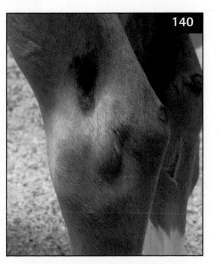

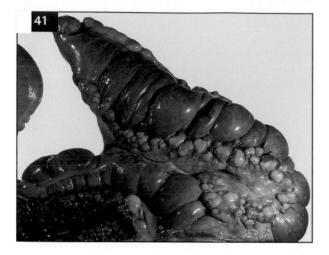

141 Typhlocolical rhodococcosis. Extensive ulcerative colitis and pyogranulomatous mesocolical lymphadenitis. Especially evident are the severely enlarged (lymphadenomegaly) pale colical lymph nodes. Rhodococcal infections are associated with a massive migration of nematode larvae, which may spread the bacterium. *Rhodococcus equi*.

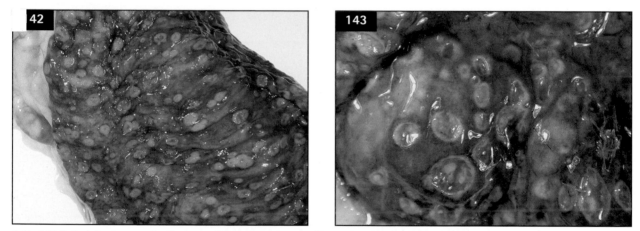

142, 143 Colical rhodococcosis. Close-up of the colon mucosa affected by typical multiple crateriform ulcerations. *Rhodococcus equi*.

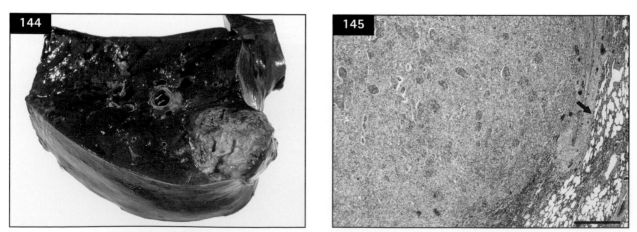

144, 145 Pulmonary rhodococcosis. **144**: Focal pyogranulomatous pneumonia/lung abscess, cut section of a pale circumscript mass of consolidated pulmonary parenchyma in otherwise hyperaemic lung tissue; **145**: corresponding micrograph depicts the nodular consolidated pulmonary parenchyma consisting of many neutrophils and macrophages enclosed by a fibrotic capsule (arrow) with adjoining still aerated alveoli. (H&E stain. Bar 500 μm.)

Diagnosis

At present, identification of *R. equi* from the respiratory tract via transtracheal aspirates is the only method for diagnosing the disease definitively *in vivo* (van der Kolk *et al.* 1999). However, only 62% of foals with positive *R. equi* cultures post-mortem yielded *R. equi* on culture of tracheal aspirates (Hillidge 1987). In addition, radiography and/or ultrasonography revealing pulmonary abscesses as well as increased total protein and gamma-globulin content of blood support the tentative diagnosis of *R. equi* pneumonia.

Pathology

R. equi infections can cause a (typhlo)colitis with typical multiple ulcerative crateriform lesions, particularly in the gut-associated lymphoid tissue (GALT) covering mucosa (**141–143**). Lesions can expand to the associated lymph nodes. Other tissues frequently affected are lungs (**144–149**), joints (**150**, *overleaf*), and muscle (**151**, *overleaf*) in foals. The intestinal and pulmonary forms usually co-occur. The lung lesions can vary from a suppurative bronchopneumonia to (multifocal) pyogranulomatous pneumonia.

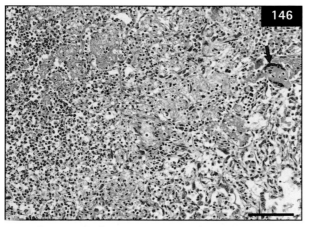

146 Pulmonary rhodococcosis. Pyogranulomatous pneumonia, numerous neutrophils and macrophages including multinucleated giant cells (arrow) occupy the alveolar spaces. (H&E stain. Bar 100 µm.)

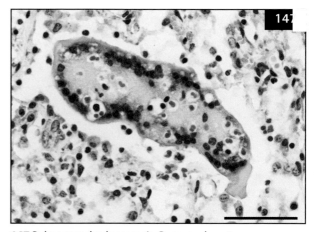

147 Pulmonary rhodococcosis. Pyogranulomatous pneumonia, a large multinucleated giant cell shows phagocytosis of neutrophils and cellular debris. (H&E stain. Bar 50 µm.)

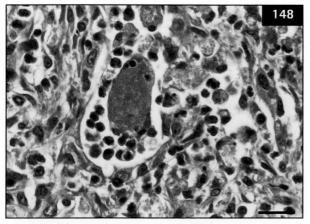

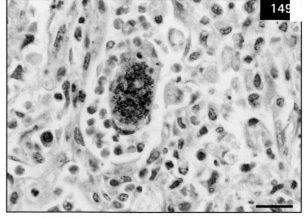

148, 149 Pulmonary rhodococcosis. Pyogranulomatous pneumonia, close-up of a multinucleated giant cell laden with cocci, especially evident in a Gram stain (**149**). The bacterium can resist and multiply in the macrophage cytoplasm when phagocytosed. (**148**: H&E stain. Bars 20 µm.)

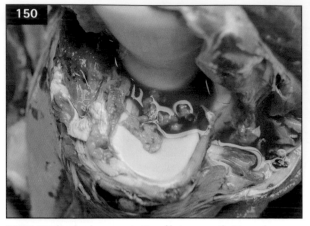

150 Articular rhodococcosis. Serofibrinous arthritis and tendovaginitis. The carpometacarpal joint and periarticular bursae contain a serofibrinous exudate. *Rhodococcus equi*.

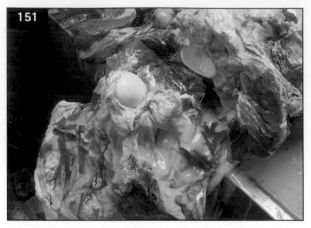

151 Rhodococcosis. Extensive muscular abscessation. In this foal the proximal hindlimb was markedly swollen due to massive amounts of intramuscular pus surrounding the hip joint. *Rhodococcus equi*.

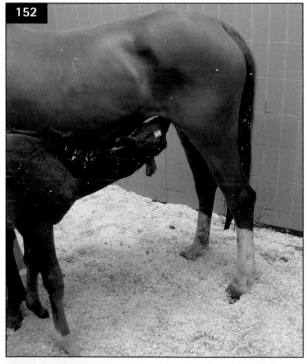

152 Acute (fatal) colitis associated with *Clostridium difficile* in mares has been reported when their foals are treated with erythromycin and rifampicin for *Rhodococcus equi* pneumonia.

Microscopically, the pyogranulomata or abscesses are composed of caseous masses of macrophages, neutrophils, multinucleated giant cells, and necrotic debris. Similar inflammatory infiltrates affect the colical mucosa, submucosa, and lymph nodes. The pathogen can readily be seen in the cytoplasm of macrophages and multinucleated giant cells in additional histochemical stains such as Gram or Giemsa.

Management/Treatment

Severe radiographic changes should not be used as a criterion for euthanasia, as foals may recover despite massive abscess formation (Sweeney *et al.* 1987). In one study, 85% of foals with radiographic evidence of lung abscessation survived (Hillidge 1987).

The combination clarithromycin (7.5 mg/kg BW PO bid)–rifampicin (rifampin) (5 mg/kg BW PO bid or 10 mg/kg BW PO bid or 10 mg/kg BW PO sid) was regarded as superior to azithromycin–rifampicin (rifampin) or erythromycin stearate–rifampicin (rifampin) for the treatment of pneumonia caused by *R. equi* in foals in a referral population associated with an overall survival rate of 69%. The odds of short-term treatment success were 12 times higher and the odds of long-term treatment success were 21 times higher in foals treated with clarithromycin compared to foals treated with erythromycin. The only reported adverse effect was diarrhoea that was mild and self-limiting in most cases (Giguère & Prescott 1997, Giguère *et al.* 2004). However, *Clostridium difficile* associated with acute colitis has been reported in mares when their foals were treated with erythromycin and rifampicin for *R. equi* (**152**) (Båverud *et al.* 1998). Preliminary findings indicate that tulathromycin (2.5 mg/kg BW IM once weekly) might be an attractive alternative treatment with reported side-effects being self-limiting diarrhoea, transient elevated temperature, and moderate swellings at the injection site (Venner 2009). However, the importance of microbiological culture and antimicrobial susceptibility testing in foals with pneumonia caused by *R. equi* has been emphasized, as the survival proportion of foals infected with resistant *R. equi* isolates (25%) was significantly less than the survival proportion of foals that received the same antimicrobial treatment from which antimicrobial-susceptible isolates were cultured (70%) (Giguère *et al.* 2010).

It has been stated that the incidence of the disease should decrease with good husbandry and helminth control (Bain 1963, Prescott *et al.* 1984). Vaccination of mares and their foals with virulence-associated protein antigen did not protect the foals and may even have enhanced *R. equi* pneumonia in them (Prescott *et al.* 1997). In addition, administration of *R. equi* hyperimmune plasma at 2 days of age decreased the severity of radiographic lesions and prolonged time to increased respiratory effort due to *R. equi*-induced pneumonia (Caston *et al.* 2006). However, the difference in incidence of pneumonia caused by *R. equi* observed between foals that received plasma and control foals was not significant (Giguère *et al.* 2002).

It has been shown that the time required to achieve a 1 $\log_{10}$ reduction in *R. equi* populations (D-value) are 17.1 h (±1.47) at 45°C, 8.6 h (±0.28) at 50°C, 2.9 h (±0.04) at 55°C and 0.7 h (±0.04) at 60°C, temperatures potentially encountered during horse manure composting (Hébert *et al.* 2009).

Public health significance

R. equi is an important cause of aquired immune deficiency syndrome (AIDS)-associated pneumonia in human immunodeficiency virus (HIV) infected humans (Meijer & Prescott 2004).

Chlamydophila spp.

Phylum BXVI Chlamydiae/Class I
Chlamydiae/Order I Chlamydiales/Family I
Chlamydiaceae/Genus I *Chlamydia*

Definition/Overview

The most important animal chlamydiosis with
zoonotic character is psittacosis, a systemic disease in
psittacine birds of acute, protracted, chronic, or
subclinical manifestation. The analogous infection in
domestic and wild fowl is known as ornithosis.
Avian strains of *Chlamydophila* (previously
Chlamydia) *psittaci* can also infect humans, the
symptoms being mainly unspecific and influenza-
like, but severe pneumonia, endocarditis, and
encephalitis are also known (Sachse & Grossmann
2002). The clinical significance of *Chlamydophila*
spp. in the development of disease in the equine
species has not yet been determined, although it has
been associated with upper respiratory and genital
tract disease, polyarthritis, hepatitis, and abortion in
horses.

Aetiology

Members of the Order Chlamydiales are obligate
intracellular bacteria that are transmitted as
metabolically inactive particles and must
differentiate, replicate, and redifferentiate within the
host cell to carry out their life cycle. Two different
forms exist, namely the elementary body and the
reticulate body. The cell wall-containing elementary
body is the spore-like infectious form, whereas the
larger intracytoplasmatic reticulate body is
associated with intracellular reproduction of the
organism (Abdelrahman & Belland 2005).

The Chlamydiales are a family of unique
intracellular pathogens that cause significant
disease in humans, birds, and a wide range of
animal hosts. Of the currently recognized species
Chlamydophila pneumoniae, unlike the other
chlamydial species, has been previously considered
to be solely a pathogen of humans, causing
significant respiratory disease, and has also been
strongly connected with cardiovascular disease
(Bodetti *et al.* 2002). The family Chlamydiaceae
now comprises two genera (*Chlamydia* and
Chlamydophila) with nine largely host-related
species and four species within the genus *Chlamydia*
(Sachse & Grossmann 2002). The presence of a
unique plasmid DNA may prove to be a useful
taxonomic marker for equine *C. psittaci* (Wills *et al.*
1990). *Chlamydophila abortus* was the agent most
frequently found in clinical samples from horses
(Pantchev *et al.* 2010), whereas *C. psittaci* or
abortus was present in the lungs of both clinically

healthy horses and those with recurrent airway
obstruction (RAO) (Theegarten *et al.* 2008).

Epidemiology

C. psittaci was isolated from 5% of nasal and
conjunctival swabs from normal horses (Mair &
Wills 1992). A seroprevalence of 15% has been
reported in light (i.e. non-draught) horses in
Japan using complement fixation antibodies, with
the 2–5 years age group having the highest
prevalence of chlamydial infections (Miyamoto *et al.*
1993).

Pathophysiology

Two *C. psittaci* proteins capable of binding
eukaryotic cell membranes were identified as a
protein of approximately 16–18 kDa and a second
larger protein, ranging in molecular mass from 24 to
32 kDa (Baghian & Schnorr 1992).

Incubation period

Following experimental challenge with an equine
isolate into the eye, nasal cavity, or bronchial tree,
C. psittaci could be isolated from nasal and
conjunctival swabs taken from ponies for up to
17 days after challenge without evidence of clinical
disease (Mair & Wills 1992). Furthermore,
following experimental challenge, interstitial
pneumonia and focal hepatic necrosis were observed,
and subsequently *C. psittaci* was reisolated from the
lung tissues (McChesney *et al.* 1982).

Clinical presentation

The clinical significance of *C. psittaci* in the
development of respiratory disease in the horse has
not yet been determined (Wills *et al.* 1990), although
it has been associated with (fatal) respiratory disease
(Moorthy & Spradbrow 1978, McChesney *et al.*
1982). Although the absence of *Chlamydophila* as
an aetiological factor in aborting mares has been
stated (Forster *et al.* 1997), the obligate
intracytoplasmic bacterium was associated with
abortion (Henning *et al.* 2000) and chlamydiae were
isolated from 27% of fetuses originating from eight
different studs (Bocklisch *et al.* 1991). Furthermore,
chlamydiae could not be detected in swab samples
taken from the uteri of mares showing reproductive
disorders (Szeredi *et al.* 2003). Chlamydiae were
demonstrated in 3.4% of stallion ejaculates without
a relationship between their presence and impaired
functional and morphological quality of ejaculates
(Vězník *et al.* 1996). Similarly, no chlamydiae were
isolated from synovial fluids from horses with acute
polyarthritis (Moorthy & Spradbrow 1978),
although a *Chlamydophila* sp. was associated with

polyarthritis in a foal (McChesney *et al.* 1974).

However, conjunctivitis and serous to mucopurulent rhinitis in Trakehner foals and older horses at a stud farm were attributed primarily to monoinfection with *Chlamydophila caviae* and subsequent aggravation by *Streptococcus equi* subsp. *zooepidemicus* (Gaede *et al.* 2010).

Differential diagnosis

The differential diagnosis predominantly includes various causes of abortion and fever (see p. 263).

Diagnosis

Although the equine species appears peculiarly resistant to infection, it is possible that this scarcity of information more accurately reflects the failure to consider chlamydia in diagnosis (Shewen 1980). A six species Chlamydiaceae-specific real-time PCR assay is available now to identify the chlamydial species involved (Pantchev *et al.* 2010).

Pathology

Following post-mortem examination, chlamydiae were not isolated from any equine lower respiratory tract (Blunden & Mackintosh 1991). Reported lesions in horses include keratoconjunctivitis, rhinitis, bronchointerstitial pneumonia, polyarthritis, enteritis, hepatitis, abortion, and encephalitis. The obligate intracellular organism can be detected microscopically as two types of cytoplasmic inclusions, the reticulate body and the elementary body (infectious form); they are composed of membrane-bound Gram-negative bacteria (Jubb *et al.* 2007, McGavin & Zachary 2007). In general, *C. psittaci* can infect respiratory epithelial cells, endothelial cells, and leucocytes, and spread to various organs via leucocyte trafficking.

Management/Treatment

Treatment of diseased horses is supportive.

Public health significance

C. psittaci has public health significance and its zoonotic risk should be minimized. The transmission of *C. psittaci* from birds to man is universally recognized. The disease in man may vary from inapparent infection to severe pneumonitis with septicaemia and death. Most frequently a transient influenza-like syndrome is observed with nausea, fever, vomiting, myalgia, chills, headache, and malaise. Trachoma-like follicular conjunctivitis may be the only sign. Infection is usually acquired by inhalation of dust from infected droppings, exudates, down, or other contaminated particles. There are few well-documented cases of human chlamydial infection with chlamydiae of mammalian origin (Shewen 1980).

A 20-year-old man who presented with painful inguinal and femoral masses following sexual contact with a donkey mare 14 days before was diagnosed with lymphogranuloma venereum based on the histopathological findings and a high titre of IgG (1:1400) (Khorvash *et al.* 2008).

Borrelia burgdorferi: LYME DISEASE

Phylum BXVII Spirochaetes
Family I Spirochaetaceae/Genus II *Borrelia*

Definition/Overview

Borreliosis is a multisystemic tick-borne disease (also called Lyme disease or Lyme borreliosis in humans) caused by the *Borrelia burgdorferi* sensu lato complex. Over 100 years ago, Afzelius described a patient with an expanding skin lesion, called erythema migrans, which is now known to be the initial skin manifestation of Lyme borreliosis in humans. Approximately 70 years later, in 1976, epidemiological evaluation of a cluster of children with arthritis in the city Old Lyme, Connecticut, USA led to a complete description of the infection, and the aetiological agent of the disease was discovered by Burgdorfer *et al.* (Butler *et al.* 2005, Steere 2006).

Aetiology

Borrelia spp. are Gram-negative, thin, elongated, motile bacteria with flagellar projections. The Lyme disease spirochaete contains 21 plasmids (nine circular and 12 linear) and this is by far the largest number of plasmids found in any known bacterium. Furthermore, the combination of genetic complexity (at least 132 functioning genes), intracellular localization, immune evasion, and autoregulation makes the Lyme disease spirochaete a formidable infectious agent (Qiu *et al.* 2004, Stricker *et al.* 2005).

The causative agents of borreliosis belong to the phylum of Spirochaetes and are grouped in the *B. burgdorferi* sensu lato species complex, which is divided into at least 11 different genospecies (*B. afzelii, B. garinii, B. burgdorferi* sensu stricto, *B. andersoni, B. japonica, B. lusitaniae, B. sinica, B. tanuki, B. turdii, B. valaisiana,* and *B. bissettii*) (Wang *et al.* 1999, Stanek *et al.* 2004). *B. afzelii* was the predominant genospecies in clinically normal horses in Austria (Muller *et al.* 2002).

Epidemiology

In Europe, the main vector of *B. burgdorferi* sensu lato is *Ixodes ricinus* (**153**), while in the USA it is black-legged ticks (*Ixodes scapularis*). Animals such as small rodents are known reservoirs (Gern *et al.* 1998, Humair *et al.* 1999). In addition, birds also play a role as reservoir hosts in the ecology of Lyme borreliosis (**154**) (Humair 2002), and ticks can be transported over large distances and across geographical barriers by avian hosts. The highest prevalence of tick infestation was observed in thrushes and dunnock (*Prunella modularis*) with *Ixodes ricinus* being the predominant tick, whereas *Hyalomma rufipes* and *Dermacentor* spp. were also found in Norway (Hasle *et al.* 2009). Prevalences of tick infestation in Switzerland were 6% and 18% for birds migrating northward and southward, respectively, with *Ixodes ricinus* being the dominant tick species. Among birds migrating southward, five species (*Erithacus rubecula, Turdus philomelos, T. merula, Phoenicurus ochruros,* and *P. phoenicurus*) carried *B. burgdorferi* sensu lato-infected ticks. Infection rates of examined *I. ricinus* ticks were 17% for larvae and 35% for nymphs (Marie-Angèle *et al.* 2006). It has been estimated that migratory birds disperse 50–175 million *I. scapularis* ticks across Canada each spring, implicating migratory birds as possibly significant in *I. scapularis* range expansion in Canada. However, infrequent larvae and the low infection prevalence in ticks carried by the birds raise questions as to how *B. burgdorferi* and *A. phagocytophilum* become endemic in any tick populations established by bird-transported ticks (Ogden *et al.* 2008).

Persistent infection with *Borrelia burgdorferi* sensu stricto in clinically healthy horses is likely (Chang *et al.* 2000). The seroprevalence in horses in some areas of the north-eastern USA is about 50% (Magnarelli *et al.* 2000) compared to 31–48% in France (Maurizi *et al.* 2010), 29% in Denmark (Hansen *et al.* 2010), 26% in Poland (Stefaniková *et al.* 2008), and 6% in Turkey (Bhide *et al.* 2008).In the USA, only *B. burgdorferi* sensu stricto as genospecies has been reported (Butler *et al.* 2005).

As viable *Borrelia burgdorferi* spirochaetes have been found in the urine of clinically healthy horses in an endemic region (Manion *et al.* 1998), the question has been raised if nontick transmission of *Borrelia burgdorferi* may occur by direct urine/mucosal contact comparable with a known transmission mechanism of *Leptospira* spp. (Butler *et al.* 2005).

Pathophysiology

Attachment to a receptor with an outer-coat protein called OspA displayed on the luminal side of the gut of ticks (like black-legged ticks *I. scapularis* or *I. ricinus*) allows *B. burgdorferi* to persist in the gut and avoid elimination from the time they were ingested by the tick. TROSPA is the name that has been coined for the receptor as tick receptor for OspA (Pal *et al.* 2004). The infection is usually acquired from larvae or nymphs (**155**) feeding on small to medium sized wild animals which happen to be a *B. burgdorferi* reservoir. Adult ticks only engorge successfully on larger animals like deer, sheep, cows, and horses. *B. burgdorferi* sensu lato DNA was most frequently detected in female ticks, less frequently in nymphs and larvae, and least

153 Micrograph of adult *Ixodus ricinus* tick (Ixodidae, hard ticks). Note the darker brown scutum, a hard chitinous rounded plate on the anterior dorsum, and four pairs of jointed legs. The capitulum harbours a harpoon-like hypostome, which secures the tick firmly in the host while sucking blood. These ticks are vectors of *Borrelia burgdorferi*. *Ixodus ricinus*. (Bar 500 µm.)

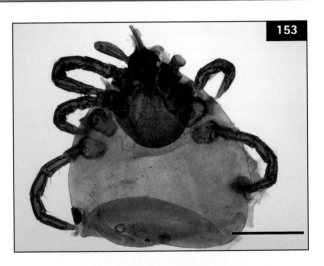

154 Migratory birds also play a role as reservoir hosts in the ecology of Lyme borreliosis. Tick (arrow) on juvenile Blyth's Reed Warbler (*Acrocephalus dumetorum*). (Courtesy Mr. B. Malmhagen.)

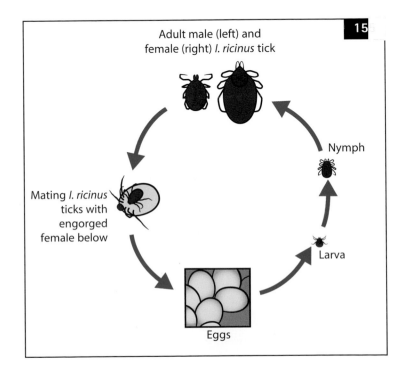

155 Schematic representation of the life cycle of the three-host tick *Ixodus ricinus*. The larvae have six legs, whereas nymphs and adults have 8 legs. The hard dorsal shield covers the entire abdomen in males, but only partly in females and nymphs. The time span from egg to adult is 2–3 years on average (range 1–6 years). The larvae, nymphs, and adults tend to feed on animals of different sizes.

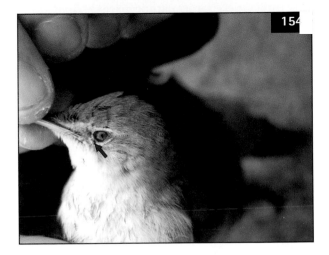

Adult male (left) and female (right) *I. ricinus* tick

Nymph

Larva

Eggs

Mating *I. ricinus* ticks with engorged female below

frequently in adult male ticks (Wodecka 2003). Once a tick attaches to a host and gets engorged, spirochaetes that are present in the tick midgut migrate through the midgut wall and haemocoel, reach the salivary glands and are inoculated with the tick saliva into the host 2–3 days after attachment (Piesman *et al.* 1987). Sometimes inoculation occurs earlier if spirochaetes are already present in the salivary glands of the infected tick (Alekseev *et al.* 1995). Although it is generally accepted that an infected tick must be attached for at least 24 hours on the mammal for *B. burgdorferi* transmission to occur (Thanassi & Schoen 2000), it has been demonstrated that *B. burgdorferi* can be transmitted to the host as early as 18 hours after attachment of an infected tick (Alekseev *et al.* 1995). Co-infection with other tick-borne pathogens like *Anaplasma phagocytophilum* is possible (Persing 1997).

B. burgdorferi predominantly migrates within connective tissue, which may protect the organism from humoral antibodies (Divers *et al.* 2001).

Incubation period
Not established in the equine species yet.

Clinical presentation
Clinical signs in horses attributed to *B. burgdorferi* include low-grade fever and lethargy (Burgess & Mattison 1987*b*, Magnarelli *et al.* 1988), lameness (Browning *et al.* 1993), arthritis (Burgess *et al.* 1986, Hahn *et al.* 1996), muscle tenderness (Divers *et al.* 2003), anterior uveitis (Burgess *et al.* 1986, Hahn *et al.* 1996), meningitis (James *et al.* 2010) encephalitis (Burgess & Mattison 1987*b*), abortion (Sorensen *et al.* 1990), and foal mortality (Burgess *et al.* 1987*a*). It should be realized that variation of the clinical manifestation in horses might be unapparent co-infection with other pathogens such as *A. phagocytophylum*. In addition, similarly to in humans, variation in clinical signs of *B. burgdorferi*-infected horses might be due to infection with different *B. burgdorferi* genospecies (Butler *et al.* 2005).

Differential diagnosis
The differential diagnosis is large not only due to the great variety of clinical signs but also associated with different *B. burgdorferi* genospecies and possible co-infection.

Diagnosis
The diagnosis of borreliosis in horses as well as in other species remains a challenge, as persistent *B. burgdorferi* infections without any clinical symptoms have also been documented in horses (Chang *et al.* 2000). Preference might be given to culture of *B. burgdorferi* from equine skin biopsies (Chang *et al.* 2000), combined with a two-step serology protocol (ELISA or IFAT supplemented by protein immunoblotting like Western blot or reverse line blot) (Trevejo *et al.* 1999, Magnarelli *et al.* 2000, Butler *et al.* 2005). The inclusion of OspF and p41-G antigens in ELISAs was most useful in the serologic diagnosis of equine borreliosis (Magnarelli *et al.* 1997). Of note, results of a PCR assay of CSF for *B. burgdorferi* DNA were positive in a 12-year-old Thoroughbred with meningitis (James *et al.* 2010).Ponies exposed to *B. burgdorferi*-infected ticks developed detectable antibodies at 5–6 weeks and the highest antibody levels were reached 3 months after exposure (Chang *et al.* 2000). An in-clinic C6 ELISA SNAP kit generated a fair sensitivity (63%) and very high specificity (100%) for horses recently infected with *B. burgdorferi*, providing equine practitioners with an inexpensive, one-step serology method to confirm infection, although its moderate sensitivity may result in a moderate chance of a false-negative test (Johnson *et al.* 2008).

Pathology
Lesions in ponies infected with *B. burgdorferi* sensu stricto were restricted to the skin and reported as perivascular and perineural lymphohistiocytic aggregates in the superficial and deep dermis (Chang *et al.* 2000).

Management/Treatment
Tetracycline (6.6 mg/kg BW IV bid for 3 weeks) has been reported to be superior to orally administered doxycycline or parenteral sodium ceftiofur in *B. burgdorferi*-infected ponies (Divers *et al.* 2003). Prevention is best achieved by avoiding tick-infested areas, and by careful grooming of the horse to remove ticks as soon as possible. Various insecticidal sprays are used to prevent tick infestation, but most are not approved for use on horses, and the efficacy of such use is as yet unproven (Butler *et al.* 2005). However, no adverse effects from the use of canine tick sprays on horses have been reported to date (Divers *et al.* 2001).

Public health significance

Borreliosis is regarded as an important tick-borne zoonosis, although the equine species is not seen as a main reservoir for human infection. However, it should be realized that viable *B. burgdorferi* spirochaetes have been found in the urine of clinically healthy horses (Manion *et al.* 1998). Lyme borreliosis is the most common human tick-transmitted disease in the northern hemisphere.

A complete presentation of the disease – in which a skin lesion results from a tick bite and is followed by heart and nervous system involvement, and later on by arthritis – is an extremely unusual observation. Late involvement of eye, nervous system, joints, and skin can also occur. The only sign that enables a reliable clinical diagnosis of Lyme borreliosis in humans is erythema migrans (**156**) (Stanek *et al.* 2004).

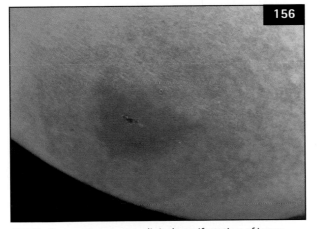

156 Erythema migrans as a clinical manifestation of Lyme disease in man.

Leptospira interrogans: LEPTOSPIROSIS
Phylum BXVII Spirochaetes
Family III Leptospiraceae /Genus I *Leptospira*

Definition/Overview
Leptospirosis is a worldwide zoonosis caused by pathogenic *Leptospira* species, for which humans are accidental hosts. Although horses are regarded as less susceptible to this pathogen, clinical symptoms in the horse include respiratory distress, renal failure, and uveitis, with the latter association already suggested in 1947 (Rimpau 1947). Urine is the chief source of infection, and apparently recovered animals intermittently pass the pathogen via the urine and are therefore regarded as carriers. The conventional tests include direct microscopy, culture, and – the most widely used reference standard method – microscopic agglutination test (MAT) (Ahmad *et al.* 2005).

Aetiology
Spirochaetes are a medically important and ecologically significant group of motile bacteria with a distinct morphology. Outermost is a membrane sheath, and within this sheath is the protoplasmic cell cylinder and subterminally attached periplasmic flagella. For spirochaetes, translational motility requires asymmetrical rotation of the two internally located flagellar bundles. Many spirochaetes, including *Treponema, Borrelia*, and *Leptospira* spp., are highly invasive pathogens (see **157–160**). Motility is likely to play a major role in the disease process (Charon & Goldstein 2002).

Leptospires are closely related to borrelias and are aquatic bacteria all classified into two species, namely *Leptospira interrogans* containing over 200 different serotypes, and the nonpathogenic *L. biflexa*. Horses are incidental hosts of several leptospiral serovars. Only serovar *bratislava* is thought to be maintained in horses (Ellis *et al.* 1983).

Epidemiology
The infection is usually transmitted via urine from reservoir hosts, e.g. small rodents such as mice and rats. High or increasing MAT titres to serovar *bratislava* have been found in foals and a closely related strain (serovar *lora*) has been isolated from a foal (van den Ingh *et al.* 1989). These observations, together with the isolation of a *bratislava* strain from the kidney of a healthy foal, indicate that horses can be infected and become carriers at a young age (Rocha *et al.* 2004). Leptospirae may persist for up to 120 days in ovine urine (Blackmore *et al.* 1982).

Serological surveys demonstrate that leptospiral infection is common in equine populations. However, most leptospiral infections in horses are subclinical (Donahue & Williams 2000). Confirmed cases of leptospiral abortion were assessed in 3% of fetuses from 5% of farms (Szeredi & Haake 2006). In addition, a bacteriological survey of kidneys from 145 abattoir horses in Portugal revealed the identification of *L. interrogans* serovar *bratislava* and *L. kirschneri* serovar *tsaratsovo* by restriction endonuclease analysis. Serology (MAT) indicated titres of 1:10 in 37% of horses. The highest percentages of titres were observed to be the *australis* (19%) and *pomona* (14%) serogroups (Rocha *et al.* 2004). Seroprevalence in clinically healthy racing horses in Korea was 25% with serovar *sejroe* being the most prevalent (77%). Seroprevalence was higher among ponies than among Thoroughbreds (Jung *et al.* 2010).

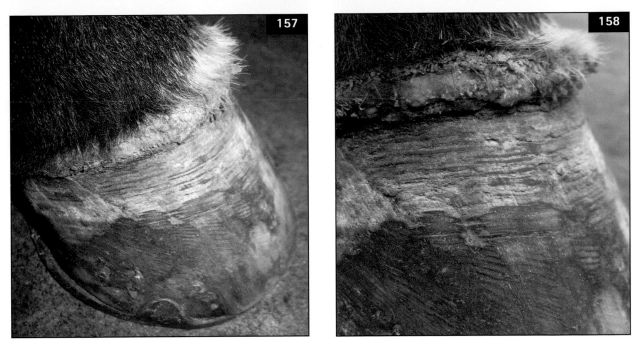

157, 158 Proliferative coronitis might be associated with intralesional spirochaetes.

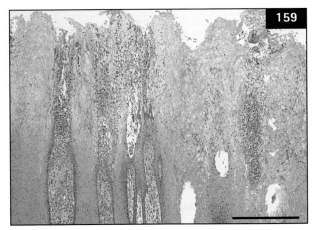

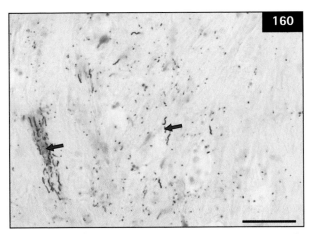

159 Proliferative coronitis associated with intralesional spirochaetes (see also Nagamine *et al*. 2005). The epidermis is thickened and hyperplastic with superficial erosions and diffuse dermal mixed inflammatory infiltrates. (H&E stain. Bar 500 μm.)

160 Close-up micrograph of proliferative coronitis associated with intralesional spirochaetes (arrows) (see also Nagamine *et al*. 2005). (Warthin–Starry silver stain. Bar 20 μm.)

Pathophysiology

It has been hypothesized that the immune component of recurrent uveitis (161–163) can be directly induced and maintained by persistent infection of the eye with *L. interrogans* (Rimpau 1947). *L. interrogans* was isolated from the vitreous humour of 52% of horses with recurrent uveitis but was not isolated from the vitreous humour of control horses. The duration of recurrent uveitis was 1 year for 38% of the horses from which the organism was isolated. Geometric mean antibody titres against *L. interrogans* in the vitreous humour and serum of horses with recurrent uveitis were 1:1,332 and 1:186, respectively. Only 76% of horses from which the organism was isolated had a fourfold or greater difference between serum and vitreous humour antibody titres (Wollanke *et al.* 2001).

Incubation period

A febrile response of 2–3 days' duration, with rectal temperatures of 39.3–40.3°C, was detected as early as 3 days and as late as 9 days after SC inoculation with *L. interrogans* serovar *pomona*, associated with alterations detected in 61% of the eyes at 133–146 weeks after inoculation (Williams *et al.* 1971). Pyrexia (39.3–40°C) occurred as early as 1 day after challenge with *L. interrogans* serovar *kennewicki* after either topical ocular or intraperitoneal injection (Yan *et al.* 2010).

Clinical presentation

It should be realized that infection without clinical signs is not uncommon in horses. Clinical symptoms caused by leptospires in horses include recurrent fever, depression, respiratory distress (164), diarrhoea, renal failure (165, 166), (recurrent) uveitis, haemoglobinuria, jaundice, stillbirth, inflammation of the umbilical cord, and abortion

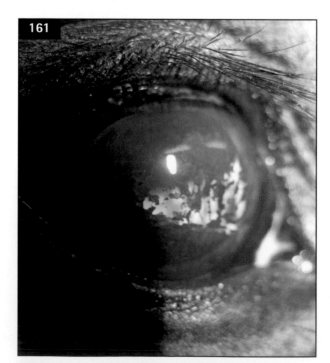

161 Equine recurrent uveitis is associated with persistent infection of the eye with *Leptospira interrogans*.

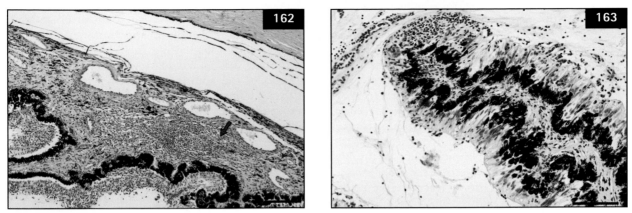

162, 163 Equine recurrent uveitis (periodic ophthalmia, moon blindness), typically a chronic lymphonodular uveitis. The iris stroma is markedly thickened by mainly lymphocytic aggregates which focally display nodule or follicle formation (arrow). Note also the intensely pigmented interior iridal epithelial lining which is covered with a more mixed inflammatory membrane. This particular case proved PCR positive for *Leptospira* sp. antigens. *L. interrogans* (*pomona* is the mostly implicated serovar). (H&E stain. Bars 200/100 μm, respectively.)

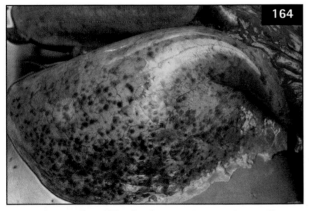

164 Widespread multifocal pulmonary haemorrhages. These haemorrhages may result from damaged blood vessels due to leptospiral cytotoxins. *Leptospira interrogans*.

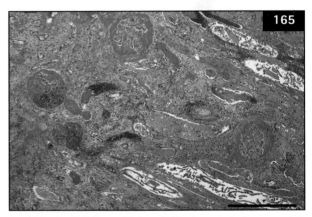

165 Acute tubulointerstitial nephritis. Acute tubular necrosis is characterized by the sloughed epithelium (top and bottom right) within the tubular lumina. There are extensive haemorrhages in glomeruli and interstitium. *Leptospira interrogans*. (H&E stain. Bar 50 μm.)

166 Acute haemorrhagic glomerulitis and tubulointerstitial nephritis. The glomerular uriniferous space of Bowman and adjoining tubuli are filled with extravasated erythrocytes and haemoglobin. Leptospiral haemolysins cause intravascular haemolysis, resulting in haemoglobinaemia and haemoglobinuria. *Leptospira interrogans*. (H&E stain. Bar 100 μm.)

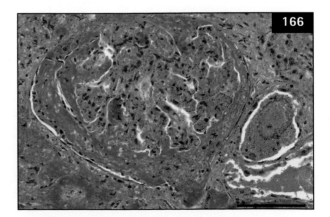

mainly in the last trimester. The most common serovar involved in equine abortion is *pomona*, but occasionally other serovars (*australis, grippotyphosa, icterohaemorrhagiae, sejroe*) have also been isolated from aborted equine fetuses (Ellis *et al.* 1983, van den Ingh *et al.* 1989, Frazer 1999, Bernard *et al.* 1993, Donahue & Williams 2000, Wollanke *et al.* 2001, Sebastian *et al.* 2005, Torfs *et al.* 2009, Whitwell *et al.* 2009). There was no significant association between clinical signs and disease and positive titres to serovar *bratislava* (except for the association between respiratory problems and fatigue and seropositivity). Overall, the age of the horse should be taken into consideration when evaluating the titre, as the average older healthy horse has a higher titre than a young horse (Båverud *et al.* 2009).

Differential diagnosis

The differential diagnosis predominantly comprises various causes for icterus and fever (see p. 262), respiratory distress (see p. 262), and abortion (see p. 263).

Diagnosis

Though dark field microscopy is useful for the diagnosis of leptospirosis it cannot be used as the sole diagnostic tool. The drawbacks of it on clinical specimens have been emphasized by stating that both false-positive and false-negative diagnoses can easily be made even in experienced hands. Though the use of culture confirms diagnosis it is impractical as it is expensive, complicated, technically demanding, time consuming – requiring prolonged incubation (minimum 1 month before declaring a sample negative) – and may not be successful (low sensitivity). Most cases of leptospirosis are diagnosed by serology (e.g. MAT or ELISA). MAT antibody titre after challenge with serovar *kennewicki* remained relatively constant for 21 days (Yan *et al.* 2010). The role of MAT in diagnosis and seroepidemiological studies is evident. However, the lack of standardization of baseline titres influences test validity and may result in overdiagnosis and overestimation of disease burden (Ahmad *et al.* 2005). In conclusion, leptospires can be detected in blood and/or urine by culture (Williams *et al.* 1971, Yan *et al.* 2010), regarded as the gold standard, or by various staining methods (Ahmad *et al.* 2005, Szeredi & Haake 2006). Leptospira can be isolated from blood while isolation from urine can occur after fever has subsided (Yan *et al.* 2010).

In addition, seroconversion (in foals as well as in the dam) might assist in diagnosis although the diagnosis of leptospirosis remains a challenge. Immunohistochemistry (91% of equine tissue samples) was more sensitive than silver staining (38% of tissue samples), and more specific than serology performed using the MAT. The primary advantage of immunohistochemistry over silver staining is the ability of immunohistochemistry to identify leptospiral antigen not only as morphologically intact spiral forms but it also enabled 1) the specific demonstration of leptospires together with light microscopic changes in tissue sections; 2) leptospires could be demonstrated not only as whole bacteria but also as intra- and extracellular granules; and 3) the samples could be easily evaluated on low magnification (100–200×) because of the good contrast of the red-stained leptospiral antigens over the blue background staining. (Szeredi & Haake 2006). Furthermore, it has been shown that a PCR assay based on the amplification of the hap1 gene represents a useful tool for specific detection of pathogenic leptospira in field samples taken from horses (Leon *et al.* 2006).

Pathology

Macroscopic lesions include swelling, yellowish discoloration and mottling of the liver, as well as swelling, perirenal oedema, and/or white radiating streaks in the renal cortex (resulting from tubular necrosis with or without inflammatory infiltrates), and cystic allantoic masses, oedema, areas of necrosis of the chorion, and necrotic mucoid exudates coating the chorion in the placenta (Poonacha *et al.* 1993, Szeredi & Haake 2006). Additionally, pinpoint greyish-white nodules in the liver corresponding to acute necrosis have been found (Szeredi & Haake 2006). Several microscopic lesions have been reported in conjunction with equine leptospiral abortion, including thrombosis, vasculitis, mixed inflammatory cell infiltration, cystic adenomatous hyperplasia, necrosis of the villi and calcification of the placenta, hepatocellular dissociation, mixed leucocytic infiltration of the portal triads, giant cell hepatopathy, multiple necrotic foci in the liver, suppurative and nonsuppurative nephritis, dilated tubules, pulmonary haemorrhages, pneumonia, myocarditis, and meningitis (Poonacha *et al.* 1993, Szeredi & Haake 2006).

Management/Treatment

Dihydrostreptomycin and tetracyclines are the antibiotics of choice for the treatment of acute diseased as well as of carrier animals. In addition, enrofloxacin (IV at 7.5 mg/kg BW sid) results in aqueous humour concentrations greater than the reported MIC for *L. interrogans* serovar *pomona* following disruption of the blood–aqueous humour barrier (Divers *et al.* 2008). Vaccine (on days 0, 28, 180, and 365 in the left lateral cervical area containing six serovars of leptospira) significantly increased days to recurrence by 40 days, but failed to slow the progression of equine recurrent uveitis. These data do not support the use of vaccination against leptospirosis as adjunct therapy for the routine treatment (consisting of a combination of anti-inflammatory agents and mydriatics to decrease pain and inflammation, minimize chronic changes, and prolong vision) of horses with equine recurrent uveitis. In addition, two new therapies have been promoted, namely 1) vitrectomy and replacement with a saline solution containing gentamicin, and 2) implantation of a sustained release cyclosporine delivery device into the vitreous through sclerotomy (Rohrbach *et al.* 2005).

Public health significance

Leptospirosis has important public health significance and its zoonotic risk should be minimized. Interestingly, patients diagnosed with Fuchs uveitis or Behçet's syndrome produced antibodies that cross-reacted with LruA and LruB, suggesting similarities of the autoimmune responses in those diseases with those of leptospiral uveitis (Verma *et al.* 2008).

Bacteroidaceae and *Fusobacteriaceae*

Phylum BXX Bacteroidetes
Class I Bacteroidetes/Order I Bacteroidales/Family I
Bacteroidaceae/Genus I *Bacteroides*

Phylum BXXI Fusobacteria
Class I Fusobacteria/Order I Fusobacteriales/ Family
I Fusobacteriaceae/Genus I *Fusobacterium*: Gram-
negative anaerobic, straight, curved, and helical rods

Definition/Overview

These obligatory Gram-negative anaerobic bacteria
are associated with opportunistic infections like
diarrhoea, pneumonia, lung abscessation with or
without pleurisy, septicaemia, cholangiohepatitis and
cholelithiasis, ulcerative keratitis, and paraoral,
endodontical, and apical molar dental diseases.
Animals that fail to respond to penicillin may benefit
from treatment with metronidazole (Carlson &
O'Brien 1990, Bienert *et al.* 2003).

Aetiology

Gram-negative, anaerobic, nonsporulating rods
phenotypically resembling *Fusobacterium
necrophorum* were isolated from the normal oral
cavities and oral disease-associated cavities of horses.
However, a novel species, *Fusobacterium equinum*
sp. *nov.* is proposed, with strain VPB 4027T
(= NCTC 13176T = JCM 11174T) as the type strain,
as a distinct member of the genus *Fusobacterium*
(Dorsch *et al.* 2001).

Epidemiology

Bacteroides spp. (10% of bacteria cultured) *fragilis,
tectum,* and *heparinolyticus* (Bailey & Love 1991)
and *Fusobacterium* spp. (2%) were isolated from the
pharyngeal tonsillar surface of normal horses. Of the
bacteria isolated from horses with lower respiratory
tract or paraoral bacterial infections, obligate
anaerobes accounted for ca. 70% of isolates,
facultative anaerobes for ca. 30% of isolates, and
obligate aerobes for 0.7% of isolates. The Gram-
negative rods comprised *B. fragilis* (5%), *B.
heparinolyticus* (5%), asaccharolytic pigmented
bacteroides (3%) and other bacteroides (13%), while
a so far unnamed species of *Fusobacterium* (7%),
and Gram-negative corroding rods (3%) were
isolated. Among the facultatively anaerobic isolates,
Streptococcus equi subsp. *zooepidemicus* accounted
for 31% of isolates, followed by *Pasteurella* spp.
(19%), *Escherichia coli* (17%), *Actinomyces* spp.
(9%), and *Streptococcus* spp. (9%) (Bailey & Love
1991).

Carbohydrate-induced laminitis in horses is
characterized by marked changes in the
composition of the hindgut microbiota, from a
predominantly Gram-negative population to one
dominated by Gram-positive bacteria. However,
bacteria such as lactobacilli, *Bacteroides fragilis*,
and *Clostridium difficile* did not establish
significant populations in the hindgut before the
onset of equine laminitis, in contrast to streptococci
of the *Streptococcus bovis/equinus* complex
(Milinovich *et al.* 2007).

Pathophysiology

The diversity of iron substrates utilized by
Porphyromonas gingivalis and the observation that
growth was not affected by the bacteriostatic effects
of host iron-withholding proteins, which it may
encounter in the periodontal pocket, may explain
why *P. gingivalis* is such a formidable pathogen in
the periodontal disease process (Bramanti & Holt
1991). The most likely source of bacteria involved
in lower respiratory tract and paraoral infections is
flora from the oral cavity (Bailey & Love 1991).

Incubation period

Not established in the equine species yet.

Clinical presentation

Clinical signs include diarrhoea (Myers *et al.* 1987),
pneumonia and lung abscessation with or without
pleurisy (Carlson & O'Brien 1990, Mair 1996,
Racklyeft & Love 2000), septicaemia, cutaneous
nodules (Carlson & O'Brien 1990),
cholangiohepatitis and cholelithiasis (Peek & Divers
2000), ulcerative keratitis (Ledbetter & Scarlett
2008), and paraoral, endodontical and apical molar
dental diseases (Bienert *et al.* 2003).

Obligate anaerobic bacteria were present within
the intralesional flora of ulcerative keratitis in 13%
of horses, the most frequent isolates being
Clostridium spp., *Peptostreptococcus* spp.,
Actinomyces spp., *Fusobacterium* spp., and
Bacteroides spp. (Ledbetter & Scarlett 2008).
Enterotoxigenic *Bacteroides fragilis* (ETBF) was
isolated from the faeces of 25% of Thoroughbred
foals in general up to 7 days old with naturally
acquired diarrhoea. Clinical or haematologic
differences were not evident between foals infected
with ETBF only and those infected with ETBF and
another recognized enteric pathogen. 10% of
ETBF-infected foals died (Myers *et al.* 1987).

Diffuse pneumonia from which *Streptococcus equi* subsp. *zooepidemicus* and *B. melaninogenicus* were isolated was reported following treatment with systemic corticosteroids for another disease (Mair 1996). Obligately anaerobic bacteria (such as anaerobic cocci, *B. tectum*, *Prevotella heparinolytica* and *Fusobacterium* spp.) and the facultatively anaerobic species *Escherichia coli*, were recovered more commonly from horses with pneumonia, lung abscessation, and necrotic pneumonia with or without pleurisy that died or were euthanized than from those that survived (Racklyeft & Love 2000).

In horses with molar dental disease in the upper or lower jaw the most common bacteria isolated were *Prevotella* spp. (80%) and *Fusobacterium* spp. (75%) (Bienert *et al*. 2003).

Diagnosis

Diagnosis should depend on the detection of obligatory anaerobic bacteria combined with appropriate clinical signs. Multiple anaerobic organisms, including *Bacteroides* spp. and *Fusobacterium* spp., might be isolated from blood and transtracheal aspirates (Carlson & O'Brien 1990) and liver biopsy material (Peek & Divers 2000).

Pathology

The outcome of pathological examination depends on the localization of lesions (**167**).

Management/Treatment

The treatment of diseased horses is supportive. Animals with anaerobic bacterial infections that fail to respond to penicillin or from which penicillin-resistant anaerobes are isolated may benefit from treatment with metronidazole (Carlson & O'Brien 1990, Bienert *et al*. 2003). In addition, supportive medical therapy with IV fluids was a critical part of the therapy of several cases suffering from cholangiohepatitis and cholelithiasis. Previous therapeutic failures may well be related to treatment periods of inadequate duration, and it has been recommended that antimicrobial therapy should be continued until gamma-glutamyl transferase (GGT) values are normal (Peek & Divers 2000).

Presurgical antibacterial therapy is recommended in horses with endodontical and apical molar dental disease, to reduce the risk of intra- and/or postsurgical bacteraemia and its serious consequences (Bienert *et al*. 2003).

Public health significance

Not convincing yet.

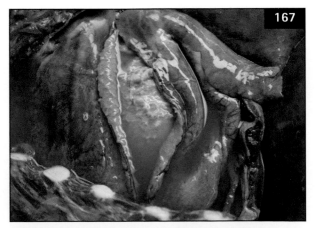

167 Bacterial serofibrinous pericarditis in a foal. The incised pericardium reveals an abundant serofibrinous exudate composed of a yellowish fibrinous irregular villous-like plaque. Gram-negative anaerobic bacteria were implicated.

BOTRYOMYCOSIS

Definition/Overview
Botryomycosis is an uncommon bacterial disease characterized by the microscopic formation of eosinophilic granules that resemble those of infection by *Actinomyces* species (Bersoff-Matcha *et al.* 1998).

Aetiology
Botryomycosis is caused by common bacterial pathogens including *S. aureus*, *E. coli*, *Proteus vulgaris*, *Streptococcus* spp., and *Pseudomonas aeruginosa*, yet the host and microbial factors that contribute to the pathobiology remain unknown (Bersoff-Matcha *et al.* 1998).

Incubation period
Not established in the equine species yet.

Clinical presentation
Commonly seen following wound contamination of limbs or scrotum. Lesions are usually firm and poorly circumscribed, with ulceration and yellowish/white granules associated with purulent discharge.

Diagnosis
The diagnosis of botryomycosis can be made when microscopic inspection and culture of the granules reveal Gram-positive cocci or Gram-negative bacilli (Bersoff-Matcha *et al.* 1998).

Pathology
Botryomycosis is defined histologically by the presence of eosinophilic material with embedded densely packed microorganisms surrounded by suppurative to pyogranulomatous inflammatory infiltrates. This characteristic pattern is known as the Splendore–Hoeppli phenomenon (**168–173**) (Bersoff-Matcha *et al.* 1998).

Management/Treatment
Successful treatment often requires a combination of both surgical debridement and long-term antimicrobial therapy (Bersoff-Matcha *et al.* 1998).

Public health significance
Although first discovered as a disease of horses (Bollinger *et al.* 1870), there have been about 90 reported cases of human botryomycosis. Human disease occurs in two broad categories: cutaneous and visceral. Cutaneous botryomycosis is more common than visceral disease, the latter having been described mainly in patients with underlying diseases (Bersoff-Matcha *et al.* 1998).

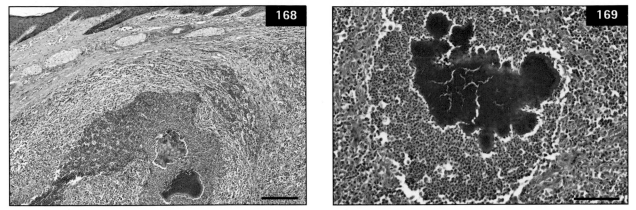

168, 169 Cutaneous botryomycosis. Focal extensive pyogranulomatous dermatitis centred upon brightly eosinophilic proteinaceous deposits with embedded causative basophilic bacteria. *Staphylococcus aureus*. (H&E stain. Bars 200/100 μm, respectively.)

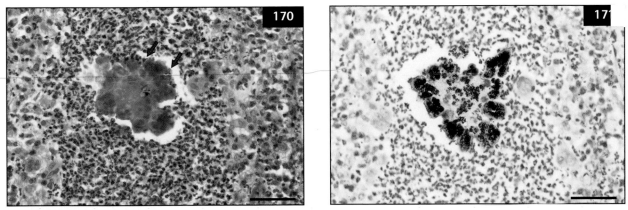

170, 171 Cutaneous botryomycosis. Close-up of the central proteinaceous mass displaying a typical irregular corrugated outline composed of club-shaped proteinaceous deposits (Splendore–Hoeppli phenomenon) (arrows) closely surrounded by numerous neutrophils and outer large macrophages which may include multinucleated giant cells. The embedded Gram-positive bacteria are especially evident in **171**. *Staphylococcus aureus*. (H&E Gram stain. Bar 50 μm.)

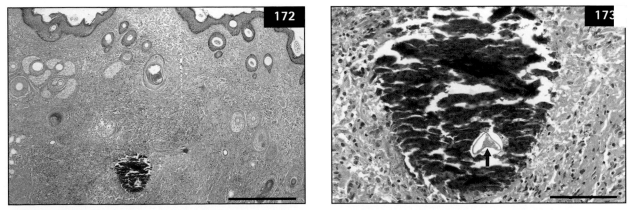

172, 173 Cutaneous habronemiasis, a differential diagnosis of cutaneous botryomycosis. Granulomatous and eosinophilic dermatitis. Poorly circumscribed granuloma present within the subcutis centred on a central dead nematode larva (arrow) surrounded by macrophages and eosinophils. Often the central focus is mineralized without Splendore–Hoeppli phenomenon. Fly intermediate hosts (*Musca* spp.) transmit the larvae. *Habronema* spp. or *Draschia* (*Habronema*) *megastoma*. (H&E, stain. Bars 500/100 μm, respectively.)

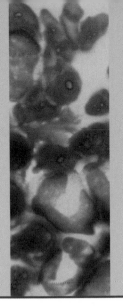

Chapter 2
Viral diseases

EQUINE ADENOVIRUS
Family Adenoviridae
Genus Mastadenovirus: double-stranded DNA

Definition/Overview
Although equine adenovirus is widespread it usually does not induce clinical signs except in immunocompromised animals. Hence, equine adenovirus is especially associated with pneumonia in Arabian foals suffering from severe combined immune deficiency (SCID).

Aetiology
Members of the family Adenoviridae are nonenveloped, icosahedral viruses that replicate in the nucleus. Their linear, double-stranded DNA molecules are 26–45 Kbp in size and rank as medium-sized among the DNA viruses. Adenoviruses fall into four recognized genera, plus possibly a fifth, which have apparently evolved with their vertebrate hosts, but have also engaged in a number of interspecies transmission events. Two genera (Mastadenovirus and Aviadenovirus) originate from mammals and birds, respectively, and the other two genera (Atadenovirus and Siadenovirus) have a broader range of hosts (Davison *et al.* 2003). Equine adenovirus is a virus with a diameter of 70–80 nm. In equine medicine two antigenically distinct equine adenovirus strains are distinguished, namely types 1 and 2 (Studdert & Blackney 1982).

Epidemiology
Despite its worldwide distribution (Giles *et al.* 2010), a matched case–control study nested within a longitudinal study of respiratory disease failed to demonstrate a significant association between clinically apparent respiratory disease in young racehorses and infection with equine adenovirus as diagnosed by subsequent seroconversion (Newton *et al.* 2003).

Pathophysiology
Adenovirus infection manifests in many ways, with respiratory and gastrointestinal symptoms associated with local production of several proinflammatory cytokines predominating in man (Moro *et al.* 2009). It is interesting to note that equine adenovirus was less sensitive to recombinant equine interferon-gamma in one study (Sentsui *et al.* 2010).

Incubation period
Not established in the equine species yet.

Clinical presentation
Clinical signs include fever, anorexia, conjunctivitis, rhinitis, and bronchopneumonia usually caused by equine adenovirus 1 (Webb *et al.* 1981, Studdert & Blackney 1982). Diarrhoea caused by equine adenovirus 1 is sometimes seen. In addition, an antigenically distinct equine adenovirus from the faeces of two foals with diarrhoea was designated equine adenovirus 2 (Studdert & Blackney 1982, Corrier *et al.* 1982). In Arabian foals with primary SCID, equine adenovirus 1 causes a progressive bronchopneumonia and generalized infection that is a major contributing cause of death in this syndrome (McChesney *et al.* 1974). The syndrome is inherited as a simple, recessive, autosomal gene (Thompson *et al.* 1975). In addition, intestinal infection by coronavirus (besides adenovirus infection) and cryptosporidia was also identified in an Arabian foal suffering from primary SCID (Mair *et al.* 1990).

Differential diagnosis

The differential diagnosis includes various causes of acute febrile upper airway disease and diarrhoea in foals (see p. 262).

Diagnosis

The diagnosis should be based on the demonstration of equine adenovirus in nasopharyngeal, conjunctival or rectal swabs combined with the presence of characteristic clinical signs and seroconversion.

Pathology

At necropsy, cranioventral pulmonary consolidation indicative of a broncho(interstitial)pneumonia is evident. Histological evaluation reveals bronchiolar epithelial necrosis with sloughing and typical intranuclear basophilic viral inclusion bodies, which may also be found in pneumocytes (**174–176**). Alveolar septa are swollen with increased numbers of septal and intra-alveolar macrophages and neutrophils (**177**). The affected lung is soon infected by secondary bacterial invaders.

Management/Treatment

Treatment of diseased foals is supportive with special reference to improvement of antibody status by means of the administration of hyperimmune serum. There is no effective vaccine available yet.

Public health significance

Zoonotic transmission cannot be excluded (Phan *et al.* 2006).

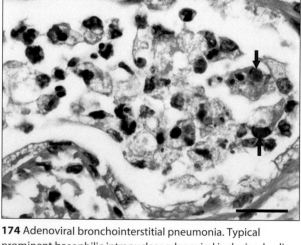

174 Adenoviral bronchointerstitial pneumonia. Typical prominent basophilic intranuclear adenoviral inclusion bodies (arrows) are present within exfoliated bronchiolar epithelial cells. Equine adenovirus. (H&E stain. Bar 20 μm.)

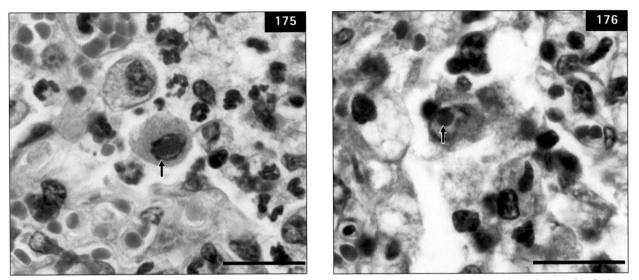

175, 176 Adenoviral bronchointerstitial pneumonia. Close-up of the typical prominent basophilic intranuclear adenoviral inclusion bodies (arrows) present within exfoliated bronchiolar epithelial cells. Equine adenovirus. (H&E stain. Bars 20 µm.)

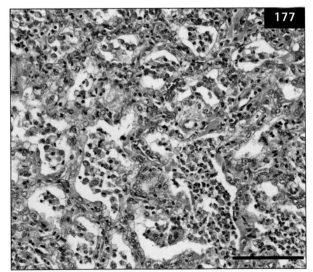

177 Adenoviral bronchointerstitial pneumonia. Alveolar septa are thickened, necrotic exfoliated alveolar and bronchiolar epithelial cells are sloughed within the respiratory lumina admixed with neutrophils. Equine adenovirus. (H&E stain. Bar 200 µm.)

EQUINE HERPESVIRUS

Family Herpesviridae
Subfamily Alphaherpesvirinae/Genus
Varicellovirus: double-stranded DNA

Definition/Overview

An acute febrile upper airway disease is caused by equine herpesvirus (EHV). EHV-1 is a highly prevalent equine respiratory pathogen that can cause abortion during the third trimester of pregnancy and neonatal foal death as well as neurological disease (Perkins *et al.* 2008). In cases of EHV-1 abortion, mares usually show no other clinical signs. Clinicians should presume that the majority of horses are latently infected with EHV-1 (Lunn *et al.* 2009). There is no evidence that current vaccines can prevent naturally occurring cases of equine herpes myeloencephalopathy (van Maanen 2002, Lunn *et al.* 2009). Quarantine of EHV-1-infected horses should be up to 3 weeks post infection to ensure that animals are no longer shedding the agent (Perkins *et al.* 2008).

Aetiology

Herpesviridae is a large family of DNA viruses that is subdivided into three subfamilies (α, β, and γ). Eight herpesviruses have been identified in equids: five in the Alphaherpesvirinae subfamily and three in the Gammaherpesvirinae subfamily. Of those eight viruses, five naturally infect the domestic horse and three infect the donkey (Patel & Heldens 2005). EHV-1 and EHV-4 are members of the family Herpesviridae, subfamily Alphaherpesvirinae, genus Varicellovirus, and are characterized by a double-stranded DNA genome. EHV-1 strains are associated with respiratory disease, abortion, and paresis/paralysis, whereas EHV-4 strains are predominantly associated with respiratory disease. Up to 4% of EHV-induced abortions were caused by EHV-4. It has been stated that at least some EHV-4 strains appear to be able to induce viraemia with potentially the same sequelae as EHV-1. On the other hand, genetic variation in EHV-1 and EHV-4 isolates is limited (van Maanen *et al.* 2000) although of the viral factors determining clinical signs specifically, the occurrence of the DNA_{pol} SNP seems to be of importance (Lunn *et al.* 2009). It has been proposed that EHV-1 viruses carrying the D_{752} variant of DNA_{pol} have a higher risk of causing neurological disease than those with the N_{752} marker. However, it is also clear that N_{752} isolates can cause neurological disease. On the other hand, in naturally occurring abortions, the association with the N_{752} strain variant is very strong (Nugent *et al.* 2006, Goodman *et al.* 2007, Lunn *et al.* 2009) with co-infection with both strains being a common observation (Lunn *et al.* 2009). Equine multinodular pulmonary fibrosis has been associated with EHV-5 infection (Williams *et al.* 2007), whereas EHV-2 infection has been associated with keratoconjunctivitis (**178**) (Borchers *et al.* 1998).

Epidemiology

The majority of horses show serological evidence of exposure to these viruses and as a consequence the seroprevalence of EHV-1/4 is very high. Of interest, both EHV-2 and EHV-5 are common in horses in Iceland (Thorsteinsdóttir *et al.* 2010). However, most serological tests cannot differentiate between EHV-1 and EHV-4 antibodies due to the extensive antigenic cross-reactivity. When using a type-specific serological assay in random samples of Thoroughbreds before 1977 all horses were positive for EHV-4, whereas only 9% were positive for EHV-1 (Crabb & Studdert 1993). In another report, the seroprevalence of EHV-1 was 30%, whereas the seroprevalence of EHV-4-specific antibodies was still 100% (Crabb *et al.* 1995). Information about persistence of type-specific antibodies after primary or repetitive respiratory infections is poor (van Maanen 2002). It has been suggested that EHV-1 has phylogenetically been derived from a donkey virus, and that donkeys may remain an alternative host for EHV-1 and as a consequence may serve as a reservoir to infect horses (Browning *et al.* 1988, Crabb & Studdert 1995). As all α–herpesviruses, EHV-1 and EHV-4 appear to establish lifelong latent infections. Latency has been demonstrated for both viruses in lymphoid tissues and peripheral leucocytes (Welch *et al.* 1992, Carvalho *et al.* 2000) as well as in trigeminal ganglia (Slater *et al.* 1994, Borchers *et al.*

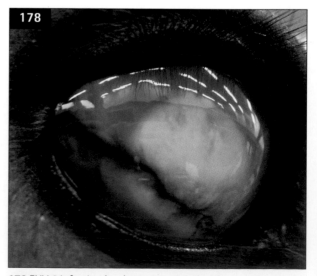

178 EHV-2 infection has been associated with keratoconjunctivitis (Borchers *et al.* 1998).

1999). Reactivation and shedding of both EHV-1 and EHV-4 creates the opportunity for transmission to other horses, which is considered important in the epidemiology and might explain why these diseases occur in closed populations (Welch et al. 1992). Previous studies have reported latency rates of 47% in the USA (Holmes et al. 2006), and 80–88% in the UK and Australia (Edington et al. 1994, Gilkerson et al. 1999). Furthermore, serological studies have demonstrated that EHV-1 infection is maintained in the population as a subclinical infection of foals and young horses (Gilkerson et al. 1997).

Pathophysiology

EHV-1 can enter disparate cell types by at least two distinct mechanisms (endocytic/phagocytic or direct fusion) and productive infection is dependent upon activation of the serine/threonine Rho kinase ROCK1 (Frampton et al. 2007). Endotheliotropism seems to be associated with abortigenic and neurogenic potential, but until now no genetic markers have been elucidated accounting for differences in endotheliotropism (van Maanen 2002). Even the propensity of certain EHV-1 isolates to induce myeloencephalitis does not reflect specific neurotropism but rather a marked endotheliotropism (Jackson et al. 1977). EHV-1 is transported by circulating peripheral blood mononuclear cells to the CNS vasculature, causing endothelial cell infection, and cell-to-cell spread of EHV-1 infection from leucocytes to brain endothelial cells has been shown in vitro (Goehring et al. 2011). On the other hand, a specific mutation in the amino acid sequence of the EHV-1 polymerase gene was linked in 85% of cases to an increased likelihood of the virus isolate coming from a case of neurological disease (Nugent et al. 2006). However, foals infected with a neuropathogenic strain of EHV-1 had an enhanced magnitude and duration of leucocyte-associated viraemia compared to foals infected with non-neuropathogenic, or abortigenic, strains of EHV-1 (Allen & Breathnach 2006).

Incubation period

The incubation period is highly variable, with references to abortion ranging from 9 days to 4 months (Allen et al. 1998), whereas the incubation period of encephalomyelitis is 6–10 days (Dinter & Klingeborn 1976, Thein 1981). The viraemia can persist for at least 14 days (Lunn et al. 2009).

Clinical presentation

For both viruses, mild or subclinical infections are common. Acute respiratory disease is predominantly caused by EHV-4 and is seen mainly in foals, weanlings, and yearlings after primary infection.

Symptoms include fever, anorexia, enlargement of lymph nodes, and serous nasal discharge. With EHV-1, about 95% of abortions occur in the last 4 months of pregnancy (Allen et al. 1998). Infection of pregnant mares often passes unnoticed with sometimes anorexia and oedema of the lower limbs (van Maanen 2002). Mares infected in late gestation may deliver a living foal often with signs of weakness, jaundice, and respiratory distress. These foals usually die within a few days (Murray et al. 1998). The clinical signs in the neurological form vary from mild ataxia to tetraparalysis, often including paralysis of the tail and urinary bladder with incontinence and sometimes perineal hypalgia or anaesthesia (Allen et al. 1998, van Maanen 2002). Typically some 10% of infected horses develop neurological signs during equine herpes myeloencephalopathy, with older horses being more susceptible (Goehring et al. 2006). The prognosis for complete recovery from equine herpes myeloencephalopathy for recumbent horses is poor (van Maanen 2002).

Differential diagnosis

The differential diagnosis predominantly includes various causes of abortion and fever (see p. 263). With reference to clinical signs and the multifocal hepatic coagulative necrosis in neonatal foals, Clostridium piliforme infection is the most important differential diagnosis at necropsy.

Diagnosis

Virus culture and isolation is considered the gold standard test for making a laboratory diagnosis of EHV-1 and should be attempted especially during epidemics of equine herpes myeloencephalopathy, concurrently with rapid diagnostic testing (PCR), in order to be able to biologically and molecularly characterize the virus isolate retrospectively (van Maanen 2002, Slater 2007, Lunn et al. 2009) and/or identify seroconversion. Nasal rather than nasopharyngeal swabs should be taken, preferably in the early febrile phase of the disease, and transported as soon as possible in sterile, cold transport medium to the laboratory (van Maanen 2002, Pusterla et al. 2008). For nasal swabs, PCR appears to be more sensitive than virus isolation (van Maanen et al. 2001) and some laboratories prefer ethylenediaminetetraacetic acid (EDTA) as an anticoagulant, as heparin may interfere with PCR reactions (Lunn et al. 2009). In cases of abortion, the fetus is the specimen of choice for diagnosis and EHV-1/4 infection can be demonstrated directly by immunofluorescence test (IFT) or via virus isolation and PCR (Mackie et al. 1996, Allen et al. 1998, van Maanen 2002). Isolation from CSF is rarely successful and swab samples should preferably be taken from febrile in-contact horses in cases with the neurological form (Wilson 1997). For isolation of virus from buffy coat, several passages are often required, which makes diagnosis rather laborious and time consuming (van Maanen 2002). Real-time quantitative PCR (qPCR) detected virus up to day 21 after challenge, whereas virus isolation detected virus only to day 5 in one study. It has been suggested that fast (35 min) qPCR of nasal swab samples should be chosen for diagnosis and monitoring of herpesvirus-induced disease in horses (Perkins *et al.* 2008). A method for the differentiation of neuropathogenic and non-neuropathogenic strains of equine herpesvirus-1 has been described based on the primer-probe energy transfer (PriProET) technique (Malik *et al.* 2010).

Pathology

Vasculitis (**179**) and thrombosis of small blood vessels in the spinal cord and/or brain are consistent histopathological changes associated with equine herpes myeloencephalopathy (**180–182**) (Lunn *et al.* 2009). Multifocal hepatic coagulative necrosis in neonatal foals (**183–187**) is regarded as pathognomonic for EHV-1 abortion.

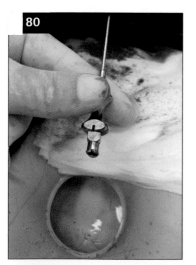

179 Herpesviral cerebral lymphohistiocytic vasculitis. A small cerebral arteriole shows swollen endothelial cells (arrow) and a cell-poor perivascular cuffing by lymphocytes and histiocytes expanding the Virchow–Robbins space (arrowhead). Equine herpesvirus-1. (H&E stain. Bar 50 μm.)

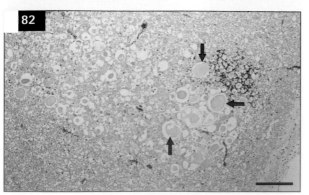

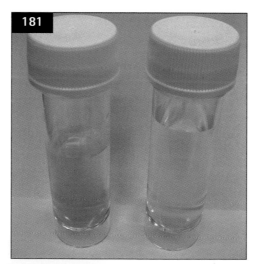

180, 181 Collection of cerebrospinal fluid (**180**) revealing xanthochromia (**181** left tube) is usually supportive of equine herpes myeloencephalopathy as well as increased protein concentration. However, equine herpesvirus isolation itself from cerebrospinal fluid is rarely successful.

182 Herpesviral myelomalacia. The affected spinal cord contains numerous variably-sized swollen eosinophilic axons (spheroids) within distended myelin sheaths (arrows). The neuropil is furthermore characterized by necrosis, proliferation of microglial cells (microgliosis), and haemorrhages (middle right). No diagnostic inclusion bodies were encountered. PCR analyses proved positive for equine herpesvirus-4 in this particular case. (H&E stain. Bar 200 μm.)

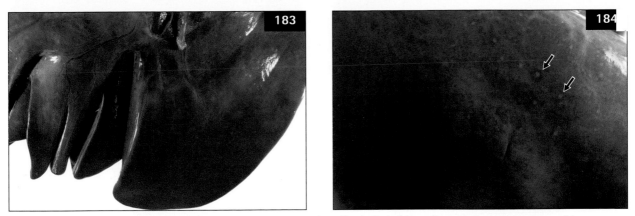

183, 184 Herpesviral multifocal miliary hepatic necrosis. Scattered small pale foci of necrosis and inflammation (arrows) in an aborted foal. Equine herpesvirus-1.

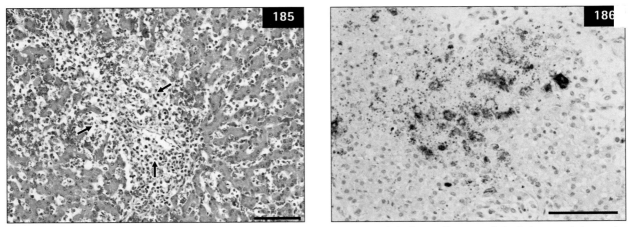

185, 186 Herpesviral acute focal necrosuppurative hepatitis. **185**: A pale eosinophilic focus of hepatocellular lytic necrosis (arrows) with adjacent infiltrated neutrophils (H&E stain.); **186**: micrograph of the same focus stained immunohistochemically for equine herpesvirus-1. The virus-infected cells and debris reveal a strongly positive brown granular staining. (Immunoperoxidase stain for EHV-1. Bars 100 μm.)

187 Herpesviral acute focal necrotizing hepatitis. At the border of necrotic hepatocytes (top right corner) and viable hepatocytes there is a hepatocytic intranuclear eosinophilic viral inclusion body (arrow) consistent with a herpesviral infection. Equine herpesvirus-1. (H&E stain. Bar 20 μm.)

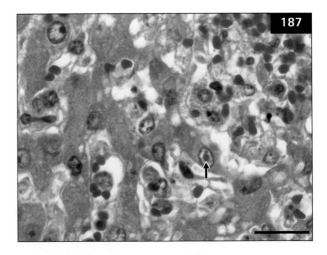

Similar multifocal parenchymal necrosis with intraepithelial viral inclusion bodies may be present in the lungs (bronchointerstitial pneumonia) (188–192) and kidneys (193). In addition, there may be lymphocyte loss (lymphocytolysis) affecting the thymus, resulting in gross shrinkage (that may be obscured by oedema) and in a histological cellular paucity. Viral inclusion bodies may be present within

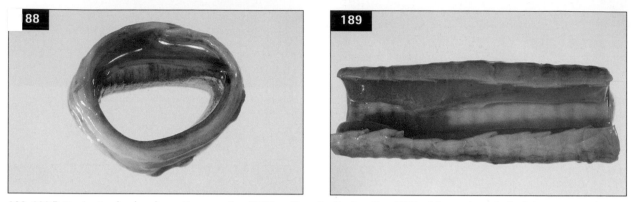

188, 189 Extensive tracheal oedema. Cross-section (**188**) and longitudinal section (**189**) of the trachea of a foal show a severely compromised luminal diameter and subsequent air flow by a gelatinous expansion of the dorsal tracheal lamina propria. Equine herpesvirus-1.

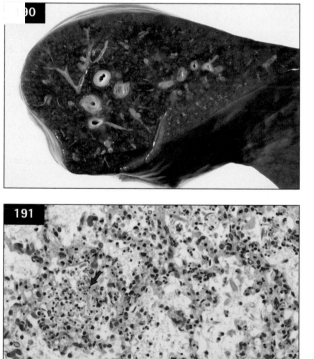

190 Herpesviral multifocal pulmonary necrosis. Both pleural and cut surface of lung parenchyma of a foal show multiple small pale foci of necrosis and inflammation. Note the intrabronchial fibrin casts (arrow). Equine herpesvirus-1.

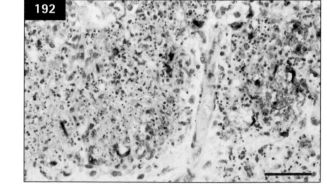

191, 192 Herpesviral multifocal pulmonary necrosis. **191**: Multiple coalescing foci of alveolar necrosis. The necrotic tissues are comprised of eosinophilic cellular debris with irregular condensed basophilic nuclear remnants (karyopycnosis and karyorrhexis indicated by arrow). Equine herpesvirus-1 (H&E stain.); **192**: micrograph of the same location stained immunohistochemically for equine herpesvirus-1. The virus-infected cells and debris reveal a strongly positive brown granular staining. (Immunoperoxidase stain for EHV-1. Bars 50 µm.)

thymic reticular epithelia (**194**). A multifocal necrotizing vasculitis may be present in other organs as well. Occasionally, in adult horses a multifocal haemorrhagic ulcerative necrotizing enterocolitis due to EHV-1 infection is reported (**195, 196**). A consistent finding in aborted fetuses is pulmonary oedema with occasional fibrin casts in the bronchial lumina (**190, 197**) (Jubb *et al* 2007).

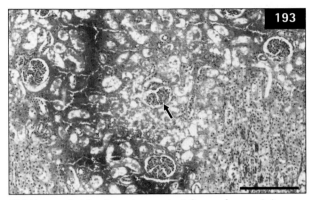

193 Herpesviral focal renal necrosis. A focus of necrosis in the kidney cortex indicated by pale eosinophilia and fading of cellular detail with, in the centre, a glomerular remnant (arrow) and a surrounding zone of haemorrhage. Equine herpesvirus-1. (H&E stain. Bar 200 μm.)

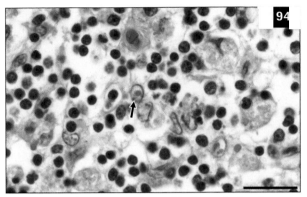

194 Herpesviral necrotizing thymusitis. Sporadic thymic reticular epithelial cells contain an eosinophilic intranuclear herpesviral inclusion body (arrow). Furthermore, this thymus was characterized by extensive necrosis of lymphocytes and subsequent lymphodepletion (not depicted in this micrograph). Equine herpesvirus-1. (H&E stain. Bar 20 μm.)

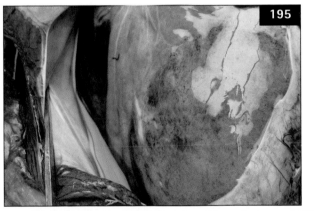

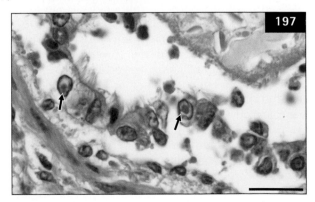

195, 196 Multiple epicardial (**195**) and small intestinal serosal (**196**) petechiae. Equine herpesvirus-1.

197 Herpesviral necrotizing bronchiolitis. Virus-infected epithelial cells are degenerated and sloughed into the bronchiolar lumen. Several of them contain spherical eosinophilic intranuclear herpesviral inclusion bodies (arrows) displacing the basophilic chromatin against the nuclear margins (chromatin margination). Note also the presence of eosinophilic intraluminal keratin squames originating from aspirated amniotic fluid (top right corner). Equine herpesvirus-1. (H&E stain. Bar 20 μm.)

Gross lesions seen in equine multinodular pulmonary fibrosis consisted of multiple nodules of fibrosis throughout the lungs. Histologically, there was marked interstitial fibrosis, often with preservation of an 'alveolar-like' architecture, lined by cuboidal epithelial cells with the airways containing primarily neutrophils and macrophages. Rare macrophages contain large eosinophilic intranuclear viral inclusion bodies (Williams *et al.* 2007). A total of 63% trigeminal ganglia were PCR-positive for the gB gene of EHV-1 and 30% harboured either latent non-neurotropic or neurotropic EHV-1 strains (Pusterla *et al.* 2010).

Management/Treatment

The three key principles for control of spread of EHV-1 are to: 1) subdivide horses into small, epidemiologically isolated closed groups, 2) minimize risks of exogenous and endogenous (stress-induced viral reactivation) introduction of EHV-1, and 3) maximize herd immunity through vaccination (Lunn *et al.* 2009, Goehring *et al.* 2010*a*).

Treatment of diseased horses is supportive. To prevent secondary bacterial infections prophylactic antibiotics can be administered and high fever can be treated palliatively with antipyretics with reference to respiratory disease. In cases of neurological disease patients may need rectum evacuation and bladder catheterization with appropriate measures to prevent cystitis and decubitation. EHV abortion is usually associated with complete expulsion of both fetus and placenta. As a consequence, no therapy is required regarding retentio secundarium (van Maanen 2002).

Oral administration of the antiviral drug valacyclovir to ponies 1 hour before EHV inoculation induced similar clinical signs, viral shedding, and viraemia in treated and control ponies (Croubels 2009). Both an attenuated EHV-1 (Jesset *et al.* 1998) and an inactivated carbomer-adjuvanted EHV-1/4 vaccine (van Maanen 2001) reduced respiratory disease, although the antibody response was low (Holmes *et al.* 2006). In addition, the inactivated carbomer-adjuvanted EHV-1/4 vaccine did provide effective protection against abortion, in spite of failing to reduce frequency or duration of viraemia (Flore *et al.* 1998, Heldens *et al.* 2001). Protection by vaccines against EHV neurological disease has never been demonstrated (van Maanen 2002, Lunn *et al.* 2009). However, vaccinations administered at intervals of 27 and 70 days followed by challenge infection 24 days later significantly reduced clinical disease after challenge with greater reduction in the MLV vaccine group (Goehring *et al.* 2010*b*).

Quarantine of EHV-1 infected horses should be up to 3 weeks post infection to ensure that animals are no longer shedding the agent (Perkins *et al.* 2008) and serial testing with PCR may be a useful adjunct to determine when the risk of transmission has been minimized (Goehring *et al.* 2010*a*).

Public health significance

Not convincing yet.

SUID HERPESVIRUS 1
Family Herpesviridae
Subfamily Alphaherpesvirinae/Genus
Varicellovirus: double-stranded DNA

Definition/Overview
Suid herpesvirus 1, also known as Aujeszky's disease virus (ADV) or pseudorabies virus (PRV) can cause a very rare, fatal, acute neurological disease in horses with signs including excessive sweating, muscle tremors, and periods of mania (Kimman *et al*. 1991).

Aetiology
Suid herpesvirus 1 is a member of the family Herpesviridae of swine, a member of the Alphaherpesvirinae subfamily, and the aetiological agent of Aujeszky's disease, characterized by a double-stranded DNA genome.

Epidemiology
The role of porcine animals in equine Aujeszky's disease remains unclear.

Incubation period
This is 4–7 days as assessed following experimental inoculation into the conjunctiva and nostrils of ponies (van den Ingh *et al*. 1990, Kimman *et al*. 1991).

Clinical presentation
A case in point is that of a 3-year-old gelding admitted because of abnormal behaviour and lack of coordination. Four days earlier, the horse had a high fever that lasted for 2 days, at which point signs of nervousness and blindness appeared. On admission, the horse had muscle tremors and a spastic gait; it stumbled and fell down and had unpredictable fits of mania when struggling to its feet again. Periods of mania alternated with exhaustion, disorientation, and depression, during which the horse was unresponsive to stimuli. Intermittent nystagmus was observed. The pupils of the eyes were dilated. The rectal temperature (37.8°C) was normal and remained so during the following days. Although nonporcine animals susceptible to spontaneous Aujeszky's disease usually die within 48 hours after appearance of the first clinical signs, the horse was sick for 7 days (van den Ingh *et al*. 1990).

In comparison, two ponies developed fever 7 days after inoculation and subsequently started to behave abnormally, showing severe neurological signs on the ninth day after inoculation. One pony became excited and the other was depressed. One pony died on the ninth day after inoculation and the other was euthanized on the tenth day (Kimman *et al*. 1991).

Differential diagnosis
The differential diagnosis predominantly includes various causes of acute neurological disease (see p. 262).

Diagnosis
The diagnosis can be established by immuno-histochemistry, DNA-*in situ* hybridization and serology by means of a virus neutralization test, in a blocking ELISA against the glycoprotein I, in an indirect double sandwich ELISA, and with colloidal gold immunoelectron microscopy (van den Ingh *et al*. 1990). Neutralizing antibodies directed against ADV were detected in the sera of two ponies from day 7 post inoculation on. Serum titres peaked at days 14 and 16 (log10 titres 1.95 and 2.65). However, sera were negative in the gI-ELISA (van den Ingh *et al*. 1990).

Pathology
Post-mortem findings indicated a nonsuppurative meningoencephalitis especially in the grey matter, with neuronal degeneration and gliosis. ADV antigen and ADV DNA were detected in neurons of the cerebrum (van den Ingh *et al*. 1990). CSF analysis revealed 0.62 G/l WBC (normal < 0.005 G/l), consisting of 55% neutrophils and 45% mononuclear cells, indicating severe meningitis (van den Ingh *et al*. 1990).

Management/Treatment
Not appropriate given the fatal outcome.

Public health significance
Not convincing yet.

BOVINE and EQUINE PAPILLOMAVIRUS
Family Papovaviridae
Genus Epsilonpapillomavirus: double-stranded DNA

Definition/Overview
In addition to causing warts in cattle, bovine papillomaviruses 1 and 2 (BPV-1 and BPV-2) are both involved in neoplastic lesions, namely equine sarcoid tumours and urinary bladder tumours in cattle, respectively (Yuan *et al.* 2007). However, the early viral proteins are expressed, but virion is not produced in the equine species (Yuan *et al.* 2007). Equine sarcoids are benign fibroblastic neoplasms which might grow progressively.

Aetiology
BPVs infect cattle and cause papillomas of cutaneous or mucosal epithelium. To date, six types of BPVs have been characterized and classified into three genera. BPV-1 and -2 belong to the genus Delta-papillomavirus (de Villiers *et al.* 2004). Although papillomaviruses are strictly species specific, BPV-1 DNA, and less commonly BPV-2 DNA, is frequently found in fibroblastic skin tumours of equids termed sarcoids, and is believed to be the causative factor of this type of tumour (Lancaster *et al.* 1979). Rolling circle amplification demonstrated that BPV-1 genome exists as a double-stranded, episomal, circular form, whereas BPV-1 E5 open reading frame showed sequence variation in equine sarcoids (Yuan *et al.* 2007). Furthermore, BPV-1 and -2 DNA were present in sarcoid-affected Cape mountain zebras (*Equus zebra zebra*) (van Dyk *et al.* 2009).

Besides equine sarcoid, at least three conditions supposedly induced by papillomavirus have been described in horses, namely classical equine papillomas, genital papillomas, and aural plaques. Novel equine papillomaviruses (EcPVs) in the two latter disorders were detected and designated as EcPV-2 and EcPV-3. As the three EcPVs share less than 60% of nucleotide identities in L1, they may be regarded as belonging to different genera (Lange *et al.* 2011).

Epidemiology
Equine sarcoid is more prevalent in young horses without a gender or breed predilection. Latent EcPV-2 infections have been shown in normal genital (including cervical) and ocular equine mucosa (Vanderstraeten *et al.* 2011).

Pathophysiology
The molecular events leading to equine sarcoids are poorly understood. It is not known how horses become infected by BPV, primarily BPV-1, and equine sarcoid is the only documented natural infection of a heterologous host by a papillomavirus. Infection of horses is believed to be abortive, with BPV DNA establishing itself as a multicopy plasmid and viral genes, including E5, are expressed (Carr *et al.* 2001). The sarcoid appears to be a tumour due not to cell hyperproliferation but to lack of apoptosis, as the markers of cell proliferation (such as cyclins and their respective kinases) are not different from normal skin, whereas the tumour suppressor and promotor of apoptosis p53 is nonfunctional in sarcoids (Nixon *et al.* 2005). It has been hypothesized that peripheral blood mononuclear cells may serve as host cells for BPV-1/-2 DNA and contribute to virus latency (Brandt *et al.* 2008).

Mitochondrial changes seem to be dynamically linked to the healing process and, additionally, may reflect prognosis (Hallamaa 2008). The proposed pathway of BPV infection in the horse comprises a first step of keratinocyte infection, followed by migration of viral material towards the dermis, resulting in infection of subepidermal fibroblasts and their fully transformed phenotype. Co-existence of a dermal BPV-1 and an epidermal BPV-2 infection in the same lesion has been shown, indicating that horses can harbour infection with more than one BPV type at the same time (Bogaert *et al.* 2010).

Incubation period
Not established in the equine species yet.

Clinical presentation
Based on clinical appearance four different types of equine sarcoid are distinguished, namely the fibroblastic type (**198–200**), the verrucose type (**201, 202**), the mixed type, and the occult type. The fibroblastic type might be preceded by either the verrucose or the occult type, especially following repeated trauma. The clinical behaviour of an equine sarcoid could not be explained on the basis of differences in BPV activity (Bogaert *et al.* 2007), although there was a highly significant correlation between intralesional viral load and disease severity (Haralambus *et al.* 2010). The most important sequela of equine sarcoids is their recurrence.

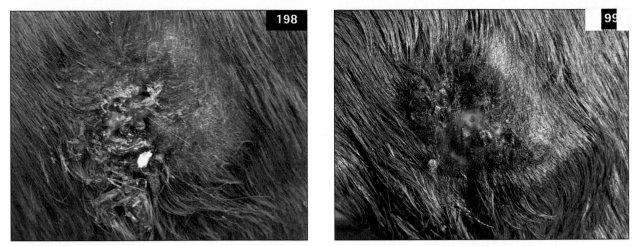

198, 199 Sarcoid (fibroblastic type) in a 16-year-old Warmblood gelding before (**198**) and after (**199**) intralesional administration of BCG.

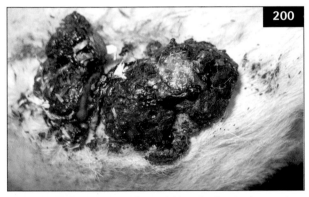

200 This fibroblastic type of sarcoid in a donkey is ulcerated with a serohaemorrhagic exudate. Bovine papillomavirus 1 and 2.

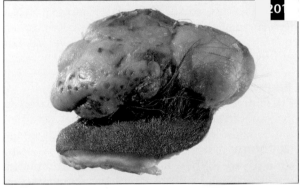

201 Equine sarcoid. Formalin-fixed specimen of a localized firm, pale, alopecic, irregular, exophytic, verrucose neoplastic nodule of haired skin. They are the most frequently diagnosed skin tumours in equines and are commonly found on the face, legs, and trunk, and are associated with sites of skin trauma and bovine papillomavirus infections. Bovine papillomavirus-1 and -2.

202 Sarcoid (verrucose type) in an 8-year-old Quarter Horse mare.

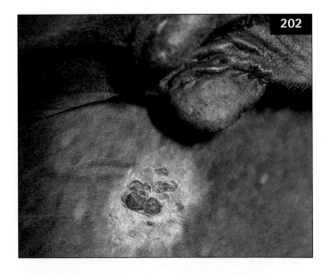

Differential diagnosis

Equine sarcoids should be differentiated from dermatophytosis, papillomatosis (203), chronic dermatitis, and various neoplasms as well as from equine sarcoidosis. Equine sarcoidosis is a rare disorder characterized by granulomatous chronic inflammation of various organs, predominantly skin (204, 205). The disorder resembles human sarcoidosis although the disease in man is predominantly characterized by lung involvement. In comparison, Whipple's disease is a rare multisystem disorder, caused by infection with the bacterium *Tropheryma whipplei* in humans. Whipple's disease should always be considered in the differential diagnosis of human sarcoidosis, particularly when apparent sarcoidosis does not respond to treatment (Dzirlo *et al.* 2007). Diagnostic tests regarding Whipple's disease include staining with periodic acid-Schiff (PAS), electron microscopy, immunohistochemistry, and PCR, which detects species-specific bacterial ribosomal RNA (Relman *et al.* 1992, Marth & Raoult 2003). In the equine species the pathology of *T. whipplei* has not yet been confirmed.

Diagnosis

A definitive diagnosis of equine sarcoids is based on histopathological examination of biopsies.

Pathology

Sarcoids are locally invasive dermal fibroblastic tumours caused by BPVs. Histologically interwoven neoplastic spindle cells with abundant amounts of intercellular collagenous matrix material distort the dermal histological architecture by compression atrophy of epidermal adnexa such as hair follicles and glands. Typically neoplastic cells show an interaction with the overlying hyperplastic epidermis forming long thin rete pegs and perpendicular alignment to the basement membrane. Sarcoids are usually poorly circumscribed and gradually invade locally, generally without distant metastasis. The overlying epidermis may be hyperkeratotic, elevated, and ulcerated with subsequent exudative inflammation (206–210). EcPV-2 DNA was present in equine genital squamous cell carcinoma as well as in other genital lesions and in ocular squamous cell carcinomas (Vanderstraeten *et al.* 2011).

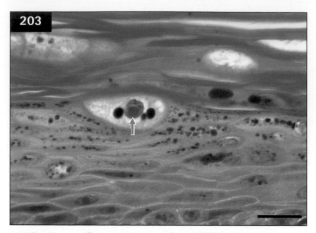

203 Equine papillomatosis. A rare basophilic intranuclear viral inclusion body (arrow) within a keratinocyte of a penile papilloma. Note the hypergranulosis within the adjoining keratinocytes' cytoplasm and the overlying intense eosinophilic hyperkeratosis. (H&E stain. Bar 20 μm.)

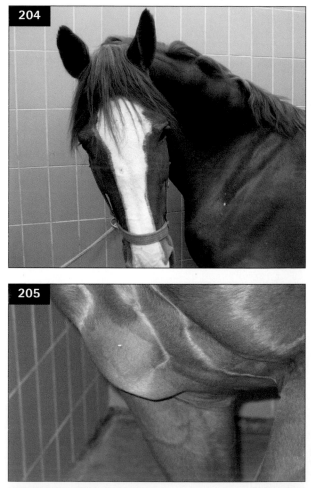

204, 205 The differential diagnosis of equine sarcoids includes multiple firm dermal and subcutaneous nodules in the neck and pectoral region, as seen in generalized sarcoidosis in this 10-year-old Warmblood gelding.

206 Equine sarcoid. Spindle cell skin tumour in which a hypercellular dermal proliferation of neoplastic fibroblasts and an irregular hyperplastic and hyperkeratotic overlying epidermis are present. Typically long, thin, epidermal rete pegs formation is seen (arrows). Bovine papillomavirus-1 and -2. (H&E stain. Bar 200 μm.)

207, 208 Equine sarcoid. The expanding hypercellular neoplastic mass induces compression atrophy of the adnexa, remnants of a sebaceous gland (**207**) and hair follicle (**208**); **208**: close-up micrograph is a long rete peg comprised of a compressed atrophic hair follicle and tumour cells positioned perpendicular to the basement membrane (arrows); this distinctive growth pattern in sarcoids is known as 'picket fencing'. Bovine papillomavirus-1 and -2. (H&E stain. Bar 200 μm.)

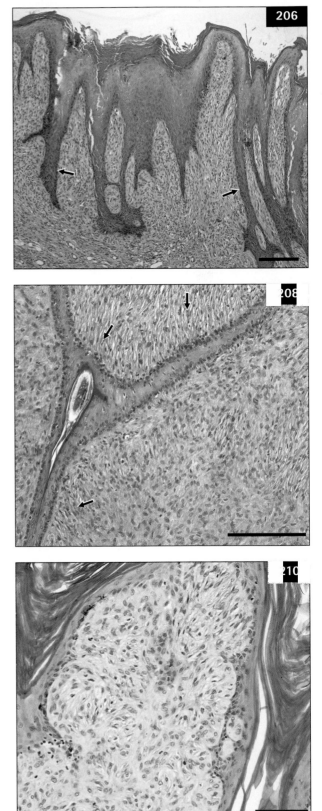

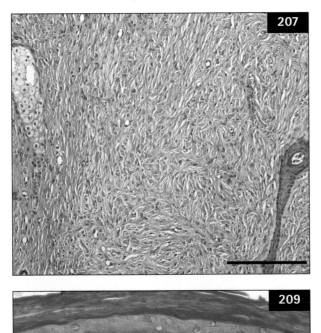

209, 210 Equine sarcoid. Close-up micrograph of the interwoven whirling neoplastic spindle cells, with abundant intercellular collagenous matrix, which show a characteristic interaction with the overlying epidermis, developing small thin weedy rete pegs. Note the extensive eosinophilic superficial orthokeratotic hyperkeratosis. Bovine papillomavirus-1 and -2. (H&E stain. Bars 100 μm.)

Management/Treatment

Treatment options largely depend on sarcoid type and localization and include surgical excision, cryotherapy, intralesional administration of bacillus Calmette–Guérin (BCG), and the use of radioactive implants. Of interest, small interfering RNA treatment of sarcoids might be feasible clinically in future (Gobeil *et al.* 2009).

The occurrence of active granulomata has been reported as a side-effect following intralesional administration of BCG (van den Boom *et al.* 2008).

Public health significance

Not convincing yet regarding equine sarcoids. In addition, EcPV-2 is not related to high-risk human papillomaviruses causing cervical cancer (Vanderstraeten *et al.* 2011).

HORSEPOX VIRUS

Family Poxviridae
Subfamily Chordopoxvirinae/Genus Orthopoxvirus: linear double-stranded DNA

Definition/Overview

A slow, mild, self-limiting progressive skin disease is caused by horsepox virus. Horsepox is differentiated clinically from two other poxviral diseases of horses, equine molluscum contagiosum and Uasin Gishu disease. Other orthopoxviruses (OPVs), as being similar to vaccinia virus (VACV), are zoonotic and significant for human health, including monkeypox virus (MPXV) and cowpox virus (CPXV) (Tulman *et al.* 2006).

Aetiology

The genus Orthopoxvirus includes members of the family Poxviridae, including human variola virus, the aetiological agent of smallpox, and vaccinia virus. Phylogenetic analysis of the conserved region has indicated that horsepox virus is closely related to sequenced isolates of vaccinia virus and rabbitpox virus, clearly grouping together these vaccinia virus-like viruses (Tulman *et al.* 2006).

Epidemiology

Although common before the 20th century, horsepox is rare today to the point of being considered extinct (Tulman *et al.* 2006).

Pathophysiology

Post translational polypeptide tagging by conjugation with ubiquitin and ubiquitin-like (Ub/Ubl) molecules is a potent way to alter protein functions and/or sort specific protein targets to the proteasome for degradation. Many poxviruses interfere with the host Ub/Ubl system by encoding viral proteins that can usurp this pathway (Zhang *et al.* 2009).

Incubation period

Not established in the equine species yet.

Clinical presentation

Multiple clinical forms of horsepox have been described, including a benign, localized form involving lesions in the muzzle (**211**) and buccal cavity known previously as contagious pustular stomatitis and a generalized, highly contagious form known as equine papular dermatitis. Horsepox has also been associated with an exudative dermatitis of the pasterns described as 'grease' or grease heel, a clinical syndrome also associated with other infectious and environmental agents (Tulman *et al.* 2006).

CPXV infection associated with a streptococcal septicaemia was diagnosed in a weak German Warmblood filly, born 29 days prematurely, and humanely destroyed on the sixth day of life. At necropsy, ulcerative lesions in the alimentary tract, colitis, polyarthritis, and nephritis were observed. Transmission electron microscopical examination of specimens from ulcerative lesions revealed typical OPV virions. CPXV was unequivocally identified by virological and molecular biological methods (Ellenberger *et al.* 2005).

Differential diagnosis

The differential diagnosis includes equine molluscum contagiosum (**212–214**), Uasin Gishu disease (Tulman *et al.* 2006), immune-mediated disorders, and vesicular stomatitis virus infection. Uasin Gishu

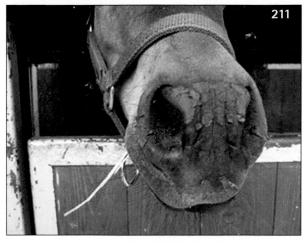

211 Horsepox is a slow, mild, self-limiting progressive skin disease caused by horsepox virus. Multiple clinical forms of horsepox have been described including a benign, localized form involving lesions in the muzzle. (Courtesy of Dr D. Kersten.)

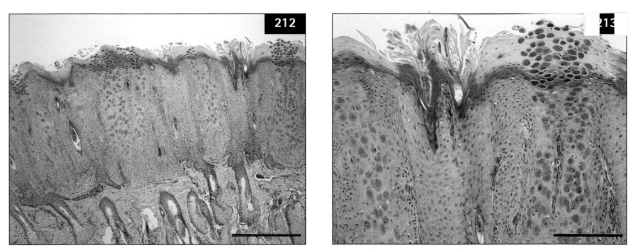

212, 213 Molluscum contagiosum. Marked epidermal hyperplasia and hyperkeratosis, usually without dermal inflammatory infiltrates. The epidermis is thickened and contains abundant large intracytoplasmic basophilic viral inclusion bodies or molluscum bodies. Molluscipoxvirus, equine molluscum contagiosum virus. (H&E stain. Bars 500/200 μm, respectively.)

214 Molluscum contagiosum. Close-up micrograph of the epidermal intracytoplasmic molluscum bodies which displace and compress the keratinocyte nucleus to the cell margins. The viral inclusion bodies exhibit an increase in condensation and basophilia upwards in the stratum corneum, where they are intensely purple. Molluscipoxvirus, equine molluscum contagiosum virus. (H&E stain. Bar 50 μm.)

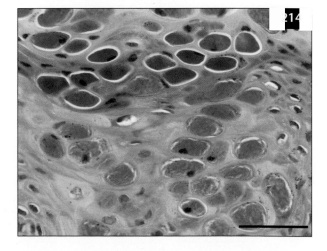

disease has been described in nonindigenous horses of eastern Africa and is associated with a poorly characterized OPV. However, generalized skin lesions are proliferative and papillomatous and the disease may be chronic in nature (Thompson *et al.* 1998, Tulman *et al.* 2006). Equine molluscum contagiosum is a mild, self-limiting cutaneous disease similar to the human disease and is associated with a virus similar to molluscum contagiosum virus. Lesions are usually seen on the chest, shoulders, medial and lateral aspects of the fore- and hindlimbs, the face, fetlocks, pasterns, on the lateral surfaces of the body, and genitalia, associated with marked scrotal oedema. The lesions vary from 4 to 20 mm in diameter, are hairless but covered by soft keratin projections which, when removed, leave a raw elevated base tightly adherent to the epidermis. These lesions bled profusely when the animals were groomed. Older lesions were well circumscribed, raised above the surface, devoid of hair, and after removal of grey-white keratin flakes had a depigmented waxy appearance (Lange *et al.* 1991, Rensburg *et al.* 1991).

Diagnosis

Electron microscopical examination might reveal the presence of typical pox virions in affected epidermal cells (Kaminjolo *et al.* 1974).

Pathology

Macroscopic lesions in the muzzle and buccal cavity are multiple and ulcerative to typical pocks. In papular dermatitis firm papules 5 mm in diameter become crusted and leave alopecic spots (Jubb *et al.* 2007). Histology characteristically exhibits both hyperplastic and degenerative to necrotizing epithelial lesions. Mixed inflammatory dermal infiltrates may vary. Pathognomonic are the large round to ovoid intraepithelial cytoplasmic inclusion bodies containing pox virions.

Management/Treatment

Not appropriate as a self-limiting skin disease, although treatment of diseased horses might be supportive.

Public health significance

Horsepox virus has no public health significance. In comparison, molluscum contagiosum occurs in 2–8% of children. This infection is among the most common viral skin infections in children. The lesions will resolve spontaneously by puberty (Scheinfeld 2007). No single intervention has been shown to be convincingly effective in treating human molluscum contagiosum (van der Wouden *et al.* 2006).

WEST NILE VIRUS/KUNJIN VIRUS

Order Mononegavirales
Family Flaviviridae/Genus Flavivirus/Japanese encephalitis virus group: linear, positive-sense, single-stranded RNA

Definition/Overview

Encephalomyelitis in an extremely broad vertebrate host range is caused by West Nile virus (WNV), which is widely distributed in South Africa (Venter & Swanepoel 2010) and identified as emerging in Europe (Vorou *et al.* 2007). Since its introduction to the western hemisphere in 1999, WNV had spread across North America, Central and South America and the Caribbean, although the vast majority of severe human cases have occurred in the USA and Canada (Murray *et al.* 2010). WNV is transmitted to susceptible mammals by mosquito vectors primarily from the genus *Culex*. It has important public health significance and is a reportable disease.

Aetiology

WNV is a member of the genus Flavivirus, family Flaviviridae, and has an extremely broad vertebrate host range. Infection of common species of birds has defined those with high *vs.* low potential to serve as amplifying hosts for the virus. In general, mammals (primates, horses, companion animals) are dead-end hosts for WNV, although some circumstances (e.g. immunosuppression) may allow individuals to become capable of transmitting the virus to mosquitoes. Some mammals (rodents, rabbits, squirrels) and reptiles (alligators) have been found to develop a viraemia of sufficient magnitude to predict at least low competence for infecting feeding mosquitoes (Bowen & Nemeth 2007). Lineage two of WNV may be significantly underestimated as a cause of neurological disease in man and animals in South Africa (Venter & Swanepoel 2010).

Epidemiology

WNV has been isolated from a range of mosquito species, primarily from the genus *Culex* (Ward *et al.* 2004). Some birds may be important reservoirs of WNV or amplifying hosts, because viraemia in birds may reach sufficient levels to infect feeding mosquitoes (Hubálek & Halouzka 1999). Furthermore, trans-Saharan migrant bird species had both higher prevalences and antibody titres than resident and short-distance migrants (López *et al.* 2008). In contrast, viraemia in naturally and experimentally infected equids is transient and at a low level (Schmidt & El Mansoury 1963). It is highly unlikely that a horse infected with WNV would transmit the virus to humans or other species in typical circumstances (Snook *et al.* 2001, Bunning *et al.* 2002).

During outbreaks, seroprevalence in horses without clinical signs of encephalomyelitis can reach 8% (Cantile *et al.* 2000, Trock *et al.* 2001). On the other hand, in one study, the proportion of equids serologically positive for natural exposure to WNV was 64% (Epp *et al.* 2007). WNV was first detected in the USA in 1999 (Trock *et al.* 2001), whereas human and equine WNV infections have recently been described in France and Portugal (Zeller & Schuffenecker 2004, Vorou *et al.* 2007) and in northeastern Italy (Barzon *et al.* 2009, Monaco *et al.* 2010). During late summer and autumn 2000, a West Nile fever outbreak in southern France resulted in 76 equine clinical cases, of which 21 horses died. It has been suggested that WNV is not endemic in the affected Camargue area, as sporadic outbreaks are separated by long silent periods (Durand *et al.* 2002). Simulated incidences are mainly determined by host and vector population dynamics, virus transmission, and herd immunity (Laperriere *et al.* 2011).

Pathophysiology

Infection of primary human brain microvascular endothelial cells can facilitate entry of cell-free virus into the CNS without disturbing the blood–brain barrier, and increased cell adhesion molecules may assist in the trafficking of WNV-infected immune cells into the CNS, via a 'Trojan horse' mechanism, thereby contributing to WNV dissemination in the CNS and associated pathology (Verma *et al.* 2009).

Virtually all of the associated OAS1 polymorphisms were located within the interferon-inducible promoter, suggesting that differences in OAS1 gene expression may determine the host's ability to resist clinical manifestations associated with WNV infection (Rios *et al.* 2010).

Incubation period

Experimental infections of horses with WNV by subcutaneous inoculation or mosquito feeding has only rarely resulted in overt clinical disease (Davis *et al.* 2001, Minke *et al.* 2004, Bowen & Nemeth 2007). Only one horse (a 13-year-old mare) out of 12 showed neurological signs, beginning 8 days after infection and progressing to severe clinical disease within 24 hours (Bunning *et al.* 2002).

Clinical presentation

The most common clinical signs are ataxia, hindlimb paresis, and muscle tremors and fasciculations, whereas fever is not commonly detected (**215**) (Trock *et al.* 2001). The case fatality rate in horses with clinical disease may exceed 23–30% (Porter *et al.* 2003, Ward *et al.* 2004), although infection of horses with WNV usually does not result in the development of clinical signs (Trock *et al.* 2001). Nielsen *et al.* found that the annual incidence of clinical and subclinical WNV infection in nonvaccinated horses was 16%, with an apparent to inapparent ratio of 1:4 among infected horses (Nielsen *et al.* 2008).

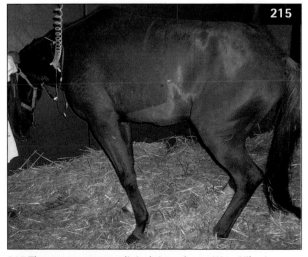

215 The most common clinical signs due to West Nile virus are ataxia, hindlimb paresis, and muscle tremors and fasciculations, whereas fever is not commonly detected. Treatment of diseased horses is supportive. Vaccination is an effective, practical method of prevention of clinical disease. (Courtesy of Dr M. Aleman, University of California, Davis, USA.)

Differential diagnosis

The differential diagnosis predominantly includes various causes of acute neurological disease (see p. 262).

Diagnosis

The tentative diagnosis is supported by positive results of serological tests such as the virus neutralization test or IgM antibody capture ([MAC]-ELISA) (Ostlund *et al.* 2001, Trock *et al.* 2001). Neutralization antibody titres ≥1:10 were detected between days 7 and 11 post infection (Bunning *et al.* 2002). Case confirmation requires virus isolation or a fourfold or greater increase in titre of the plaque reduction neutralization test (PRNT). In addition, detection of both IgM anti-WNV antibody and an increased titre (≥1:10) in the PRNT in a single serum sample may be used. The presence of clinical signs and positive results of MAC-ELISA in a single serum sample are sufficient criteria to suspect a probable case of encephalomyelitis caused by WNV (Ostlund *et al.* 2001). The induction of antibodies to the WN19 epitope during WNV infection of horses is generally associated with E protein glycosylation of the infecting viral strain (Hobson-Peters *et al.* 2008). It should be realized that diagnosis of WNV infection in Japanese encephalitis virus (JEV)-immunized horses requires serological tests for NtAb and IgM titres to both WNV and JEV (Shirafuji *et al.* 2009).

Pathology

Gross lesions may be present and consist of spinal cord malacia and haemorrhage. Histological lesions of a nonsuppurative encephalomyelitis mostly affect the brainstem and spinal cord grey matter; they consist of thin lymphoplasmacytic cuffs, glial nodules, and occasional neuronal degeneration. Axonal distension with formation of spheroids is seen (Jubb *et al.* 2007).

Management/Treatment

Treatment of diseased horses is supportive. Vaccination is an effective, practical method of prevention of clinical disease (Davis *et al.* 2001, Minke *et al.* 2004, Bowen & Nemeth 2007). Nonvaccinated equids were 23 times more likely to develop clinical disease than those vaccinated (Epp *et al.* 2007). The estimate of vaccine efficacy in a field study was 96% (Epp *et al.* 2007). WNV vaccination with an inactivated product with a series of three vaccines at 3-week intervals effectively induced an antigen-specific antibody response, as well as CD4+ and CD8+ lymphocyte activation (Davis *et al.* 2008). WNV vaccine-induced NS1 antibodies were detected by blocking ELISA and a complement-dependent cytotoxicity (CDC) assay and affected the ability of these assays to differentiate WNV from JEV infections (Kitai *et al.* 2011). Furthermore, it is of importance to decrease exposure of horses to infected mosquitoes.

Public health significance

WNV has important public health significance and is a reportable disease. Persistent movement disorders, cognitive complaints, and functional disability may occur after WNV neuroinvasive disease. WNV poliomyelitis may result in limb weakness and ongoing morbidity that is likely to be long term. Although further assessment is needed, the long-term neurological and functional sequelae of WNV infection are likely to represent a considerable source of morbidity in human patients long after their recovery from acute illness (Sejvar 2007).

Corvids can be a sensitive indicator for WNV prevalence and are a component of many WNV surveillance program. An improved sampling procedure using a bilateral intraocular cocktail has been developed for testing corvid carcasses for WNV. This new procedure is substantially faster than harvesting internal organs, requires less specialized equipment and training, and yields excellent diagnostic sensitivity (Lim *et al.* 2009).

Kunjin virus (KUN) is a flavivirus also within the Japanese encephalitis antigenic complex that was first isolated from *Culex annulirostris* mosquitoes captured in northern Australia in 1960. It is the aetiological agent of a human disease characterized by febrile illness with a rash or mild encephalitis and, occasionally, of a neurological disease in horses. It has been designated as a subtype of WNV. KUN shares a similar epidemiology and ecology with the closely related Murray Valley encephalitis virus, the major causative agent of arboviral (arthropod-borne) encephalitis in Australia (Hall *et al.* 2001).

JAPANESE ENCEPHALITIS VIRUS/MURRAY VALLEY ENCEPHALITIS VIRUS

Order Mononegavirales
Family Flaviviridae/Genus Flavivirus/Japanese encephalitis virus group: linear, positive-sense, single-stranded RNA

Definition/Overview

An acute, rapidly progressive, fatal neurological disease of horses and humans is caused by Japanese encephalitis virus (JEV) or Murray Valley encephalitis virus (MVE). Horses are considered to be dead-end hosts for JEV (Lam *et al.* 2005) and MVE (Kay *et al.* 1987).

Aetiology

Flaviviruses are among the most important emerging viruses known to man. Most are arboviruses (arthropod-borne), being transmitted by mosquitoes or ticks. They derived from a common ancestor 10,000–20,000 years ago and are evolving rapidly to fill new ecological niches. JEV is numerically the most important cause of epidemic encephalitis; its geographical area is expanding despite the availability of vaccines. JEV comprises five genotypes. Other mosquito-borne neurotropic flaviviruses with clinical and epidemiological similarities are found across the globe. These include St Louis encephalitis virus and WNV, which recently reached the Americas for the first time (Solomon & Mallewa 2001). KUN shares a similar epidemiology and ecology with the closely related MVE (Hall *et al.* 2001). JEV from an equine case was classified into genotype I by nucleotide sequence analysis of the viral envelope gene (Yamanaka *et al.* 2006).

Epidemiology

WNV is now distributed worldwide, except in most areas of Asia, where JEV is distributed (Kitai *et al.* 2007). Seroprevalence against JEV was 50% for Thoroughbred horses tested in Korea (Yang *et al.* 2008) and 50% in horses in Nepal (Pant *et al.* 2006). The natural infection rate in epizootic seasons, which was determined by a significant increase in NS1 antibody level, was 4–27% in Ibaraki and 0–41.7% in Shiga, indicating that high levels of JEV activity still exist in central Japan (Konishi *et al.* 2006). Horses are unlikely to be efficient amplifiers of MVE virus and do little to incriminate it as an important pathogen (Kay *et al.* 1987). Remarkably, the circulation of Usutu virus (USUV), a flavivirus also of the JEV complex, has been demonstrated in northeastern Italy (Lelli *et al.* 2008).

Pathophysiology

Following replication at the site of infection and haematogenous spread it may cross the blood–brain barrier causing encephalitis. Mortality most probably results from a combination of CNS pathology and systemic inflammatory and stress responses (Hayasaka *et al.* 2009).

Incubation period

Horses inoculated with MVE either by intravenous injection or by the bite of *Culex annulirostris* or *Aedes vigilax* orally-infected mosquitoes, induced circulation of trace amounts of MVE virus for 1–5 days postinoculation, with some horses developing mild pyrexia and transient clinical signs (Kay *et al.* 1987).

Clinical presentation

In equines, JEV/MVE causes a spectrum of disease ranging from subclinical to acute (lethal) encephalitis. Following recovery, residual neurological signs are sometimes seen as sequelae. It should be realized that Japanese encephalitis has been reported in a horse that had been vaccinated against Japanese encephalitis, suggesting the possibility that the horse might have been infected with a recombinant between genotype I and genotype II viruses (Lam *et al.* 2005).

Following inoculation with MVE in one study, most horses remained normal, although some developed mild pyrexia and transient clinical signs (Kay *et al.* 1987).

Differential diagnosis

The differential diagnosis predominantly includes various causes of acute neurological disease (see p. 262).

Diagnosis

No pathognomonic clinical signs distinguish JEV from MVE infection. Definitive diagnosis of the disease requires serology and/or virus isolation from blood and CSF. An ELISA to detect antibodies to JEV nonstructural 1 (NS1) protein is available and is able to detect subclinical natural infections in vaccinated equine populations (Konishi *et al.* 2004). In addition, an epitope-blocking ELISA has been described able to differentiate WNV from JEV infections in equine sera (Kitai *et al.* 2007). However, in serosurveillance of WNV, JEV-vaccinated horses can produce false-positive results in WNV IgG-ELISA, haemagglutination inhibition (HI) and PRNT (Hirota *et al.* 2010).

Pathology

Microscopically a nonsuppurative encephalitis of the cerebral hemispheres is characterized by marked perivascular lymphoplasmacytic cuffing, gliosis, and malacia (Jubb *et al.* 2007).

Management/Treatment

A single intramuscular immunization of a DNA recombinant plasmid vector vaccine of JEV protected horses from virus challenge (Chang *et al.* 2001), and the risk of JEV death was lowered and the symptomatic period of survivors shortened with inactivated JEV vaccination (Satou & Nishiura 2007).

Public health significance

JEV is estimated to cause 30,000–50,000 cases of encephalitis every year predominantly in rural Asia, associated with thalamic lesions seen on computed tomography (CT) and/or magnetic resonance imaging (MRI) (Dung *et al.* 2009). MVE is the major causative agent of arboviral encephalitis in Australia (Hall *et al.* 2001).

EQUINE ARTERITIS VIRUS

Order Nidovirales
Family Arteriviridae/Genus Arterivirus: linear positive-sense, single-stranded RNA

Definition/Overview

Equine arteritis virus (EAV) can cause panvasculitis, inducing oedema, haemorrhage, and abortion (Doll *et al.* 1957a, Doll *et al.* 1957b, Jones *et al.* 1957). The virus neutralization test is considered the gold standard serological screening test for the detection of antibodies to EAV (Duthie *et al.* 2008). Case confirmation requires virus isolation from nasopharyngeal and conjunctival swabs, blood, urine (**216**), semen, or placental and fetal fluids. Mares and geldings eliminate the virus within 60 days, but 30–60% of acutely infected stallions will become persistently infected. Identification of carrier stallions is crucial to control the dissemination of EAV (Glaser *et al.* 1997, Pronost *et al.* 2010).

Aetiology

EAV is caused by an enveloped, spherical, positive-stranded RNA virus with a diameter of 50–70 nm. The virus is a nonarthropod-borne virus classified as a member of the order Nidovirales, including also the bigeneric family Coronaviridae, within the family Arteriviridae. As a consequence, EAV is similar to coronaviruses (Cavanagh *et al.* 1994). Genetic diversity with reference to EAV is recognized among field isolates (Belak *et al.* 1999).

Epidemiology

Serological investigations indicate that EAV has a worldwide distribution and that its prevalence is increasing (Glaser *et al.* 1997). Affected stallions may become long-term carriers and may shed EAV in their semen. In one study, 27% of seropositive stallions were identified as presumptive shedders of EAV in semen (Newton *et al.* 1999). As a consequence, stallions shedding EAV in their semen serve as a reservoir for the virus within the equine population, which has resulted in restrictions for international transport of horses and semen (Timoney *et al.* 1987). The carrier stallion can be a source of genetic diversity of EAV, and outbreaks of EAV can be initiated by the horizontal aerosol transmission of specific viral variants that occur in the semen of particular carrier stallions (Balasuriya *et al.* 1999, Zhang *et al.* 2010). EAV can also be associated with epidemic abortion (Timoney & McCollum 1993).

Pathophysiology

The vascular system is the principal, but not the only target. Following colonization of macrophages, the virus spreads systemically using circulating monocytes and enters the endothelium and tunica media of blood vessels, histiocytes, and dendrite-like cells. Eventually, the virus multiplies within renal tubular cells (Del Piero 2000). Data indicate that EAV-induced, macrophage-derived cytokines may contribute to the pathogenesis of EAV in horses, and that the magnitude of the cytokine response of equine endothelial cells and macrophages to EAV infection reflects the virulence of the infecting virus strain (Moore *et al.* 2003). It has been stated that testosterone plays an essential role in the establishment and maintenance of the carrier state (McCollum *et al.* 1994). On the other hand, EAV is sensitive to inhibition by recombinant equine interferon-gamma (Sentsui *et al.* 2010).

Incubation period

Geldings were febrile for varying periods from 2 to 10 days after intranasal inoculation. Viraemia occurred from day 2 onwards, for periods varying from 9 to at least 19 days. Nasal shedding of virus began 2–4 days after inoculation and persisted for 7–14 days (McCollum *et al.* 1994).

Clinical presentation

Clinical signs may be absent or may include pyrexia, depression, anorexia, limb oedema, stiffness of gait, rhinorrhoea and epiphora, conjunctivitis, and rhinitis. Oedema of the periorbital and supraorbital areas, midventral regions, scrotum, prepuce (**217–220**), and

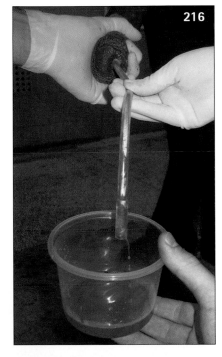

216 EAV virus can be demonstrated in urine following virus multiplication within renal tubular cells.

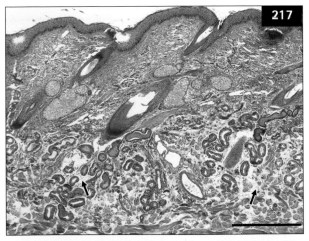

217 Chronic perivascular lymphocytic dermatitis and vasculitis with oedema. Haired skin of the prepuce which shows oedema of the mid-dermis (arrows) and perivascular lymphocytic infiltrates in the deep dermis consistent with equine arteritis virus infection. (H&E stain. Bar 500 μm.)

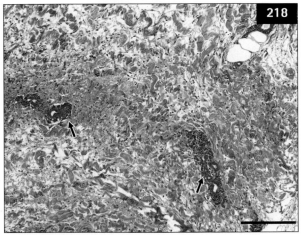

218 Perivascular lymphocytic dermatitis and vasculitis with oedema of the prepuce. Multifocal perivascular accumulations of lymphocytes within the deep dermis (arrows); lesions consistent with equine arteritis virus infection. (H&E stain. Bar 500 μm.)

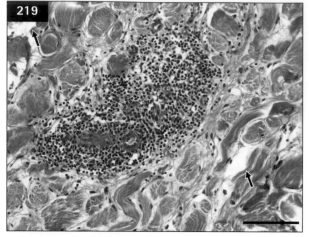

219 Perivascular lymphocytic dermatitis and vasculitis with oedema of the prepuce. Extensive perivascular lymphocytic infiltrate within the deep dermis accompanied by interstitial oedema (arrows) consistent with equine arteritis virus infection. (H&E stain. Bar 100 μm.)

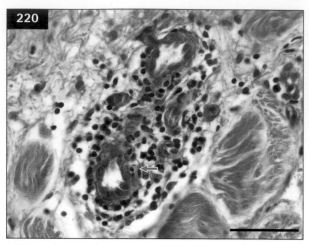

220 Lymphocytic dermatitis and vasculitis of the prepuce. Higher magnification of deep dermal arterioles lined by swollen endothelial cells and cuffing with lymphocytes, few lymphocytes infiltrate the vessel walls (arrow). Note the paleness, indicative of oedema, of the surrounding interstitium with distension of the dermal collagen fibres. Lesions consistent with equine arteritis virus infection. (H&E stain. Bar 50 μm.)

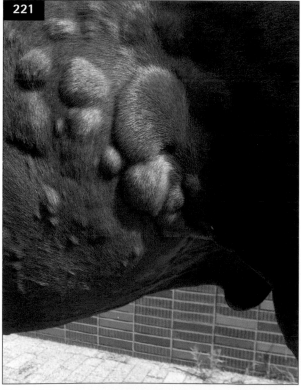

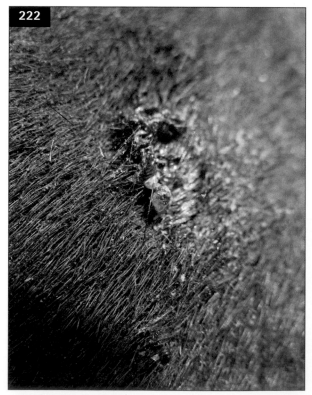

221, 222 Clinical signs may include urticarial rash (**221**) with serum oozing from the skin (**222**).

mammary gland, urticarial rash (**221, 222**), and abortion also occur. Less frequently, severe respiratory distress, ataxia, mucosal papular eruptions, submaxillary lymphadenopathy, and intermandibular and shoulder oedema may be observed (Doll *et al.* 1957*a*, Doll *et al.* 1957*b*, Timoney & McCollum 1993, Del Piero 2000). EAV is occasionally fatal in adult horses and more frequently fatal in foals (Vaala *et al.* 1992, Timoney & McCollum 1993, Wilkins *et al.* 1995).

Differential diagnosis

Differential diagnoses includes EHV, equine adenovirus, influenza, equine infectious anaemia, African horse sickness (AHS), Hendra disease, Getah virus of the alphavirus subgroup of the Togaviridae, purpura haemorrhagica, and the toxic plant hoary alyssum (*Berteroa incana*) (Del Piero 2000).

Diagnosis

The diagnosis of EAV is based on demonstration of lesions and the aetiological agent and/or seroconversion. The detection of seroconversion with complement-dependent virus neutralization performed using the Bucyrus strain in EAV-infected animals is a reliable method for identifying EAV infection in horses. Geldings seroconverted to EAV by day 11, with serum neutralization titres ranging from 8 to 64. The titres ranged from 8 to 32 after 4 weeks (McCollum *et al.* 1994). Post suckle testing may be invalid because of passive transfer of maternal immunity in seroconverted mares.

Tissue culture cell lines generally used to isolate EAV are RK-13 cells, Vero cells, and equine lung cells (Timoney & McCollum 1993, Del Piero 2000). In addition, reverse transcription (RT-)PCR has been used to detect EAV antigen (Del Piero 2000).

Pathology

EAV has a variable presentation, including interstitial pneumonia, panvasculitis (inflamed veins, lymphatics, and arteries) with oedema, thrombosis (lungs and intestines) and haemorrhage, lymphonodular lymphoid necrosis, renal tubular necrosis, abortion, and inflammation of male accessory genital glands. Microscopic lesions consist of arterial fibrinoid necrosis and mainly lymphocytic mural and perivascular infiltrates with or without thrombosis and perivascular interstitial oedema. Infarctions and necrosis may be present in the large intestine and adrenals. EAV antigen can be demonstrated within the cytoplasm of epithelial cells such as alveolar pneumocytes, enterocytes, adrenal cortical cells, trophoblasts, thymus stroma, renal tubular cells, and male accessory genital gland cells. It can also be demonstrated within endothelia, in vascular, myometrial, and cardiac myocytes, macrophages, dendrite-like cells of lymphoid organs, and chorionic mesenchymal stromal cells. Lesions are uncommon in the aborted fetus. If present, they are mild and EAV antigen is frequently not detectable within fetal tissues and placenta. At day 10 post-infection, the most severe damage occurs to blood vessels associated with abortion (Del Piero 2000).

Low concentrations of EAV were detected in the kidney and blood of one gelding killed 30 days after inoculation and in the blood of another killed after 57 days (McCollum *et al.* 1994). Infective EAV is no longer detectable in most tissues 28 days after experimental infection, except in the reproductive tracts of some stallions (Fukunaga *et al.* 1981, Neu *et al.* 1987, McCollum *et al.* 1994, Fukunaga *et al.* 1997).

Management/Treatment

As affected stallions may become long-term carriers, preference should be given to semen from stallions that are seronegative for EAV or that have been shown not to shed virus in their semen. Both inactivated and attenuated virus vaccines are available (Fukunaga *et al.* 1997, Glaser *et al.* 1997). However, vaccination will complicate EAV monitoring, whereas it does not prevent virus shedding via semen. EAV infection is readily prevented through serological and virological screening of horses, coupled with sound management practices that include appropriate quarantine and strategic vaccination (MacLachlan & Balasuriya 2006).

Public health significance

Not convincing yet.

EQUINE INFLUENZA VIRUS
Family Orthomyxoviridae
Genus Influenza A: linear negative-sense, single-stranded RNA

Definition/Overview
An economically important, severe, self-limiting respiratory infection is caused by equine influenza virus. When horses return to training too soon, sequelae such as myocarditis and chronic obstructive pulmonary disease may occur following influenza infection. Vaccination strategies are the core of preventive management of the disease. However, a widespread outbreak of equine influenza in the UK during 2003 in vaccinated Thoroughbred racehorses challenged the current dogma on vaccine strain selection. Furthermore, several new developments in the first decade of the 21st century, including transmission to and establishment in dogs, a presumed influenza-associated encephalopathy in horses, and an outbreak of equine influenza in Australia, serve as a reminder of the unpredictable nature of influenza viruses (Daly et al. 2010).

Aetiology
Equine influenza virus belongs to the family Orthomyxoviridae comprising enveloped, single-stranded, negative-sense RNA viruses, genus Influenzavirus A and B, species influenza A virus. Some influenza A viruses cause disease in species of veterinary importance, whereas influenza B and C viruses are restricted to humans. Two clusters of glycoproteins project from the envelope: the rod-shaped haemagglutinin (H) and the mushroom-shaped neuraminidase (N). Only the subtypes H7N7 and H3N8 have been reported in equines, although the former has not been isolated since 1979. The H3N8 isolate was originally designated influenza A/equine/2/Miami/63, whereas the H7N7 isolate was originally designated influenza A/equine/1/Prague/56 (van Maanen & Cullinane 2002). The phylogenetic diversity of type A influenza viruses has been published based on the viral external HA and NA gene sequences and their six internal genes (PB2, PB1, PA, NP, MP, and NS) with all the influenza A viruses isolated from human, horses, pigs, or birds showing more or less time difference. The time difference among human and equine influenza viruses was more obvious than that of swine influenza viruses, i.e. some swine influenza viruses were similar to each other, even though they were isolated in different time periods (Chen et al. 2009).

Epidemiology
Although aerosols are considered most important in transmission of equine influenza, personnel and contaminated transport vehicles can contribute to a rapid and wide distribution as well (Mumford 1990, van Maanen & Cullinane 2002), whereas avian fomite transmission cannot be excluded (Spokes et al. 2009). Equine influenza virus is still transmitted by subclinically-infected vaccinated horses (Mumford 1990, van Maanen & Cullinane 2002). Since 1963, antigenetic drift of equine H3N8 viruses has developed along a single lineage with a rate of 0.8 amino acid substitutions per year, regularly compromising vaccine efficacy (Daly et al. 1996).

Influenza virus, subtype H3N8, was transmitted from horses to greyhound dogs in 2004 and subsequently spread to pet dog populations. The co-circulation of H3N8 viruses in dogs and horses makes bidirectional virus transmission between these animal species possible. Analysis of a limited number of equine influenza viruses suggests substantial separation in the transmission of viruses causing clinically apparent influenza in dogs and horses (Rivailler et al. 2010).

Pathophysiology
The virus spreads through the respiratory tract within 1–3 days, causing desquamation and denudation of respiratory epithelial cells, and clumping of cilia. Impairment of clearance mechanisms can be profound, resulting in significantly reduced tracheal clearance rates for up to 32 days after infection (Willoughby et al. 1992). Regeneration of the respiratory epithelium takes at least 3 weeks (van Maanen & Cullinane 2002).

Incubation period
Equine influenza virus is contracted by inhalation and is extremely contagious. The short incubation period (1–5 days) and the persistent coughing that characterizes influenza in horses, contribute to the rapid spread of the disease (van Maanen & Cullinane 2002).

Clinical presentation

Equine influenza virus can cause a severe, self-limiting respiratory infection characterized by a distinctive harsh cough, serous nasal discharge (**223**), pyrexia, tachycardia, hyperaemia of nasal and conjunctival mucosae, limb oedema (**224**), and muscle soreness and stiffness. Prolonged fever and mucopurulent nasal discharge (**225**) indicate secondary bacterial infection. Pregnant mares may abort or resorb the fetus as a result of fever. Young susceptible foals may develop a rapidly fatal pneumonia and donkeys are more susceptible to influenza than horses (van Maanen & Cullinane 2002). In vaccinated racehorses poor performance is frequently reported with or without cough and nasal discharge (Mumford & Rossdale 1980). Unusual clinical signs of enteritis and pneumonia were associated with an H3N8 strain closely resembling an avian H3N8 virus during an epidemic in China (Webster & Guo 1991). When horses return to training too soon, sequelae such as myocarditis and chronic obstructive pulmonary disease may occur (Gerber & Lohrer 1966, Rooney 1966, Chambers *et al.* 1995).

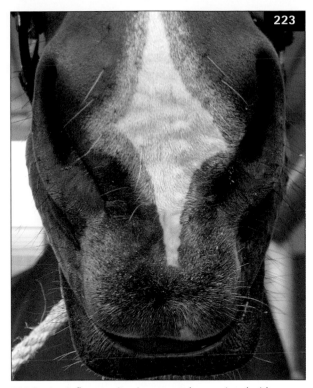

223 Equine influenza virus is commonly associated with serous nasal discharge (arrow).

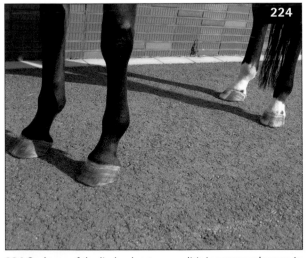

224 Oedema of the limbs due to vasculitis is commonly seen in various viral infections, such as influenza, of horses.

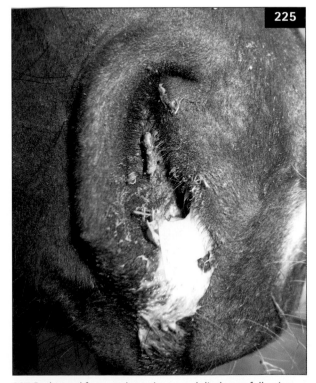

225 Prolonged fever and purulent nasal discharge following equine influenza indicate secondary bacterial infection.

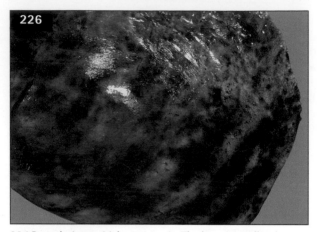

226 Bronchointerstitial pneumonia. The lung is swollen (note the rib imprints), hyperaemic, and heavy with multiple haemorrhages. Lesions consistent with equine influenza virus infection.

Differential diagnosis

The differential diagnosis includes various causes of fever and dyspnoea (see p. 262).

Diagnosis

After influenza infection, naive horses may shed virus in nasopharyngeal secretions for 7–10 days. Nasopharyngeal swabs should be taken preferably within 24 h after the appearance of fever, and transported in cool transport medium to the laboratory within 24 h (Mumford *et al*. 1998). In addition to virus isolation, tests to detect the nucleoprotein, one of the type-specific antigens of type A influenza viruses, appeared to be a valuable adjunct to virological diagnosis and were at least as sensitive as virus isolation, with results of these tests available within hours (van Maanen 2001). Furthermore, direct sequencing of the HA gene after RT-PCR on nasal swab extracts can yield valuable information for surveillance of antigenic drift (Ilobi *et al*. 1998), but for complete surveillance virus isolation remains essential to provide isolates for antigenic analysis and cross-protection studies (van Maanen & Cullinane 2002).

Since many horses have been vaccinated or have been previously infected, acute and convalescent sera should be taken for serological diagnosis of influenza virus infections, and a significant increase in titre should be demonstrated. HI, virus neutralization (VN), and single radial haemolysis (SRH) tests can be used (van Maanen & Cullinane 2002). In HI- and VN-tests a fourfold increase in titre, and in SRH tests an increase of 50% (or 25 mm^2) is considered evidence of infection (Wood *et al*. 1994, Mumford *et al*. 1995). Also an ELISA based on a haemagglutinin protein is available for serodiagnosis (Sugiura *et al*. 2001). During the Australian epidemic of equine influenza in 2007, tens of thousands of horses were infected. From the resulting field data, the commonly used bELISA for influenza A under field conditions was evaluated. Sensitivity and specificity of the test were 0.992 and 0.967, respectively (Sergeant *et al*. 2009). In addition, four blocking/competitive ELISAs performed well in the detection of influenza A antibodies in horses (Kittelberger *et al*. 2011).

Pathology

Grossly the lungs may be swollen with alveolar oedema and haemorrhages (**226**). On histology there is necrosis of bronchiolar epithelium with influx of neutrophils, macrophages, and lymphocytes. Frequently opportunistic secondary pathogenic bacterial invaders (*Streptococcus equi* subsp. *equi*, *Streptococcus equi* subsp. *zooepidemicus*, *Staphylococcus aureus*, *Bacteroides* spp.) complicate the viral bronchointerstitial pneumonia and a suppurative bronchopneumonia prevails (Jubb *et al*. 2007, McGavin & Zachary 2007).

Management/Treatment

Treatment is largely symptomatic with antibiotic treatment and anti-inflammatory drugs used only if necessary (van Maanen & Cullinane 2002). An essential component of recovery from equine influenza is stall rest. A guideline is, that horses should be stall-rested for as many weeks as the number of days they suffered fever (Wilson 1993, Chambers *et al*. 1995). With reference to myocarditis as a sequela, the administration of corticosteroids should be considered.

Management procedures reducing the level of virus in the environment, e.g. the removal and isolation of horses in the early stage of infection, markedly reduce the likelihood of disease spread (Mumford 1991, 1992). Virucidal products such as quaternary ammonium compounds, phenolic disinfectants, formalin or chlorine-based products should be used for disinfection of putatively contaminated stables, equipment, and transport vehicles (Wilson 1993).

Vaccination strategies (using either inactivated virus vaccine or an intranasal cold-adapted modified live virus vaccine) are the core of preventive management (van Maanen & Cullinane 2002, van de Walle *et al*. 2010). An influenza vaccine based on a carboxypolymer-based adjuvant was associated with superior ability to produce antibodies after vaccination in comparison with other commercial influenza vaccines (Holmes *et al*. 2006). Vaccination with either an ISCOM-based or a canarypox-based vaccine partially protected against infection with A/eq/Sydney/2888-8/07-like strains and limited the spread of disease in a vaccinated horse population (Bryant *et al*. 2009). Aged horses had higher IgGa and IgGb influenza antibody titres before vaccination than younger horses, but similar titres after vaccination (Muirhead *et al*. 2008). Maternally-derived antibodies clearly interfered with vaccination, and foals from regularly vaccinated mares should not be vaccinated before 24 weeks of age (van Maanen *et al*. 1992). Modifications introduced into the viral NS1 gene via reverse genetics have resulted in attenuated influenza viruses with promising vaccine potential. As a consequence, NS1-modified viruses could represent a new generation of improved influenza virus vaccines (Richt & García-Sastre 2009).

Horses intending to participate in Fédération Equestre Internationale (FEI) competitions must have at least received an initial primary course of two vaccinations, given between 21 and 92 days apart. Thereafter, a third dose (referred to as the first booster) must be given within 6 months + 21 days after the date of administration of the second primary dose, with at least annual boosters given subsequently (i.e. within 365 days of the last dose). If the horse is scheduled to take part in an FEI competition, the last booster must have been given within 6 calendar months + 21 days of arrival at the FEI event. No vaccination shall be given within 7 days of the day of arrival at the FEI event (FEI equine influenza vaccination rule prior to 1st January 2005).

Public health significance

Not convincing yet.

HENDRA VIRUS (HEV)

Order Mononegavirales
Family Paramyxoviridae/Subfamily
Paramyxovirinae/Genus Henipavirus: linear
negative-sense, single-stranded RNA

Definition/Overview

An acute interstitial pneumonia can be caused by
Hendra virus (HeV) (formerly called equine
morbillivirus) reported in horses in Australia with
possible horse-to-human transmission (Field *et al.*
2000, Barker 2003). HeV and Nipah virus (NiV)
form a separate genus, Henipavirus, within the
family Paramyxoviridae. Both viruses emerged from
their natural reservoir during the last decade of the
20th century, causing severe disease in humans,
horses, and swine, and infecting a number of other
mammalian species (Weingartl *et al.* 2009).
Emergence of HeV is a serious medical, veterinary,
and public health challenge (Playford *et al.* 2010).

Aetiology

Members of the Paramyxoviridae family are large,
enveloped viruses and the family is divided into two
subfamilies, namely the Paramyxovirinae and
Pneumovirinae. The Paramyxovirinae subfamily is
divided into three genera, namely rubulavirus,
morbillivirus, and respirovirus (Pringle 1998).
A recently emerged zoonotic paramyxovirus
responsible for fatal disease in horses and humans in
Queensland, Australia, NiV has ultrastructural,
serological, and molecular similarities to HeV (Black
et al. 2001). However, gene sequencing of the
enveloped NiV revealed that one of the genes had
21% difference in the nucleotide sequence with
about 8% difference in the amino acid sequence
from HeV isolated from horses in Australia (Uppal
2000). HeV and NiV both comprise the genus
Henipavirus within the family Paramyxoviridae. It
has been suggested that HeV is of low infectivity
(Selvey *et al.* 1995, Williamson *et al.* 1998).

Epidemiology

Fruit bats (flying foxes) were found to have a
prevalence of antibody to HeV, indicating that they
may be a wildlife reservoir of the virus (Young *et al.*
1996). On the other hand, Grey-headed fruit bats
(*Pteropus poliocephalus*) seroconvert and develop
subclinical disease when inoculated with HeV
(Williamson *et al.* 1998). Although it seems
improbable that a reservoir of infection for horses
other than flying foxes (suborder *Megachiroptera*,
genus *Pteropus*) exists, the possibility of an
unidentified intermediate host or vector cannot be
discounted while the mode of transmission from
flying fox to horse remains unknown (Field *et al.*
2000). Furthermore, it is possible to transmit HeV
from cats to horses. Transmission from Grey-headed
fruit bats to horses could not be proven and neither
could transmission from horses to horses or horses
to cats (Williamson *et al.* 1998). Recently swine has
been suggested as a potential host (Li *et al.* 2010).

The isolation of virus from the spleen of a
recovered horse following inoculation, at 21 days
postinoculation, in the presence of a high antibody
titre, demonstrates that HeV can persist in
recovered horses for some time after the initial
infection. The question still remains open about
persistence of virus and the carrier state
(Williamson *et al.* 1998). It has been suggested that
the Australian paralysis tick, *Ixodes holocyclus*,
which has apparently only recently become a
parasite of flying foxes, may transmit HeV and
perhaps other related viruses from flying foxes to
horses and other mammals (Barker 2003).

Pathophysiology

Horses can be infected by oronasal routes and can
excrete HeV in urine and saliva (Williamson *et al.*
1998).

Incubation period

Experimentally challenged horses developed clinical
disease in less than 11 days following oral
inoculation or by subcutaneous or intranasal
injection (Williamson *et al.* 1998).

Clinical presentation

Clinical signs include anorexia, depression combined with restlessness, fever (up to 41.0°C), tachycardia, dyspnoea, profuse sweating, large amounts of blood-stained frothy secretions issuing from the nose, neurological signs (including convulsions and ataxia), and oedema of the face, lips, and neck (Selvey *et al.* 1995, Williamson *et al.* 1998, Field *et al.* 2000, Hanna *et al.* 2006, Field *et al.* 2010).

Differential diagnosis

The differential diagnosis includes various causes of fever and dyspnoea (see p. 262).

Diagnosis

Serum samples can be tested for specific neutralizing antibody by serum neutralization test (SNT) and by an indirect ELISA. Samples for histological analysis can be examined for HeV antigen using indirect immunoperoxidase staining using a high-titre, polyclonal rabbit serum to inactivated HeV (Williamson *et al.* 1998). In addition, the presence of virus might be shown in nasal discharge, saliva and/or urine of infected horses (Barker 2003).

Pathology

At necropsy, following subcutaneous or intranasal inoculation, high titres of HeV were detected in the kidneys, in the urine, and the mouth, but not in the nasal cavities or tracheas (Williamson *et al.* 1998). The predominant histological findings are interstitial pneumonia and severe vascular degeneration, and HeV could be isolated from the lung, kidney, spleen, urine, and saliva. No virus was isolated from the brain, prescapular lymph nodes, blood, faeces, or nasal cavity following inoculation (Williamson *et al.* 1998). Since HeV is endotheliotropic, lesions arise from vascular damage. Grossly affected lungs are severely oedematous with distended pleura and subpleural lymph vessels, petechiae, and intratracheal froth. In addition, microscopic lesions include vasculitis, thrombosis, and typical multinucleated syncytial cells within the endothelium of small pulmonary blood vessels. Viral inclusion bodies are not seen in horses (Jubb *et al.* 2007, McGavin & Zachary 2007).

Management/Treatment

As the virus has important public health significance treatment is not appropriate. Vaccination might be an option in theory, but no vaccine is available as yet.

Public health significance

HeV infection should be suspected in someone with close association with horses or bats who presents acutely with pneumonia or encephalitis (potentially after a prolonged incubation period) in an endemic area (McCormack & Allworth 2002). Several humans have been killed by the virus after respiratory and renal failure and relapsing encephalitic disease (Field *et al.* 2001, Field *et al.* 2010). In addition, a veterinarian became infected after managing a terminally ill horse and performing a limited autopsy with inadequate precautions. Seven days after performing the autopsy, she developed a dry cough and sore throat, associated with cervical lymphadenopathy and fever lasting 4 days. The illness continued for about 8 days with generalized body aches. Nevertheless, she remained well 2 years after her initial illness (Hanna *et al.* 2006, Prociv 2007). Furthermore, a horse-trainer developed pneumonitis, respiratory failure, renal failure, and arterial thrombosis, and died from a cardiac arrest 7 days after admission to hospital (Selvey *et al.* 1995).

There is a reasonably strong hypothesis for horse-to-human transmission: transmission of virus via nasal discharge, saliva, and/or urine. In contrast there is no strong hypothesis for flying fox-to-human transmission (Barker 2003).

BORNA DISEASE VIRUS
Order Mononegavirales
Family Bornaviridae/Genus Bornavirus: linear negative-sense, single-stranded RNA

Definition/Overview
A sporadically occurring infectious meningo-encephalomyelitis affecting horses and sheep in central Europe is caused by Borna disease virus (BDV), which has important public health significance (Richt et al. 2000).

Aetiology
The aetiological agent is the Borna disease virus (BDV), an enveloped, nonsegmented negative-stranded RNA virus with strict neurotropism classified in the virus family Bornaviridae (Mononegavirales order). The Mononegavirales order also includes Filoviridae (Marburg and Ebola viruses), Paramyxoviridae (measles and mumps viruses) and Rhabdoviridae (rabies and vesicular stomatitis viruses) (Dauphin et al. 2002). Until the discovery of avian bornavirus (ABV) associated with proventricular dilatation disease (PDD) in parrots, the Bornaviridae family consisted of a single species, classical BDV (Staeheli et al. 2010).

Epidemiology
Clinical cases of horses and sheep have very rarely been reported outside the endemic region (Germany, Austria, and Switzerland). The average seroprevalence of BDV-specific antibodies is 12% in clinically healthy horses (Herzog et al. 1994), while this seroprevalence ranges from 23% (Richt & Rott 2000) to 50% (Dieckhöfer 2008) in the endemic region. Approximately 40% of infected horses were clinically healthy and approximately 43% were clinically ill (Dieckhöfer 2008). BDV is probably shed in nasal, salivary, and conjunctival secretions. The natural source of infection is still unknown, but rodents are regarded as a potential reservoir and vector (Dauphin et al. 2002) as well as the bicoloured white-toothed shrew, Crocidura leucodon (Puorger et al. 2010).

Pathophysiology
An olfactory route of transmission from horse to horse has been proposed, either by direct contact or through contaminated food or water (Herzog et al. 1994, Dauphin et al. 2002), and vertical transmission has also been reported in horses (Hagiwara et al. 2000).

Incubation period
The experimental disease is possible in several warm-blooded mammals and birds, including primates. The incubation period is variable, between 2 weeks and a few months (Richt et al. 2000, Dauphin et al. 2002).

Clinical presentation
BDV infections in horses are often clinically inapparent (Richt et al. 2000, Dieckhöfer 2008). However, sporadically simultaneous or consecutive disorders in behaviour, sensitivity, and locomotion are seen. During the initial phase, nonspecific signs such as fever, anorexia, and colic are observed. During the acute phase, neurological signs result from meningo-encephalitis, namely abnormal posture, ataxia, proprioceptive deficit, and repetitive movements (bruxism, circular ambulation, trismus, nystagmus, strabismus, myosis). These signs can be associated with abnormal reactions to external stimuli such as hyperexcitability, aggression, lethargy, somnolence, and stupor. In the final phase, paralysis can occur, followed by convulsions. Death usually occurs after 1–3 weeks and the death rate in horses is above 80% (50% in sheep). In chronic infection, recurrent episodes with depression, apathy, somnolence, and fearfulness might occur (Grabner & Fischer 1991, Dürrwald & Ludwig 1997, Richt & Rott 2000). Life-long viral persistence without apparent disease has also been described (Jordan & Lipkin 2001).

Differential diagnosis
The differential diagnosis predominantly includes various causes of acute neurological disease (see p. 262).

Diagnosis
Borna disease can be diagnosed by serology, viral isolation, antigen detection, and RT-nested PCR, but none of these methods is yet sensitive and specific enough to be used alone for a sure diagnosis. Antibody detection in blood and/or CSF is possible by means of Western blot, ELISA, and immunofluorescence assay (IFA), the latter method being the most reliable. Low antibody titres are detectable in nearly all animals suffering from acute disease, whereas in the subacute and chronic disease they are hardly detectable. BDV can be easily cultivated on monkey kidney (Vero) and dog kidney cells (MDCK) (Dauphin et al. 2002).

Pathology
Gross lesions are not present. Histologically there is a nonsuppurative meningoencephalitis with prominent lymphocytic perivascular cuffing and

lymphoplasmacytic foci in the neuropil. Predilection sites include grey matter of the olfactory bulbs, hippocampus, basal ganglia, and brainstem (**227–230**) (Jubb *et al.* 2007). Joest–Degen inclusion bodies located in the nuclei of infected neurons have been used as specific markers, but they are not systematically observed (Gosztonyi & Ludwig 1995).

Management/Treatment

Horses with a tentative diagnosis of Borna disease should be isolated to prevent possible human exposure. Treatment should not be attempted, as the virus has important public health significance and it is a reportable disease. For prevention of disease, an attenuated virus vaccine is available.

Public health significance

Borna disease has important public health significance. The disease can affect a large number of warm-blooded animal species, including humans. In humans, BDV could be responsible for psychiatric disorders such as schizophrenia, autism, chronic fatigue syndrome, or chronic depression (Dauphin *et al.* 2002). BDV infection in Australia particularly involved multitransfused human patients (Flower *et al.* 2008).

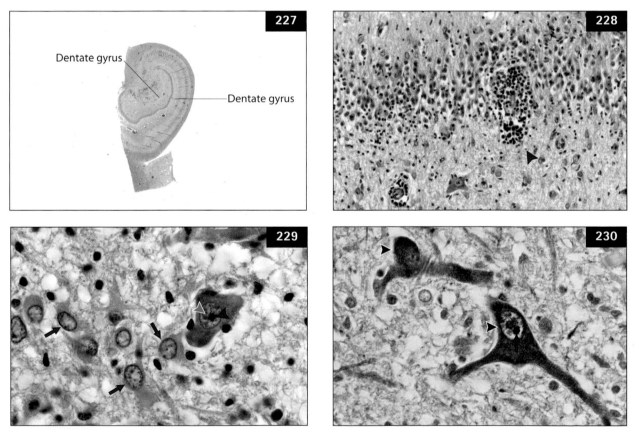

227–230 Borna disease virus. **227**: Low-power field image of an affected hippocampus with coalescing infiltrates seen in the hilus of the dentate gyrus (DG) (H&E stain); **228**: close-up of the granule cell layer and hilus of the dentate gyrus showing multifocal perivascular lymphohistiocytic infiltrates (arrowhead) as well as a diffuse microglial activation, astrocytosis, and astrogliosis; **229**: high-power field image of the hilus of the dentate gyrus showing a neuron with a viral amphophilic round intranuclear inclusion body (Joest–Degen body) (green arrowhead) next to the more basophilic nucleolus (red arrowhead). The image also shows extensive astrocytosis and astrogliosis with predominance of protoplasmic phenotypes (arrows); **230**: investigation for viral nucleoprotein p40 showing diffuse cytoplasmic immunopositivity in the perikarya of large multiple neurons (black arrowheads) as well as a single positive intranuclear inclusion body (arrow). (Courtesy of Professor K. Matiasek, University of Munich, Germany.)

EQUINE RHINITIS VIRUS
Family Picornaviridae/Genus Rhinovirus: linear positive-sense, single-stranded RNA

Definition/Overview
An acute febrile upper-airway disease can be caused by equine rhinitis virus (formerly named equine rhinoviruses). Equine rhinitis A virus (ERAV) is an important respiratory pathogen of horses and is of additional interest because of its close relationship and common classification with foot-and-mouth disease virus (FMDV) (Li *et al.* 1997, Stevenson *et al.* 2003). Although these viruses are considered to cause respiratory disease in horses and are potentially infectious for humans, little is known about their prevalence and pathogenesis (Mori *et al.* 2009).

Aetiology
Equine rhinitis A and B viruses (ERAV and ERBV) are respiratory viruses of horses belonging to the family Picornaviridae (Mori *et al.* 2009). ERAV is classified as a member of the genus Aphthovirus, whereas ERBV is classified as the sole member of the new genus Erbovirus. The genus Erbovirus currently comprises three serotypes: ERBV1, ERBV2, and the proposed ERBV3 (Huang *et al.* 2001, Black & Studdert 2006).

Epidemiology
ERAV infection occurs worldwide with the incidence of neutralizing antibody varying according to the age of the horse. Sixteen percent of horses 6–12 months of age were seropositive, rising to 53% in some populations comprising horses more than 12 months old (Studdert & Gleeson 1978). Seroprevalence against ERBV2 was 24% for horses tested in Australia (Huang *et al.* 2001). The prevalence of ERAV, ERBV1, and ERBV2 serum neutralizing antibodies was 37%, 83%, and 66%, respectively (Black *et al.* 2007). Mixed viral infections are not uncommon (Dynon *et al.* 2007).

Horse sera neutralized ERAV and ERBV1, by 90% and 86%, respectively, whereas only 2.7% and 3.6% of human veterinary sera showed weak neutralizing activity to ERAV and ERBV1, respectively, indicating that the risk of acquiring zoonotic infection among veterinarians appears low (Kriegshäuser *et al.* 2005).

Pathophysiology
Sialic acid acts as a receptor for ERAV binding and infection (Stevenson *et al.* 2004).

Incubation period
Not established in the equine species yet.

Clinical presentation
Disease is characterized by fever, anorexia, nasal discharge (**231**), coughing, pharyngitis, and lymphadenitis of the head and neck (Plummer 1963). However, a matched case–control study nested within a longitudinal study of respiratory disease failed to demonstrate a significant association between clinically apparent respiratory disease in young racehorses and infection with ERAV as diagnosed by subsequent seroconversion (Newton *et al.* 2003). On the other hand, ERBV was detected in 16% of nasal swabs collected from horses with respiratory disease (Mori *et al.* 2009).

Of note, ERAV was isolated from aborted dromedary (*Camelus dromedarius*) fetuses during an 'abortion storm' (Wernery *et al.* 2008).

Differential diagnosis
The differential diagnosis includes various causes of fever and dyspnoea (see p. 262).

Diagnosis
Diagnosis usually depends on the detection of viral antigen and/or seroconversion combined with clinical signs. However, it has been stated that the relative importance of ERBV1 as a cause of acute febrile respiratory disease in horses has been underestimated due to failure in many instances to isolate the virus by conventional cell culture methods (Li *et al.* 1997), due to inefficient growth and lack of cytopathic effect in cell cultures. Therefore, molecular assays should be considered as the method of choice for the detection of infection in symptomatic or apparently healthy horses. A real-time duplex TaqMan PCR has been developed as an useful new diagnostic method for the rapid detection and differentiation of ERAV and ERBV as well as to detect viral RNA in cell culture supernatants and nasal swabs, and lung and urine (Mori *et al.* 2009). Virus neutralization (VN) has been the standard method for the detection of ERAV antibody in horse serum (Kriegshäuser *et al.* 2009).

Pathology

Unless complicated by secondary infections, inflammatory lesions of the upper respiratory tract are usually mild and transient (McGavin & Zachary 2007).

Management/Treatment

Treatment of diseased animals is supportive.

Public health significance

Horses with a tentative diagnosis of equine rhinitis virus should be isolated to prevent possible human exposure, given infection and disease in man (Plummer 1962, Kriegshäuser *et al.* 2005).

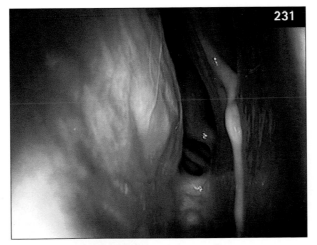

231 Sinusitis as a sequela from respiratory disease as illustrated by purulent discharge oozing from the left apertura naso-maxillaris (arrow).

AFRICAN HORSE SICKNESS VIRUS

Family Reoviridae/Genus Orbivirus: linear double-stranded RNA

Definition/Overview

African horse sickness (AHS) is a noncontagious, infectious insect-borne disease caused by African horse sickness virus (AHSV), associated with serous effusion and haemorrhage in various organs and tissues. Oedema is never seen in the lower limbs. Although zebra and donkeys rarely exhibit clinical signs (232), the effects of the disease, particularly in susceptible populations of horses, can be devastating and mortality rates for this species may exceed 90% (Mellor & Hamblin 2004).

Aetiology

AHSV is a member of the genus Orbivirus in the family Reoviridae and as such is morphologically similar to other orbiviruses such as bluetongue virus of ruminants and equine encephalosis virus. The double-stranded RNA virus is transmitted by at least two species of biting midge (*Culicoides*), the most important of which is the Afro-Asiatic species *C. imicola*. The bluetongue virus utilizes the same vector species of *Culicoides* (Mellor & Hamblin 2004). To date, nine different serotypes have been described (Sánchez-Vizcaíno 2004). The presence of three distinct S10 phylogenetic clades (alpha, beta, and gamma) has been reported. Some serotypes (6, 8, and 9 in alpha; 3 and 7 in beta; 2 in gamma) were restricted to a single clade, while other serotypes (1, 4, and 5) clustered into both the alpha and gamma clades (Quan *et al.* 2008). In naive horses the form of disease expressed is a property of the AHSV inoculum. For instance, AHS/4SP consistently caused the pulmonary form of AHS with 100% mortality, AHS/9PI resulted in the cardiac form of AHS with 70% mortality, and AHS/4PI produced mild to subclinical disease in horses without mortality (Laegreid *et al.* 1993). The virus is acid sensitive, being readily inactivated at pH values below 6.0, but remains relatively stable at more alkaline pH values (pH 7.0–8.5). It is resistant to lipid solvents and relatively heat resistant (Mellor & Hamblin 2004).

Epidemiology

It has been assumed that *C. imicola* is exophilic and, consequently, that stabling should provide effective protection against AHS. However, the mean catch of *C. imicola* inside stables in Spain was consistently higher than that outside (Calvete *et al.* 2009).

Zebras are considered the natural vertebrate host and reservoir of AHSV. This species rarely exhibits clinical signs (Mellor & Boorman 1995). The capability of zebra to maintain AHSV is clearly illustrated by the continuing infections during every month of the year, with a peak period in winter (Barnard 1993). Though susceptible to infection, the donkey is unlikely to be a long-term reservoir for AHSV, as reflected by the absence of virus in any of the tissues collected at 14–19 days post-inoculation (Hamblin *et al.* 1998). Dogs have died from AHSV, contracted by the consumption of uncooked meat from the carcass of a horse that had died from the disease, respiratory embarrassment being the main clinical sign (van Rensberg *et al.* 1981).

The nine serotypes of AHSV have been described in eastern and southern Africa. Only AHSV serotypes 9 and 4 have been found in west Africa, from where they occasionally spread into countries surrounding the Mediterranean, for example, in the Middle East (1959–1963), in Spain (serotype 9, 1966, serotype 4, 1987–1990), in Portugal (serotype 4, 1989) and Morocco (serotype 4, 1989–1991) (Sánchez-Vizcaíno 2004).

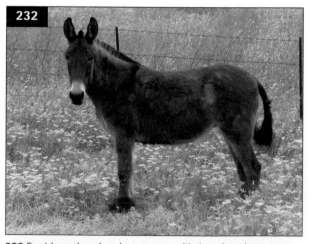

232 Equidae other than horses are unlikely to be a long-term reservoir for AHSV.

It has been predicted that climate change will increase the risk of incursions of AHSV into Europe from other parts of the world, with West Nile virus (WNV) being less affected (Gale *et al.* 2010).

Pathophysiology

Serous effusion and haemorrhage in various organs and tissues is seen due to infection of target organs and cells, namely the lungs, spleen, and other lymphoid tissues and endothelial cells following initial multiplication of AHSV in the regional lymph nodes and subsequent dissemination throughout the body via the blood. Virus multiplication in these tissues and organs gives rise to a secondary viraemia (Mellor & Hamblin 2004). A role for intravascular coagulation in the pathogenesis of AHS has been suggested (Skowronek *et al.* 1995).

Incubation period

Control ponies developed clinical signs typical of AHS and died within 9 days of challenge inoculation (House *et al.* 1994) or within 3–6 days after onset of fever (Mellor & Hamblin 2004).

Clinical presentation

The extent and severity of the clinico-pathological findings have been used to classify the disease into four forms. In ascending order of severity these are horse sickness fever (which usually affects only mules, donkeys, and partially immune horses), the subacute or cardiac form, the cardio-pulmonary or mixed form, and the peracute or pulmonary form (Laegreid *et al.* 1993, House *et al.* 1994, Mellor & Hamblin 2004). Horse sickness fever is invariably mild, usually involving only mild to moderate fever and oedema of the supraorbital fossae without mortality. The cardiac form is characterized by fever and the main clinical finding is subcutaneous oedema, particularly of the head, neck, and chest but also of the supraorbital fossae (**233**). Oedema is never seen in the lower limbs. The mixed form is often the most common form and is a combination of the cardiac and pulmonary forms of disease. The pulmonary form is associated with marked depression and fever followed by severe dyspnoea. Terminally quantities of frothy fluid may be discharged from the nostrils (Mellor & Hamblin 2004). Clinical AHS occurred more frequently in horses than donkeys and mules and 16% of the equines died and 14% were slaughtered. Of these, 81% were horses, 11% were donkeys, and 8% were mules (Portas *et al.* 1999).

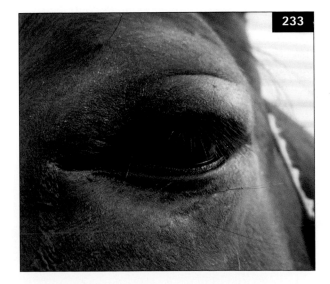

233 The cardiac form of AHS is characterized by fever and the main clinical finding is subcutaneous oedema, particularly of the head, neck, and chest but also of the supraorbital fossae.

Differential diagnosis

The differential diagnosis includes equine encephalosis virus (Howell *et al.* 2008), and other causes of fever and dyspnoea.

Diagnosis

Currently, diagnosis of AHS is based on typical clinical signs and lesions, a history consistent with vector transmission, and confirmation by laboratory detection of virus and/or anti-AHSV antibodies (Laegreid 1994). Clinical signs and lesions may be sufficient for a tentative clinical diagnosis, but AHS must be confirmed by isolation and identification of the virus. Intracerebral inoculation of 2–4-day-old suckling mice is the preferred method for primary isolation of AHSV, although the virus will adapt and grow in embryonated hens' eggs following intravenous inoculation. Several mammalian-derived cell lines including baby hamster kidney, African green monkey (Vero), and monkey kidney cells are available for AHSV isolation, all of which usually show cytopathic effects within 7 days (Erasmus 1963, Erasmus 1964). AHSV can also be identified directly using molecular probes and RT-PCR, although indirect sandwich ELISA is also extremely useful for the rapid identification of AHSV antigen, as well as complement fixation and direct and indirect fluorescence (Davies & Lund 1974).

An assay that uses Hamblin antiserum in a basic avidin–biotin complex detection system provides a robust diagnostic tool for the detection of AHSV in formalin-fixed tissues. The only cross-reactivity observed was in the lungs of two negative cases infected with *Rhodococcus equi*. The assay gave good results on tissues that had been fixed in formalin for up to 365 days (Clift *et al.* 2009). Application of a nested RT-PCR resulted in direct detection of AHSV double-stranded RNA from blood and a variety of tissue samples collected from equines infected experimentally and naturally (Aradaib 2009). In addition, an ELISA for the detection of AHSV antigens and antibodies has been described (Rubio *et al.* 1998).

Pathology

The pathological findings vary in accordance with the disease. With the pulmonary form the most remarkable finding is interlobular oedema of the lungs and hydrothorax. Ascites can occur in abdominal and thoracic cavities and the mucosa of the stomach may be hyperaemic and oedematous. In the cardiac form the most prominent lesions are gelatinous exudate in the subcutaneous, subfascial, and intramuscular tissues and lymph nodes. Hydropericardium is seen and haemorrhages are found on the epicardial and/or endocardial surfaces. As in the pulmonary form ascites may occur but oedema of the lungs is either slight or absent. The histopathological changes are a result of increased permeability of the capillary walls and consequent impairment in circulation (Mellor & Hamblin 2004). The only gross pathological changes observed in donkeys post-mortem were increased fluid accumulation in the serosal lined compartments, particularly the peritoneal cavity, and petechial (see **234**) and ecchymotic haemorrhages on the left hepatic ligament (Hamblin *et al.* 1998). Virus was localized to target cells (predominantly heart and lung) with morphological features compatible with endothelium in all organs except the spleen, where it was found in both endothelium-like cells and large mononuclear cells, these being the main target cells for virus replication (Brown *et al.* 1994, Clift & Penrith 2010).

Management/Treatment

There is no specific treatment, and secondary infections should be treated appropriately. AHSV is noncontagious and can only be spread via the bites of infected vector species of *Culicoides* and as a consequence vector control is of importance. A limited number of vaccines are available for AHS (Roth & Spickler 2003). Polyvalent or monovalent attenuated vaccines provide solid immunity when administered twice in the first and second years of life, and annually thereafter (Mellor & Hamblin 2004). Serial vaccination of naive horses with the polyvalent AHS-attenuated live virus vaccine generated a broad neutralizing antibody response to all vaccine strains as well as cross-neutralizing antibodies to serotypes 5 and 9. Booster vaccination of horses with monovalent vaccine vAHSV6 or vAHSV8 induced an adequate protective immune response to challenge with homologous and heterologous virulent virus. *In vivo* cross-protection between AHSV6 and AHSV9 and AHSV8 and AHSV5, respectively, was demonstrated (von Teichman *et al.* 2010).

Vaccination with an inactivated recombinant canarypox virus vectored vaccine might also be useful for the protective immunization of equids against AHS (Guthrie *et al.* 2009). Furthermore, the immunogenicity of recombinant modified vaccinia Ankara (MVA) vectored AHSV vaccines, in particular MVAVP2, indicates that further work to investigate whether these vaccines would confer protection from lethal AHSV challenge in the horse is justifiable (Chiam *et al.* 2009). Assumptions of virulence or reversion to virulence of attenuated live vaccine reassortants post-vaccination in horses could not be substantiated (von Teichman & Smit 2008).

Portugal was declared free of AHS 1 year after ending vaccination. The cost of eradication was US$11.5 per Portuguese equine (Portas *et al.* 1999).

Public health significance

Encephalitis and uveochorioretinitis with predominant temporal lobe involvement was associated with an airborne transnasal route of infection of the neurotropic AHSV released in dried powder form, secondary to the accidental breaking of vaccine bottles (van der Meyden *et al.* 1992).

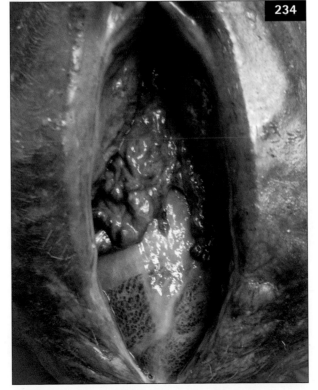

234 Mucosal petechiation on the surface of the vagina.

EQUINE INFECTIOUS ANAEMIA VIRUS

Family Retroviridae/Subfamily Orthoretrovirinae/Genus Lentivirus: positive-sense, single-stranded RNA

Definition/Overview

The disease equine infectious anaemia (EIA) is caused by equine infectious anaemia virus (EIAV), and is characterized clinically by intermittent fever, depression, emaciation, and oedema, with anaemia appearing in the chronic stages of infection. As an arbovirus it is transmitted by arthropods and the disease is also known as swamp fever. Treatment should not be attempted as EIA is a reportable disease.

Aetiology

The causative agent is a RNA virus, a member of the Retroviridae family and of the Lentivirus genus with an almost worldwide distribution. Among lentiviruses, EIAV is unique in that, despite a rapid virus replication and antigenic variation, most infected animals progress from a chronic stage characterized by recurring peaks of viraemia and fever to an asymptomatic stage of infection (Leroux et al. 2004). As with all lentiviruses, EIAV has been shown to have a high propensity for genomic sequence and antigenic variation of approximately 40%, especially in its envelope (Env) proteins (Craigo et al. 2009). The EIAV strain isolated from the 2006 outbreak in Ireland shared 85% identity with a Canadian strain, 82–83% with USA strains, and 82% with a strain from China (Mooney et al. 2006).

Epidemiology

Inapparent carriers remain infective for life. The main route of transmission is by haematophagous insects of the Tabanidae family. However, iatrogenic and close-contact transmission should also be considered (Menzies & Patterson 2006, More et al. 2008a, 2008b). The virus is carried on the mouthparts of the horsefly. EIA is considered a worldwide disease but due to its transmission by insect vectors, it is predominant in warm climates (Leroux et al. 2004). While susceptible to infection, donkeys do not develop clinical EIA, and lower amounts of plasma-associated virus and/or viral nucleic acids are observed in donkeys compared to ponies infected with the same strain of EIAV (Cook et al. 2001). Analysis suggested most Italian isolates were geographically restricted, somewhat reminiscent of the 'clades' described for human immunodeficiency virus 1 (HIV-1) (Cappelli et al. 2011).

Pathophysiology

EIAV retains the ability to use equine lentivirus receptor 1 for entry which suggests that this virus can interact with an additional, unidentified receptor to superinfect equine dermis cells (Brindley et al. 2008). The concept of 'pathogenic threshold' postulates that the level of viral replication must reach a critical level to induce disease. Clearance of the primary infectious plasma viraemia correlates with the emergence of EIAV-specific CD8+ cytotoxic T lymphocytes and non-neutralizing antibodies (Leroux et al. 2004). U3 regions in the viral long terminal repeat (LTR), surface envelope protein, and the accessory S2 gene strongly influence acute disease expression (Payne & Fuller 2010).

Incubation period

Not established in the equine species yet although EIAV infection results in a high-titre, infectious plasma viraemia within 3 weeks post infection (Leroux et al. 2004). In addition, serological data suggest an incubation/seroconversion period of approximately 37 days, but it may be more than 60 days in a few cases (Cullinane et al. 2007).

Clinical presentation

EIAV is responsible for a persistent infection in horses characterized by recurring cycles of fever associated with viraemia, depression, weakness, oedema, wasting symptoms, and haemorrhage (either dysentery or nasal discharge). Based on experimental infection, acute, chronic, and asymptomatic stages are classified. Acute disease is characterized by hyperthermia concomitant with severe decrease in the platelet number. The acute episode usually subsides within a few days, then the animal enters the chronic stage of disease characterized by the recurrence of clinical cycles. If clinical episodes are frequent, the animal may develop classic clinical disease with anaemia, weight loss, and oedema. In EIAV-infected equids, there is a transition from a chronic to an asymptomatic state, in which the animals remain free of clinical symptoms, but remain infected for the rest of their life (Leroux et al. 2004, Menzies & Patterson 2006, More et al. 2008a, 2008b). Neurological disease occurs sporadically in horses infected with the EIAV (Oaks et al. 2004).

Differential diagnosis

The differential diagnosis includes various causes of fever and anaemia (see p. 263).

Diagnosis

Blood analysis might reveal thrombocytopenia, the presence of band form neutrophils, elevated bilirubin, elevated glutamate dehydrogenase (GLDH) activity, anaemia, leukopenia, and hypoalbuminaemia (More *et al.* 2008*a*, 2008*b*). The diagnosis of EIA is based on demonstration of lesions and the aetiological agent and/or seroconversion. The 'Coggins Test' (a serological test based on agar gel immunodiffusion (AGID) using p26 antigen) is regarded as the standard diagnostic test for EIAV infection (Leroux *et al.* 2004, More *et al.* 2008*a*, 2008*b*). However, both PCR and RT-PCR demonstrate potential to detect acutely infected horses earlier using plasma than some of the official tests. In addition, ELISA is an excellent premovement screening test for EIAV (Cullinane *et al.* 2007). A single-band Western blot using recombinant p26 capsid protein of EIAV is a reliable confirmatory diagnostic tool to be used as a complementary test after an ELISA or AGID test yielding doubtful results (Alvarez *et al.* 2007).

Pathology

Horses that die in an acute haemolytic crisis consistently show hepatosplenomegaly, icterus, anaemia, and extensive haemorrhages. Mesenteric lymphadenomegaly, subcutaneous oedema, anaemia, and cachexia may be present in more chronic cases. Microscopic examination reveals systemic perivascular lymphocytic accumulations and systemic reticuloendothelial cell hyperplasia. The hepatic sinusoids are hypercellular with proliferated haemosiderin-laden Kupffer cells, and varying periportal lymphocytic infiltrates. The spleen exhibits congested hypercellular sinusoids with haemosiderin-laden macrophages and plasma cells. Within the bone marrow increased or exhausted haematopoiesis and haemosiderosis may be found. In few cases a proliferative glomerulonephritis and lymphocytic interstitial nephritis is observed. Sporadically there may be an encephalomyelitis or a lymphohistiocytic periventricular leucoencephalitis (Jubb *et al.* 2007, McGavin & Zachary 2007). Viral RNA and DNA were detected by RT-PCR and PCR in all the tissues from the infected animals examined post-mortem during the 2006 outbreak in Ireland (Cullinane *et al.* 2007).

Management/Treatment

Treatment should not be attempted as EIA is a reportable disease. EIAV-seropositive animals are either euthanized or kept in quarantine for the rest of their life depending on local regulations. EIAV vaccine trials are encouraging, but correlates of protection remain to be clearly defined yet (Leroux *et al.* 2004, Mealey *et al.* 2007). Management also relies on eradicating the haematophagous insects of the *Tabanidae* family.

Public health significance

Not convincing yet.

ROTAVIRUS
Family Reoviridae/Genus Rotavirus: linear double-stranded RNA

Definition/Overview
Acute enteritis associated with diarrhoea in neonatal foals can be caused by highly contagious rotaviruses. Rotaviruses, a genus within the family Reoviridae, are regarded as a major cause of diarrhoea in neonatal foals in contrast to equine coronavirus. The ubiquity of rotavirus infection should be considered in diagnosis (Conner & Darlington 1980).

Aetiology
Rotaviruses are among the most important aetiological agents of severe diarrhoeal illness in humans and animals worldwide (Müller & Johne 2007). The double-stranded, nonenveloped RNA rotaviruses are classified as a genus of the family Reoviridae further subdivided as group A. Worldwide, G3P[12] and G14P[12] are the most prevalent equine rotavirus strains, and G3P[12] vaccines have been developed for the prevention of rotavirus-associated diarrhoea in foals (Browning *et al.* 1992, Collins *et al.* 2008). Their genome, consisting of 11 segments of double-stranded RNA, is characterized by genetic variability including (i) point mutations, (ii) genomic reassortment, and (iii) genome rearrangements, thus leading to the considerable diversity of rotaviruses (Müller & Johne 2007).

Epidemiology
The presence of sufficient maternal antibodies against the virus in the colostrum is important for protective immunity. In a study scoring Thoroughbred foals up to 3 months of age, rotaviruses had a similar prevalence in all age groups, with an overall prevalence of 37% among diarrhoeic foals and, as a consequence, they are regarded as significant pathogens. The prevalence of cryptosporidia, potentially pathogenic *Escherichia coli*, *Y. enterocolitica*, and *C. perfringens* was similar in normal or diarrhoeic foals. Group A rotaviruses and *Aeromonas hydrophila* showed a significantly higher prevalence in diarrhoeic foals. *A. hydrophila* had an overall prevalence of 9% among diarrhoeic foals. No evidence was found of synergistic effects between rotavirus, cryptosporidia and *E. coli*. Other putative pathogens found at very low prevalence were coronavirus, the putative picobirnavirus, *Campylobacter* spp. and *Salmonella* spp. (Browning *et al.* 1991). Rotavirus was also the most frequently detected pathogen (20%) followed by *C. perfringens* (18%), *Salmonella* spp. (12%), and *C. difficile* (5%) in a population of hospitalized foals with diarrhoea; the type of infectious agent identified in the faeces or bacteraemia was not significantly associated with survival (Frederick *et al.* 2009).

Pathophysiology
Transmission of rotaviruses is via the faecal–oral route. Following infection, destruction of the proximal part of the villi of the small bowel occurs, leading to maldigestion and malabsorption. As a consequence, diarrhoea is seen due to increased osmolarity of the contents of the small bowel. The profuse diarrhoea is usually foul-smelling. Replacement of destroyed proximal epithelial cells is provided by proliferation of crypt cells. Hence, the disease is usually self-limiting.

Incubation period
Colostrum-deprived, colostrum-fed, or suckling foals were orally inoculated with foal rotavirus and enterotoxigenic *E. coli* derived from a calf. Neither agent given alone caused diarrhoea in foals aged 1 or 2 days, although with rotavirus, two of the three inoculated foals became depressed 3 days after inoculation and all three were excreting rotavirus in their faeces (Tzipori *et al.* 1982). However, the disease was produced in an experimental foal by inoculation via stomach tube of a bacteria-free faecal filtrate containing rotavirus (Conner & Darlington 1980).

Clinical presentation
Clinical signs include fever, depression, anorexia, dehydration, and foul-smelling diarrhoea (**235, 236**) (Tzipori & Walker 1978). There was an apparent age-related resistance to rotavirus diarrhoea, which developed between 2 and 3 weeks of age independently of pre-inoculation maternal antibody (Tzipori *et al.* 1982).

Differential diagnosis
The differential diagnosis includes various causes of diarrhoea in foals (see p. 262).

Diagnosis

Diagnosis usually depends on the detection of viral antigen in the faeces using either ELISA or latex agglutination assay combined with clinical signs. A comparison of diagnostic tests for rotavirus in the faeces showed electron microscopy (EM) and polyacrylamide gel electrophoresis (PAGE) to have similar sensitivity. The ELISA test kit was found to have the same sensitivity as a combination of EM and PAGE (Browning *et al.* 1991). Furthermore, a nested RT-PCR for the detection and identification of group A rotaviruses in faeces is a powerful diagnostic tool and has been shown to be applicable to rotaviruses of different origin, including equine and human sources (Elschner *et al.* 2002). A recent study also indicated very good agreement between detection of rotavirus by ELISA and by electron microscopy ($\kappa = 0.88$) in hospitalized foals with diarrhoea. Using EM as the gold standard, rotavirus ELISA had a sensitivity of 91%, specificity of 98%, and accuracy of 96% (Frederick *et al.* 2009). In addition, an RT loop-mediated isothermal amplification (RT-LAMP) has been applied to detection of equine rotavirus (Nemoto *et al.* 2010).

Pathology

Pathology is associated with replicating virus in the small intestinal epithelial cells and villous atrophy (Conner & Darlington 1980).

Management/Treatment

Although rotavirus enteritis is usually self-limiting, treatment of diseased foals is supportive, especially with regard to diarrhoea (Jones *et al.* 1989). Given the fact that rotavirus is frequently excreted via the faeces of clinically normal foals and the virus is highly resistant to external factors and can survive for several months in the environment, adequate hygiene is of utmost importance. An inactivated virus vaccine is available against equine rotaviruses for use in pregnant mares in order to improve foal protective immunity.

In comparison, nitazoxanide is a thiazolide anti-infective for treating diarrhoea caused by *Cryptosporidium parvum* and *Giardia lamblia* in humans. Interestingly, a 3-day course of nitazoxanide significantly reduced the duration of rotavirus disease in hospitalized paediatric patients (Rossignol *et al.* 2006).

Public health significance

Reciprocal cross-neutralization studies showed antigenic similarities between animal and human

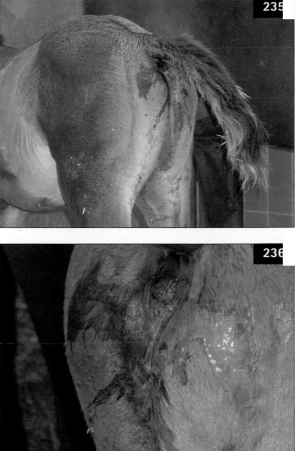

235, 236 Foul-smelling diarrhoea due to the highly contagious rotavirus enteritis.

strains including a newly defined fifth human serotype (Albert *et al.* 1987). In addition, human isolates failed to infect gnotobiotic calves and lambs (Tzipori *et al.* 1980) in contrast to viral isolates from foals (Tzipori & Walker 1978). Zoonotic transmission cannot be excluded (Steyer *et al.* 2008, Mukherjee *et al.* 2009) as animal rotaviruses are regarded as a potential reservoir for genetic exchange with human rotaviruses. There is now increasing evidence that animal rotaviruses can infect humans, either by direct transmission of the virus or by contributing one or several genes to reassortants with essentially a human strain genetic background (Müller & Johne 2007).

RABIES
Order Mononegavirales/Family Rhabdo-
viridae/Genus Lyssavirus: linear, negative-sense,
single-stranded RNA

Definition/Overview
Rabies is a lethal viral infection of the CNS
transmitted by salivary contamination of a bite
wound. Horses are moderately susceptible to rabies
and rabid horses may serve as a source of infection
for humans.

Aetiology
The aetiological agent is the rabies virus, an
enveloped, nonsegmented negative-stranded
neurotropic RNA virus classified in the virus family
Rhabdoviridae (Mononegavirales order) belonging
to the genus Lyssavirus. Lyssaviruses comprise six
distinct genotypes.

Epidemiology
Rabies is primarily a disease that affects and is
maintained by wildlife populations. The wildlife
species most frequently reported rabid are bats,
raccoons, skunks, and foxes. Rabies in bats is
epidemiologically distinct from terrestrial rabies
maintained by carnivores (Krebs *et al*. 2002). During
2009, within the USA 6,690 rabid animals and four
human rabies cases were reported, representing a
2.2% decrease from 2008. Approximately 92% of
reported rabid animals were wildlife. Compared
with 2008, numbers of rabid raccoons and bats that
were reported decreased, whereas numbers of rabid
skunks, foxes, cats, cattle, dogs, and horses that were
reported increased (Blanton *et al*. 2010).

Pathophysiology
The neurotropic virus enters the body via salivary
contamination of a bite wound. The virus replicates
at the site of the bite in striated muscle cells followed
by infection of the CNS via an ascending wave of
peripheral nerve infection. Rabies virus is shed
predominantly via saliva.

Incubation period
Average incubation period was 12.3 days and
average morbidity was 5.5 days. Naive animals had
significantly shorter incubation and morbidity
periods as compared with test-vaccinated horses
(Hudson *et al*. 1996). Bites on the head usually result
in a reduced incubation period as compared to bites
on the extremities.

Clinical presentation
The clinical signs are variable and include fever,
anorexia, ptyalism, teeth grinding, pica, ataxia, colic,
hyperaesthesia, somnolence, frequent whinnying,
automutilation (**237**), and aggressive behaviour. The
clinical signs can present with either a silent form or
a furious form dominant. Muzzle tremors were the
most frequently observed (81%) and most common
initial sign following experimentally induced rabies
in horses. Other common signs were pharyngeal
spasm or pharyngeal paresis (71%), ataxia or paresis
(71%), and lethargy or somnolence (71%). The
furious form was manifested in 43% of rabid horses
and some of these furious animals initially
manifested the silent form. The paralytic form was
not observed following experimentally induced
rabies (Hudson *et al*. 1996). Death usually occurs
within 1 week – sometimes as early as 12 hours –
after onset and is preceded by (respiratory) paralysis
(Green 1997).

Differential diagnosis
The differential diagnosis predominantly includes
various causes of acute neurological disease (see p.
262).

Diagnosis
The rabies virus is mainly contained in the saliva of
animals, but tears, urine, serum, liquor, and other
body fluids may be infectious as well. There is no
chance of treatment after the onset of clinical
symptoms (Haupt 1999). Ante-mortem laboratory
assessments are of limited diagnostic value as
negative serology does not preclude rabies as a
possible diagnosis. Isolation of the rabies virus in
equine salivary glands demonstrated the potential
risk for humans exposed to infected animals
(Carrieri *et al*. 2006).

Pathology

Histological lesions of rabies virus induced nonsuppurative encephalomyelitis. Ganglioneuritis of paravertebral ganglia may consist of perivascular lymphocytic cuffs, neuronal degeneration, and necrosis accompanied by focal microglial nodules. The severity of these changes may vary and may be scant to absent. Typically there may be presence of Negri bodies in ganglion cells and neurons within the CNS (238). In addition, immunohistochemistry of the CNS and cornea might show rabies virus. Analysis by FAT showed that there was a greater amount of viral antigen in the brainstem and cervical medullar tissues than in the hippocampus, cortical and cerebellar tissues when transmitted by the vampire bat, *Desmodus rotundus* (Carrieri *et al.* 2006). The best sites for rabies virus detection in horses are the cervical spinal cord and adjacent brainstem (Stein *et al.* 2010).

Management/Treatment

Horses with a tentative diagnosis of rabies should be isolated to prevent possible human exposure. Treatment should not be attempted as the virus has important public health significance and rabies is a reportable disease. However, an effective veterinary post-exposure prophylaxis (PEP) protocol for unvaccinated domestic animals exposed to rabies was shown to be immediate vaccination against rabies, a strict isolation period of 90 days, and administration of booster vaccinations during the third and eighth weeks of the isolation period (Wilson *et al.* 2010).

The most effective method of preventing the entry of rabies into an area free of the disease is the imposition of a quarantine period of about 6 months. For prevention of disease, preference is given to killed rabies vaccines in order to reduce the risk of potential virus spread as in the case of modified live virus vaccine.

Healthy aged horses generated a primary immune response to a killed rabies vaccine similar to that of younger adult horses. Horses receiving a booster rabies vaccine (4 weeks after initial vaccine) had titres >0.5 IU at 8 weeks after initial vaccination, although 28% of these horses had serum titres below this level at 24 weeks. As a consequence, the current rabies vaccination label recommendation of a single dose being administered on primary vaccination may need to be reconsidered (Muirhead *et al.* 2008).

Successful control of terrestrial rabies through the use of oral vaccines will have no effect on enzootic rabies in bats and the associated risk of human disease (Krebs *et al.* 2002).

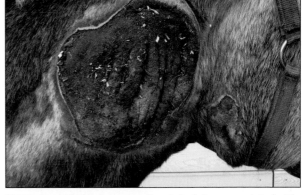

237 Automutilation is among the clinical signs associated with rabies.

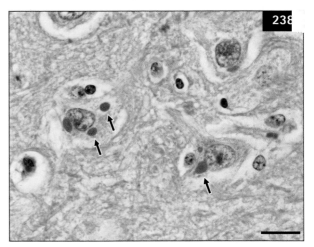

238 Rabies. Micrograph of central nervous tissue in which three neuron cell bodies contain several round to oval eosinophilic rabies viral inclusion bodies or Negri bodies (arrows). Inflammatory and degenerative changes are not depicted here but can consist of perivascular lymphocytic cuffs, neuronal degeneration, and necrosis accompanied by focal microglial nodules. Rhabdoviridae, rabies virus. (H&E stain. Bar 20 μm.)

Public health significance

Rabies has important public health significance (239) and is a reportable disease causing approximately 50,000 to 100,000 deaths per year worldwide. Most deaths occur in developing countries. Dogs are the major vector, especially in developing countries (Leung *et al*. 2007). PEP is indicated when a person is bitten by a rabid animal. Most of the persons (94%) who received PEP after contact with a rabid pony had an exposure for which PEP was indicated (Feder *et al*. 1998). Australian bat lyssavirus (ABL) is closely related genetically to rabies virus. Both the clinical manifestations and pathological changes of ABL infection in the human cases were very similar to those of rabies, with meningoencephalomyelitis and neuronal intracytoplasmic inclusions. Rabies vaccine and immunoglobulin offer significant protection against ABL (McCormack & Allworth 2002).

VESICULAR STOMATITIS VIRUS

Order Mononegavirales/Family Rhabdoviridae/Genus Vesiculovirus: linear, negative-sense, single-stranded RNA

Definition/Overview

An acute painful vesicular stomatis can be caused by vesicular stomatitis virus (VSV).

Aetiology

The aetiological agent is VSV, an enveloped, nonsegmented negative-stranded RNA virus classified in the genus Vesiculovirus of the family Rhabdoviridae (Mononegavirales order) to which cattle and swine are also susceptible. In the USA, outbreaks have been associated with two genotypically and serologically distinct serotypes: vesicular stomatitis New Jersey virus (VSNJV) and vesicular stomatitis Indiana virus (VSIV) (McCluskey & Mumford 2000, Howerth *et al*. 2006, Lee *et al*. 2009) with similar findings between the two viruses (Howerth *et al*. 2006). However, there is evidence that some outbreaks of equine stomatitis are caused by as yet unidentified infectious agents (McCluskey & Mumford 2000).

Epidemiology

Vesicular stomatitis outbreaks of unknown origin occur at 8–10-year intervals in the Southwestern USA resulting from the introduction of viral strains from endemic areas in Mexico (Rainwater-Lovett *et al*. 2007). Seroprevalence was 37% for horses and 15% for cattle following the 1995 epidemic (Mumford *et al*. 1998).

Pathophysiology

The virus enters the body via mucous membranes and abrasions of the skin. Transmission may occur by direct contact or via mosquitoes. Detection of viral RNA from tonsil and lymph nodes of the head at necropsy suggests that these tissues play a role in the pathogencsis of the disease (Howerth *et al*. 2006).

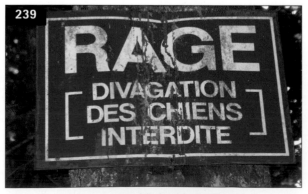

239 Rabies has important public health significance as illustrated by this sign in French.

Incubation period

Horses inoculated with VSNJV developed primary lesions at the site of inoculation as early as post-inoculation day 1 (swelling and blanching of the area due to early vesicle formation) following intraepithelial/subepithelial injection of the tongue and as early as post-inoculation day 2 after applying the virus to a scarified area on the oral mucosa (reddening, superficial necrosis, and erosion). By post-inoculation day 2, horses inoculated in the tongue had large ruptured vesicles in which the dorsal tongue epithelium was separated from the underlying submucosa and eventually sloughed, leaving a reddened superficial ulcer with ragged margins (Howerth *et al.* 2006).

Clinical presentation

Clinical signs include fever, depression, anorexia, excessive salivation associated with the formation of vesicles in the oral cavity, followed by ulceration. Formation of vesicles is also possible on the prepuce, the udder, and the coronary band. The latter is associated with lameness (Green 1993, McCluskey & Mumford 2000, Howerth *et al.* 2006). However, some horses never stopped eating. Rectal temperatures were rarely elevated above 39.0°C and never above 40.0°C following inoculation. All lesions had evidence of healing by post-inoculation day 12 (Howerth *et al.* 2006).

Differential diagnosis

Physical trauma, dietary factors, certain toxins, immune-mediated disorders, and VSV infection are known causes of stomatitis in horses (McCluskey & Mumford 2000).

Diagnosis

Viral shedding was most often from the oral cavity, followed by the nasal cavity; titres were highest from oral cavity samples. Virus was rarely isolated from the conjunctival sac and never from faeces or blood (Howerth *et al.* 2006). The definitive diagnosis is made by virus isolation and/or the presence of seroconversion using two serum samples collected 10–14 days apart. A blocking ELISA using glycoprotein (GP ELISA) exhibited 99.6% specificity for naive sera from horses from domestic farms. This GP ELISA could be a useful tool as an alternative to the VN test for detecting antibodies specific to VSV (Lee *et al.* 2009). Serum-neutralizing antibodies were first detected on post-inoculation days 6–12, depending on the virus and inoculation group, and increased over time (Howerth *et al.* 2006). In addition, a real-time PCR is available with a clinical sensitivity and specificity of 83% and 99%, respectively (Wilson *et al.* 2009).

Pathology

Intercellular oedema (spongiosis) of the stratum spinosum and dissociation of keratinocytes leads to vesicle formation. At post-mortem examination (post-inoculation days 12–15), lesions were healing, were not vesicular, and did not contain detectable virus by isolation, RT-PCR, or immuno-histochemistry. Numerous infiltrating lymphocytes and plasma cells in the lamina propria suggested that lesion resolution was partially due to local immunity. Virus was not isolated from retropharyngeal lymph node, mandibular lymph node, tonsil, or residual lesion tissue obtained at necropsy on post-inoculation days 12–15 (Howerth *et al.* 2006).

Management/Treatment

Vesicular stomatitis is a reportable disease. A DNA vaccine that expressed the glycoprotein (G) gene of VSNJV may become a useful tool for control of this disease in cattle and horses (Cantlon *et al.* 2000).

Public health significance

Vesicular stomatitis is a zoonosis similar to foot-and-mouth disease that can likewise affect humans with similar clinical manifestations, in which the presence of aphthae is highly suggestive (López-Sánchez *et al.* 2003).

EASTERN EQUINE ENCEPHALOMYELITIS VIRUS

Family Togaviridae/Genus Alphavirus: linear positive-sense, single-stranded RNA

Definition/Overview

An acute, rapidly progressive, fatal neurological disease can be caused by eastern equine encephalomyelitis virus (EEEV) (Peters & Dalrymple 1990). The transmission of the virus is by mosquitoes to vertebrates and back to mosquitoes. In wild and domestic birds, rodents, and primates, the virus induces transient viraemia without clinical signs. However, EEEV causes clinical disease in horses, deer, swine, and humans, which are presumed to be dead-end hosts. Transmission occurs throughout the year in subtropical areas. The overwintering mechanism for EEEV is unknown (Peters & Dalrymple 1990, Weaver et al. 1991).

Aetiology

The equine encephalomyelitis viruses (EEVs) are members of the genus Alphavirus, in the family Togaviridae. Three main virus serogroups represented by western (WEEV), eastern (EEEV) and Venezuelan equine encephalomyelitis (VEEV) viruses cause epizootic and enzootic infection of horses throughout the western hemisphere. All EEVs are transmitted through the bite of an infected mosquito (Roehrig 1993). It is important to note the distinction between four genetic lineages: one that circulates in North America (NA EEEV) and the Caribbean, and three that circulate in Central and South America (SA EEEV) (Brault et al. 1999, Arrigo et al. 2010). Estimates of time since divergence vary widely depending upon the sequences used, with NA and SA EEEV diverging ca. 922 to 4,856 years ago and the two main SA EEEV lineages diverging ca. 577 to 2,927 years ago. The single, monophyletic NA EEEV lineage exhibits mainly temporally associated relationships and is highly conserved throughout its geographic range. In contrast, SA EEEV comprises three divergent lineages, two consisting of highly conserved geographic groupings that completely lack temporal associations. A phylogenetic comparison of SA EEEV and VEEV demonstrated similar genetic and evolutionary patterns, consistent with the well-documented use of mammalian reservoir hosts by VEEV (Arrigo et al. 2010).

North American strains of EEEV are considered to be more virulent than South American strains of EEEV, which are rarely associated with human illness (Scott & Weaver 1989). Members of the genus Alphavirus have a spherical, enveloped virion 60–65 nm in diameter and possess a single-stranded, positive-sense RNA genome of over 11,000 nucleotides in length (Johnston & Peters 1996). It has been suggested that NA and SA EEEV should be reclassified as distinct species in the EEEV complex (Arrigo et al. 2010).

Epidemiology

The natural transmission cycles of WEEV and EEEV involve a variety of mosquito and avian species. Unusually, WEEV and EEEV can be transmitted from avian hosts to equines, free-ranging white-tailed deer, and humans, which are presumed to be dead-end hosts (Johnston & Peters 1996, Schmitt et al. 2007). The majority of EEEV activity has occurred in the Eastern USA (Johnston & Peters 1996, Larkin 2010) and Canada (Chénier et al. 2010) within the geographic range of *Culiseta melanura*, the primary mosquito vector of NA EEEV (Johnston & Peters 1996). Seroprevalence against EEE virus was 47% for horses during the 1980 epizootic in Michigan (McLean et al. 1985).

Pathophysiology

As an arbovirus it is transmitted by arthropods. Following replication at the site of infection and haematogenous spread it may cross the blood–brain barrier, causing encephalitis.

NA EEEV-infected common marmoset (*Callithrix jacchus*) either died or were euthanized due to neurological signs, but SA EEEV-infected animals remained healthy and survived. The latter infected animals developed viraemia in contrast to the NA EEEV-infected animals. In contrast, virus was detected in the brain, liver, and muscle of the NA EEEV-infected animals only (Adams et al. 2008).

Incubation period

Not established in the equine species yet, but perhaps 3 days as reported in Venezuelan equine encephalomyelitis (Fine et al. 2007).

Clinical presentation

Clinical signs show a spectrum of disease ranging from inapparent/subclinical to acute (lethal) encephalitis. No pathognomonic clinical signs distinguish EEEV from either WEEV or VEEV infection. The overall incidence of eastern equine encephalomyelitis was estimated as 17%, with a case-fatality rate of 61% during the 1981 epizootic in Argentina (Sabattini *et al.* 1991). Following recovery, residual neurological signs are sometimes seen as sequelae.

Differential diagnosis

The differential diagnosis predominantly includes various causes of acute neurological disease (see p. 262).

Diagnosis

No pathognomonic clinical signs distinguish EEEV from either WEEV or VEEV infection. Definitive diagnosis of the disease requires serology and/or virus isolation from blood and CSF. Traditionally, the identification of alphaviruses from mosquitoes and vertebrate tissues was achieved by inoculation of cell culture or suckling mouse brain, followed by identification of an isolate by IFAs. However, while these methods are reliable, they are also time-consuming and cannot be used in laboratories that do not have cell culture or animal use capabilities (Lambert *et al.* 2003). Nucleic acid sequence-based amplification (NASBA), standard RT-PCR, and TaqMan nucleic acid amplification assays are valid for the rapid detection of NA EEEV RNA. The standard RT-PCR assay for the detection of NA EEEV RNA detected <1 plaque-forming unit (PFU) of virus, whereas the NASBA and TaqMan assays were 10 times more sensitive, detecting <0.1 PFU of virus (Lambert *et al.* 2003). Furthermore, specific (including all known alphavirus species) and sensitive RT-PCR assays have been developed for the detection of EEEV, WEEV, and VEEV (Linssen *et al.* 2000). EEEV may also be isolated from the intestine and detected by DNA *in situ* hybridization (Poonacha *et al.* 1998).

Pathology

The primary lesions of EEEV infection in the horse are limited to the grey matter of brain and spinal cord, and consist of widespread areas of perivascular lymphomonocytic cuffing, focal areas of necrosis, neutrophilic infiltration, haemorrhage, neuronal degeneration, and microgliosis. Intestinal lesions in addition to changes in the CNS were found in a 6-month-old male Tennessee Walking horse. Microscopic lesions in the small intestine were mainly in the muscular layer and consisted of multifocal areas of myonecrosis and lymphomonocytic infiltration, with a few focal areas

of mild fibrous connective tissue proliferation. Occasional focal mild perivascular lymphocytic infiltration was observed in the submucosa. Hepatic changes consisted of periportal lymphocytic infiltration and mild vacuolar degeneration of hepatocytes. However, association with inadequate inactivation of vaccine virus could not be excluded (Poonacha *et al.* 1998).

Management/Treatment

Treatment of diseased horses is supportive. Control can be achieved by vector control and vaccination. Cross-protective immunity between EEEV or WEEV and VEEV has been demonstrated. Challenge infection with an equine pathogenic (epizootic) strain of VEEV produced 40% mortality in WEEV-seropositive equids, whereas all EEEV-seropositive equids survived (Walton *et al.* 1989). Inactivated vaccines are used to prevent equine infections with EEEV (Roehrig 1993). Of the horses given annual vaccination with bivalent WEEV and EEEV, 57% retained detectable serum neutralizing (SN) antibody titres for VEEV 18 months after the initial VEEV vaccination was given. In horses previously vaccinated against WEEV–EEEV and VEEV, the best SN antibody response to VEEV revaccination occurred when VEEV vaccine was given simultaneously with the bivalent WEEV–EEEV vaccine (Vanderwagen *et al.* 1975). Significant EEEV-specific antibody responses were generated over the entire period of 6 months by vaccines using different adjuvant preparations (carbopol and squalene/surfactants, respectively). However, the carbopol-based EEEV vaccine was most effective (Holmes *et al.* 2006).

Public health significance

EEEV produces the most severe human arboviral disease in North America (Adams *et al.* 2008). Surveillance for the presence of NA EEEV and WEEV in vector mosquitoes is used to assess the risk of epizootic and epidemic activity. Public health efforts include mosquito control programs and education campaigns that can be implemented to decrease the likelihood of virus transmission to vulnerable vertebrate hosts (Lambert *et al.* 2003).

WESTERN EQUINE ENCEPHALOMYELITIS VIRUS

Family Togaviridae/Genus Alphavirus: linear positive-sense, single-stranded RNA

Definition/Overview

An acute, rapidly progressive neurological disease of horses and humans (presumed to be dead-end hosts), caused by western equine encephalomyelitis virus (WEEV) transmitted through the bite of an infected mosquito.

Aetiology

The EEVs are members of the genus Alphavirus, in the family Togaviridae. Three main virus serogroups represented by western (WEEV), eastern (EEEV), and Venezuelan equine encephalomyelitis (VEEV) viruses cause epizootic and enzootic infection of horses throughout the western hemisphere. All EEVs are transmitted through the bite of an infected mosquito (Roehrig 1993). Members of the genus Alphavirus have a spherical, enveloped virion 60–65 nm in diameter and possess a single-stranded, positive-sense RNA genome of over 11,000 nucleotides in length (Johnston & Peters 1996).

Epidemiology

The natural transmission cycles of WEEV and EEEV involve a variety of mosquito and avian species. Unusually, WEEV and EEEV can be transmitted from avian hosts to equines and humans, which are presumed to be dead-end hosts (Johnston & Peters 1996). The majority of WEEV activity has occurred in the western USA, where *Culex tarsalis* is the primary mosquito vector of WEEV (Johnston & Peters 1996, Janousek & Kramer 1998). *C. tarsalis* can travel distances of 1250–1350 km in 18–24 h at heights up to 1.5 km with temperatures greater than or equal to 13°C. Landing takes place where the warm southerly winds meet cold fronts associated with rain (Sellers & Maarouf 1988). A WEEV seroprevalence of 1.2% (EEEV 6.7%) has been reported in equines of the Brazilian Pantanal area, where undiagnosed horse deaths are frequently observed (Iversson *et al.* 1993). One epizootic cycle of WEEV was illustrated as follows: pre-epizootic silence (1977–1980), epizootic (1982–1983), and residual focus plus inapparent infections during the post-epizootic period (1983–1986) (Aviles *et al.* 1993).

Pathophysiology

As an arbovirus it is transmitted by arthropods. Following replication at the site of infection and haematogenous spread it may cross the blood–brain barrier causing encephalitis. For WEEV, the viraemia level usually correlates with the strain virulence in each animal host (Bianchi *et al.* 1997).

Incubation period

Not established in the equine species yet, but perhaps 3 days as reported in VEEV (Fine *et al.* 2007).

Clinical presentation

Clinical signs show a spectrum of disease ranging from subclinical to acute (lethal) encephalitis. No pathognomonic clinical signs distinguish WEEV from either EEEV, VEEV, or Highlands J virus (HJV) (Karabatsos *et al.* 1988) infections. Many horses develop subclinical infections (Potter *et al.* 1977). Following recovery, residual neurological signs are sometimes seen as sequelae.

Differential diagnosis

The differential diagnosis predominantly includes various causes of acute neurological disease (see p. 262).

Diagnosis

No pathognomonic clinical signs distinguish WEEV from either VEEV or EEEV infection. Definitive diagnosis of the disease requires serology (Calisher *et al.* 1986) and/or virus isolation from blood and CSF. Traditionally, the identification of alphaviruses from mosquitoes and vertebrate tissues was achieved by inoculation of cell culture or suckling mouse brain followed by identification of an isolate by IFAs. However, while these methods are reliable, they are also time-consuming and cannot be used in laboratories that do not have cell culture or animal use capabilities (Lambert *et al.* 2003). Serological tests confirmed infection in 44% (haemagglutination-inhibition), 56% (complement-fixation), and 80% (neutralizing antibody) of WEEV infected horses. Use of the latter test as an adjunct to the HI and CF tests increased the likelihood of serological confirmation to 92% (Calisher *et al.* 1983).

Nucleic acid sequence-based amplification, standard RT-PCR, and TaqMan nucleic acid amplification assays are valid for the rapid detection of WEEV RNA. The standard RT-PCR assay for the detection of WEEV RNA detected <100 PFU of virus, whereas the NASBA assay was 10 times more sensitive, detecting <10 PFU of virus. The TaqMan assay for the detection of WEEV RNA was 100 times more sensitive than the NASBA assay and 1,000 times more sensitive than the standard RT-PCR assay, detecting <0.1 PFU of WEEV (Lambert *et al.* 2003). Furthermore, specific (including all known alphavirus species) and sensitive RT-PCR assays have been developed for the detection of EEEV, WEEV, and VEEV (Linssen *et al.* 2000).

Pathology

Histological lesions are those of a nonsuppurative encephalitis of the cerebral cortex grey matter and include a narrow lymphocytic perivascular cuffing, microgliosis, varying infiltrates of neutrophils, and neuronal degeneration. Endothelial cells may be swollen with intravascular thrombi and perivenular haemorrhages and oedema (Jubb *et al.* 2007).

Management/Treatment

Treatment of diseased horses is supportive. Control can be achieved by vector control and vaccination. Inactivated vaccines are used to prevent equine infections with WEEV (Roehrig 1993). Cross-protective immunity between EEEV, WEEV, and VEEV has been demonstrated. Challenge infection with an equine pathogenic (epizootic) strain of VEEV produced 40% mortality in WEEV-seropositive equids, whereas all EEEV-seropositive equids survived (Walton *et al.* 1989). In addition, the serological response of previously vaccinated horses to revaccination against EEEV and WEEV showed variable results to each antigen. Geometric mean titres peaked 2 weeks after revaccination and were significantly increased from before revaccination. However, some horses had low or undetectable antibody titres 6 months after vaccination, whereas some horses did not develop increasing titres to EEEV or WEEV despite recent vaccination. Regular vaccination against EEEV and WEEV did not interfere with testing for Saint Louis encephalitis virus (Waldridge *et al.* 2003).

Public health significance

Encephalitic alphaviruses, i.e. WEEV, EEEV, VEEV and, more rarely, Ross River virus, Chikungunya virus and HJV, are neuroinvasive and may cause neurological symptoms ranging from mild (e.g. febrile illness) to severe (e.g. encephalitis) in humans (Zacks & Paessler 2010). EEEV produces the most severe human arboviral disease in North America (Adams *et al.* 2008). WEEV might also cause a fatal infection of the CNS in humans. However, neither human vaccine nor antiviral drug is available for WEEV infection (Barabé *et al.* 2007). The incidence of WEEV infection in humans peaked during the mid-20th century and has declined to fewer than 1–2 human cases annually during the past 20 years, associated with ecological factors rather than a decline in virulence (Forrester *et al.* 2008). Surveillance for the presence of NA EEEV and WEEV in vector mosquitoes is used to assess the risk of epizootic and epidemic activity. Public health efforts include mosquito control programs and education campaigns that can be implemented to decrease the likelihood of virus transmission to vulnerable vertebrate hosts (Lambert *et al.* 2003).

VENEZUELAN EQUINE ENCEPHALOMYELITIS VIRUS

Family Togaviridae/Genus Alphavirus: linear positive-sense, single-stranded RNA

Definition/Overview

Venezuelan equine encephalomyelitis (VEE) is an acute (lethal) encephalitis in horses and humans caused by Venezuelan equine encephalomyelitis virus (VEEV) complex strains, opportunistic in their use of mosquito vectors with equines as highly efficient amplification hosts. In contrast to VEEV, both EEEV and WEEV are maintained by a bird/mosquito cycle (Gibbs 1976). VEE is an emerging infectious disease (Sharma & Maheshwari 2009). Horses with a tentative diagnosis of VEE should be isolated to prevent possible human exposure as a high-titre viraemia occurs with VEEV in the horse (Gibbs 1976).

Aetiology

The EEVs are members of the genus Alphavirus, in the family Togaviridae. Three main virus serogroups represented by western (WEEV), eastern (EEEV) and VEEV cause epizootic and enzootic infection of horses throughout the western hemisphere. All EEVs are transmitted through the bite of an infected mosquito (Roehrig 1993).

Of the New World alphaviruses, VEEV is the most important human and equine pathogen (Weaver et al. 2004b). Togaviruses are small, enveloped RNA viruses. The VEEV complex now comprises 14 subtypes and varieties and includes seven different virus species (van Regenmortel et al. 2000). Genetic studies imply that mutations in the E2 envelope glycoprotein gene are major determinants of adaptation to both equines and mosquito vectors (Weaver et al. 2004a). A small number of envelope gene mutations can generate an equine amplification-competent, epizootic VEEV from an enzootic progenitor, which underscores the limitations of small animal models for evaluating and predicting the epizootic phenotype (Greene et al. 2005). RNA viruses including alphaviruses exhibit high mutation frequencies. Therefore, ecological and epidemiological factors probably constrain the frequency of VEE epidemics more than the generation, via mutation, of amplification-competent (high equine viraemia) virus strains (Anishchenko et al. 2006).

Epidemiology

VEEV has caused periodic outbreaks of febrile and neurological disease primarily in Latin America. Epizootic subtype IAB and IC viruses may be more virulent for both humans and equines. A feature common to all major outbreaks is the role of equines as highly efficient amplification hosts. Although the vertebrate host range of epizootic VEEV strains is wide and includes humans, sheep, dogs, bats, rodents (e.g. *Liomys salvini*, *Oligoryzomys fulvescens*, *Oryzomys couesi*, and *Sigmodon hispidus*), and some birds, major epidemics in the absence of equine cases have never occurred. Although epizootic VEEV strains are opportunistic in their use of mosquito vectors, the most widespread outbreaks appear to involve specific adaptation to the black salt marsh mosquito (*Ochlerotatus taeniorhynchus*), the most common vector in many coastal areas. In contrast, enzootic VEEV strains are highly specialized and appear to utilize vectors exclusively in the Spissipes section of the *Culex* (*Melanoconion*) subgenus (Weaver et al. 2004b, Deardorff et al. 2009).

Follow-up after the major 1995 VEE epizootic/epidemic in Western Venezuela revealed natural post-epizootic persistence of genetically stable subtype virus strains (Navarro et al. 2005).

Pathophysiology

As an arbovirus it is transmitted by arthropods. Following replication at the site of infection and haematogenous spread it may cross the blood–brain barrier causing encephalitis. The mechanisms underlying the host immune response to VEEV infection in the brain are not fully understood. The upregulation of Toll-like receptors and associated signalling genes following VEEV infection of the brain has important implications for how VEEV induces inflammation and neurodegeneration (Sharma & Maheshwari 2009). Furthermore, VEEV capsid protein inhibits nuclear import in mammalian but not in mosquito cells (Atasheva et al. 2008).

Incubation period

Horses challenged SC with VEE Trinidad donkey strain became viraemic and showed classical signs of VEE beginning on day 3 post-inoculation (Fine et al. 2007).

Clinical presentation

In equines, VEEV causes a spectrum of disease ranging from subclinical to acute (lethal) encephalitis. Clinical signs include fever, tachycardia, depression, and anorexia. Most animals go on to develop encephalitis 5–10 days after infection, with signs of circling, ataxia, pruritis, and hyperexcitability. Death usually occurs about 1 week after experimental infection. Encephalitis and death correlate with the magnitude of equine viraemia, but even equine avirulent enzootic strains produce lethal encephalitis when inoculated intracerebrally (Walton et al. 1973, Johnson & Martin 1974, Gibbs 1976, Wang et al. 2001, Weaver et al. 2004a, Finc et al. 2007). Equine mortality rates during epizootics have been estimated at 19–83% (Johnson & Martin 1974). In 1993, a VEEV (subtype IE) outbreak of encephalitis among equids in coastal Chiapas, Mexico, resulted in a 50% case-fatality rate (Deardorff et al. 2009). Following recovery, residual neurological signs are sometimes seen as sequelae.

Differential diagnosis

The differential diagnosis predominantly includes various causes of acute neurological disease (see p. 262).

Diagnosis

No pathognomonic clinical signs distinguish VEEV from either WEEV or EEEV infection. Definitive diagnosis of the disease requires serology and/or virus isolation from blood and CSF. Specific (including all known alphavirus species) and sensitive RT-PCR assays have been developed for the detection of EEEV, WEEV, and VEEV (Linssen et al. 2000). Chimaeric viruses have been produced efficiently in cell culture and were as effective as the parental virus for identifying infection in humans, horses, and rodents in serological assays, e.g. PRNT, HI assay, and CF test, thereby not requiring bio-safety level 3 facilities (Ni et al. 2007).

Pathology

Pathology reveals oedema and haemorrhage of the CNS, with similar histological lesions to WEEV and EEEV of a nonsuppurative encephalitis of the cerebral cortex grey matter with neuronal degeneration (Jubb et al. 2007).

Management/Treatment

Horses with a tentative diagnosis of VEE should be isolated to prevent possible human exposure. Treatment of diseased horses is supportive. Control can be achieved by vector control and vaccination (Baker et al. 1978, Weaver et al. 2004b). Currently, both live and inactivated versions of a live-attenuated strain (TC-83) are used to vaccinate equines. The live-attenuated version (Baker et al. 1978, Ferguson et al. 1978) is far superior in areas of Latin America at high risk for VEE outbreaks owing to the faster and longer lasting immunity elicited (probably lifetime) (Weaver et al. 2004a). In addition, a new live-attenuated virus (V3526) derived by site-directed mutagenesis from a virulent clone intended for human use in protection against VEEV has been shown to be safe and efficacious in protecting horses (Fine et al. 2007). However, pre-existing antibody to EEEV and/or WEEV may modify or interfere with infection by VEEV (Calisher et al. 1973).

Public health significance

One of the largest VEE epizootics and epidemics on record, involving an estimated 75,000–100,000 people associated with an estimated human mortality rate of about 0.5%, occurred in 1995 in Venezuela and Colombia (Weaver et al. 1996). VEEV represents a continuous public health threat in the USA. It has the ability to cause fatal disease in humans and in horses and other domestic animals (Atasheva et al. 2008).

GETAH VIRUS and ROSS RIVER VIRUS: ROSS RIVER VIRUS and SAGIYAMA VIRUS

Family Togaviridae/Genus Alphavirus: linear positive-sense, single-stranded RNA

Definition/Overview

These viruses cause an acute febrile disease associated with limb oedema and urticarial rashes, especially caused by Getah virus.

Aetiology

Getah virus is an RNA virus and a member of the Alphavirus genus of the family Togaviridae. It is maintained in a cycle between mosquitoes and various vertebrate hosts (Marchette *et al.* 1978). Sagiyama virus and Ross River virus (RRV) are other members of the Alphavirus genus (Kumanomido *et al.* 1988, Jones *et al.* 2010). The difference in the capsid region is a useful marker in the genetic classification of Sagiyama virus and strains of Getah virus, and might be responsible for the serological difference in the CF test. The genomic differences among the Getah virus strains are due to time factor rather than geographical distribution (Wekesa *et al.* 2001).

Epidemiology

Getah virus is widely distributed in Southeast Asia (Brown & Timoney 1998). Seroepizootiological studies indicate that the virus ranges from Eurasia to Southeast and far Eastern Asia, the Pacific islands, and Australasia (Fukunaga *et al.* 2000). A seroprevalence of 17% has been reported in Indian horses (Brown & Timoney 1998). Serological surveys of the equine population in Japan revealed that while up to 53% of horses in some areas had been infected with the virus, the incidence of clinical disease had been much lower (Imagawa *et al.* 1981, Matsamura *et al.* 1982). Horses are unlikely to be efficient amplifiers of RRV and do little to incriminate it as an important pathogen (Kay *et al.* 1987).

Pathophysiology

Most likely due to vasculitis associated with viral infection.

Incubation period

Horses challenged experimentally with Sagiyama virus developed fever within 2–6 days for 2–6 days duration (Kumanomido *et al.* 1988). With RRV, only one of 11 horses inoculated either by intravenous injection or by the bite of *Culex annulirostris* or *Aedes vigilax* mosquitoes infected orally developed a viraemia detectable by inoculation of suckling mice, but five horses contained virus sufficient to infect 41/383 *Culex* that fed on them 3–4 days after inoculation. On primary inoculation with RRV, only two horses developed haemagglutination inhibition (HI) antibody but late responses occurred in three horses following probable naturally acquired reinfections. Most horses remained normal, although some developed mild pyrexia and transient clinical signs (Kay *et al.* 1987).

Clinical presentation

Clinical signs include depression, anorexia, pyrexia (up to 40.0°C), urticarial rashes, oedema in the hindlimbs, and enlargement of the submandibular lymph nodes (Sentsui & Kono 1980, Kumanomido *et al.* 1988) associated with lymphocytopenia (Kumanomido *et al.* 1988, Brown & Timoney 1998). Also reported are mild abdominal pain, scrotal oedema, mild icterus, and stiffness (Brown & Timoney 1998). The morbidity was 38% in one training centre, with 96% of affected horses making a full clinical recovery within 1 week without any significant sequelae (Fukunaga *et al.* 2000).

RRV was associated with clinical signs including petechial haemorrhages, lymphadenopathy, distal limb swelling, and reluctance to move at a time when a known RRV vector, the mosquito *Aedes camptorhynchus* was recorded at very high levels (El-Hage *et al.* 2008).

Differential diagnosis

The differential diagnosis includes various causes of fever and limb oedema (see p. 263).

Diagnosis

Getah virus isolation can be attempted in VERO, RK-13, BHK-21, and many other cell lines as well as in suckling mouse brain. Blood plasma collected from suspect cases of infection at the onset of pyrexia is the specimen of choice. A diagnosis of Getah virus infection can also be confirmed serologically based on testing acute and convalescent phase sera by using SN, CF, HI, and ELISA tests (Fukunaga *et al.* 2000). A specific and analytically sensitive RT-PCR for the detection of RRV is available to confirm the presence of this virus in clinical samples (Studdert *et al.* 2003).

In one study, infected horses developed SN antibody against the homologous strains of Sagiyama virus by day 5 post-inoculation. The maximum titres were observed on day 14 post-inoculation in a range of 1:256–1:1024 (Kumanomido *et al.* 1988).

Pathology

Sagiyama virus has been recovered from nasal discharge, spleen, liver, lung, and various lymph nodes (submandibular, anterior cervical, axillary, splenic, renal, mesenteric, inguinal, and internal iliac) (Kumanomido *et al.* 1988). Getah virus lesions resemble equine viral arteritis.

Management/Treatment

Treatment of diseased animals is supportive. An inactivated Getah virus vaccine is available.

Public health significance

RRV causes epidemic polyarthritis (EPA) in humans (Jones *et al.* 2010).

Chapter 3
Protozoal Diseases

Klossiella equi

Definition/Overview
Rare glomerulonephritis and multifocal non-suppurative interstitial nephritis can be caused by *Klossiella equi* (Marcato 1977).

Aetiology
Klossiella equi is a renal protozoan parasite of equids, including zebras (Suedmeyer *et al.* 2006) and donkeys (Karanja *et al.* 1995). Developmental stages include micro- and macrogametocytes in syzygy (preparing to form gametes), sporonts with multiple (20–30) oval to spindle-shaped beginning sporoblasts within parasitic vacuoles, sporoblasts containing multiple spherical to slightly ovoid 5 μm sporocysts within a sacculated tubular epithelial cell, and a late sporoblast composed of a central spherical structure (15 μm) surrounded by a rosette of 20–30 spindle-shaped structures (10 μm). Both gametogony (sexual) and sporogony (asexual) stages can be seen. However, the definitive life cycle of *Klossiella equi* is still unknown (Anderson & Picut 1988).

Epidemiology
Not established yet.

Pathophysiology
Renal pathology probably due to parasite development within kidney cells (**240–246**).

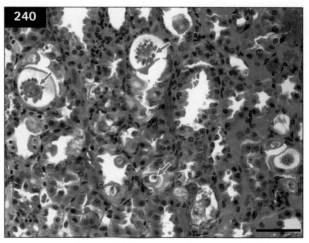

240 Renal coccidiosis. Multifocal tubulonecrosis and lymphoplasmacytic interstitial nephritis. Located within the renal tubular epithelial cells are the various developmental stages and forms of an apicomplexan coccidian parasite (arrows). The tubular epithelium shows swelling and exfoliation due to degeneration and necrosis. Note the scant associated mononuclear inflammatory infiltrate within the surrounding interstitium. *Klossiella equi*. (H&E stain. Bar 50 μm.)

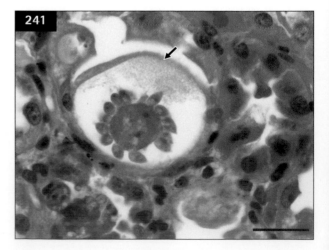

241 Renal coccidiosis. Higher magnification of a large intraepithelial sporont located within a pale parasitophorous vacuole displaying the typical outer radiating budding formation of sporoblasts. Note the severe hypertrophied swollen infected epithelial cell strained into forming a thin enveloping rim of cytoplasm that bulges in the tubule lumen (arrow). *Klossiella equi*. (H&E stain. Bar 20 μm.)

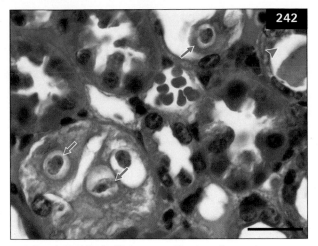

242 Renal coccidiosis. Higher magnification of several intraepithelial trophozoites (arrows) and a microgamete (arrowhead) each surrounded by a parasitophorous vacuole located in the cytoplasm of medium hypertrophied tubular epithelial cells. *Klossiella equi*. (H&E stain. Bar 20 μm.)

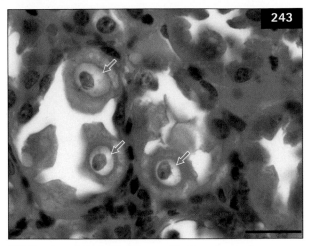

243 Renal coccidiosis. Higher magnification of several intraepithelial trophozoites (arrows), each of which contains a faint excentric basophilic nucleus. *Klossiella equi*. (H&E stain. Bar 20 μm.)

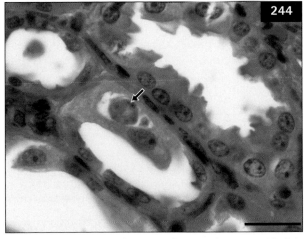

244 Renal coccidiosis. Higher magnification of an intraepithelial developing schizont containing several faint basophilic merozoites (arrow). Note the swollen adjacent nucleus of the infected host cell. *Klossiella equi*. (H&E stain. Bar 20 μm.)

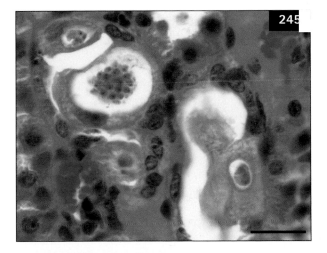

245 Renal coccidiosis. Higher magnification of an intraepithelial cluster of sporoblasts each containing developing multinucleated sporocysts (top left). On the bottom right a macrogamete is present. *Klossiella equi*. (H&E stain. Bar 20 μm.)

246 Renal coccidiosis. Higher magnification of intraepithelial free sporoblasts containing sporocysts with several basophilic dot-like nuclei. *Klossiella equi*. (H&E stain. Bar 20 μm.)

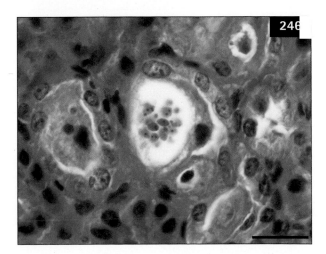

Incubation period

Not established in the equine species yet.

Clinical presentation

Clinical signs reported in a 25-year-old mixed-breed pony gelding were weight loss, hirsutism, polyuria, and polydipsia of 6 months' duration. As pituitary pars intermedia adenoma (PPIA) was detected at necropsy it is impossible to differentiate between signs attributed either to equine Cushing's disease or to *K. equi* infection (Anderson & Picut 1988).

Differential diagnosis

The differential diagnosis includes various causes of polyuria and polydipsia (see p. 263).

Diagnosis

Urinalysis might reveal multiple sporocytes (Reinemeyer *et al.* 1983, Reppas & Collins 1995).

Pathology

Necropsy reveals tubular nephrosis and multifocal nonsuppurative interstitial nephritis associated with infiltration of lymphocytes and plasma cells (Anderson & Picut 1988).

Management/Treatment

Treatment of diseased animals is supportive.

Public health significance

Not convincing yet.

Sarcocystis neurona/Neospora hughesi: EQUINE PROTOZOAL MYELOENCEPHALITIS (EPM)

Definition/Overview

Equine protozoal myeloencephalitis (EPM) is a neurological disease of horses, ponies, and sea otters (Sundar *et al.* 2008) caused by infection of the CNS with protozoan parasites. EPM due to *Sarcocystis neurona* infection is one of the most common neurological diseases in horses in the USA (Witonsky *et al.* 2008).

Aetiology

Myeloencephalitis is caused by *Sarcocystis neurona* or *Neospora hughesi* (Marsh *et al.* 1996, Wobeser *et al.* 2009) with opossums (*Didelphis virginiana*) being the definitive host for *S. neurona*.

Sarcocystis spp. (**247**) exhibit a heteroxenous life cycle in which merogony takes place in endothelial tissues of the intermediate host and gametogony takes place in the intestinal epithelium of the definitive host (Granstrom *et al.* 1994, Mullaney *et al.* 2005). Unlike *S. neurona*, *Neospora* spp. can form tissue cysts, and it has been suggested that because of this tissue cyst stage, the parasite would remain refractory to treatment (Marsh *et al.* 1996).

Epidemiology

The disease has not been reported among horses originating outside the western hemisphere (Fayer *et al.* 1990). In *Sarcocystis* spp., the intermediate hosts are usually herbivores that acquire the infection by ingesting sporulated oocysts or sporocysts. Opossums (*Didelphis* spp.) are the definitive host for the protozoan parasite *S. neurona*. Opossums shed sporocysts in faeces that can be ingested by true intermediate hosts (cats, raccoons, skunks, armadillos, and sea otters). Horses acquire the parasite by ingestion of feed or water contaminated by opossum faeces. Recently it has been stated that the horse also has the potential to act as intermediate host (Mullaney *et al.* 2005) and that cats may play a role in the natural epidemiology of EPM (Cohen *et al.* 2007). It is clear that diverse intermediate hosts share a common infection source, the opossum (*D. virginiana*) (Sundar *et al.* 2008).

Pathophysiology

Parasitaemia with *S. neurona* has been demonstrated in an immunocompetent horse (Rossano *et al.* 2005). In accord, infected horses had significantly decreased proliferation responses as soon as 2 days post-infection (Witonsky *et al.* 2008). However, it has been shown that infection of immunodeficient horses with *S. neurona* does not result in

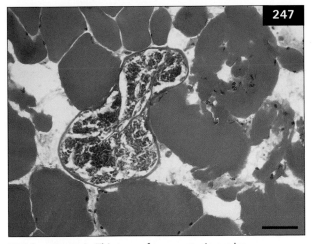

247 Sarcocystosis. This type of sarcocystosis can be encountered in equine skeletal musculature; it has no relation to EPM. Depicted is an end-stage sarcocystis cyst; it is thin walled and contains myriads of banana-shaped bradyzoites. They rarely cause any significant tissue reaction or clinical disease. Two species of sarcocystis are recognized in the horse, *S. bertrami* (*equicanis*) and *S. fayeri*, the dog being the intermediate host of both. *Sarcocystis* sp. (H&E stain. Bar 20 µm.)

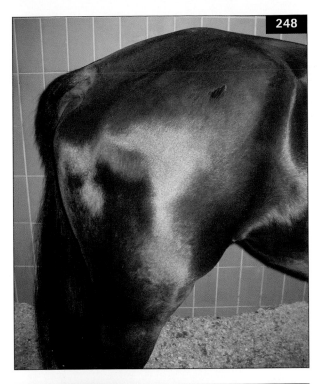

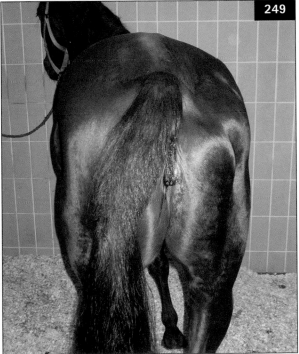

248, 249 Equine protozoal myeloencephalitis might be associated with asymmetrical signs like right gluteal muscle atrophy as seen in a 12-year-old Warmblood mare.

neurological disease (Sellon *et al.* 2004). On the other hand, the use of corticosteroids resulted in milder clinical signs than in horses inoculated with sporocysts without corticosteroid treatment, suggesting an immunopathological component to EPM (Saville *et al.* 2001).

Merozoites multiply in neurons, leucocytes and vascular endothelial cells of the CNS resulting in perivascular mononuclear cell infiltration and necrosis of the neuropil (Granstrom *et al.* 1994, Mullaney *et al.* 2005).

Incubation period
The incubation period is as short as 7–9 days (Saville *et al.* 2001, Elitsur *et al.* 2007).

Clinical presentation
Although EPM has been reported in ponies, donkeys, and most horse breeds, the greatest incidence is among Thoroughbreds, Standardbreds, and Quarter Horses. Age was most strongly associated with disease risk, with horses usually being at least 6 months old when first diagnosed with EPM (MacKay *et al.* 1992, Morley *et al.* 2008). Neurological examination findings that support a diagnosis of EPM include evidence of multifocal disease, evidence of lesions affecting both upper and lower motor neurons, muscle atrophy, or presence of asymmetric neurological signs (**248, 249**).

However, EPM has also been diagnosed in horses with symmetric signs referable to a single focus of CNS disease. Less commonly, presenting complaints can also include signs referable to brain or brainstem disease (**250**) (Furr *et al.* 2002).

Differential diagnosis
It can be difficult to distinguish EPM from West Nile viral encephalomyelitis on the basis of clinical signs. However, in contrast to horses with EPM, most horses with West Nile viral encephalomyelitis appear to have abnormal CSF cytological findings, which include a moderate mononuclear pleocytosis with increased protein concentration (Furr *et al.* 2002).

Diagnosis
Ante-mortem diagnosis is considered presumptive, as definitive diagnosis requires post-mortem examination and confirmation of *S. neurona* infection via microscopic identification, immunohistochemistry, culture, or PCR. Specialists appear to agree that the diagnosis should be the presence of compatible neurological signs and the exclusion of other potential diseases. The diagnosis must always be considered tentative in the living horse (Furr *et al.* 2002). Because some horses might not develop a vigorous antibody response to *S. neurona*, these results could be consistent with a diagnosis of EPM in some horses. A favourable response to treatment, especially when subsequently followed by a relapse of similar signs, is also supportive of a diagnosis of EPM in the living horse (Furr *et al.* 2002). However, the use of polyvalent (surface antigens) SnSAG ELISAs (Yeargan & Howe 2011) and subsequent calculation of the antibody index (AI) and C-value (Furr *et al.* 2011) might enhance the reliability of serological testing for *S. neurona* infection, which should lead to improved diagnosis of EPM.

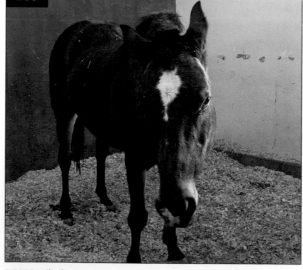

250 Vestibular ataxia associated with equine protozoal myeloencephalitis. (Courtesy of Dr M. Aleman, University of California, Davis, USA.)

Furthermore, it should be noted that 29% of CSF samples from horses seropositive to *S. neurona* are negative. A negative CSF Western blot test result provides valuable information for the veterinarian and client, who could thereby pursue further diagnostic evaluation of other neurological diseases and potentially avoid paying for costly, unnecessary antiprotozoal medication. As a consequence, this supports the practice of testing CSF of seropositive horses suspected of having EPM (Rossano *et al.* 2003).

A diagnosis of EPM associated with *N. hughesi* can be made on the basis of the presence of gait abnormalities or ataxia, elimination of other causes of neurological disease, and a positive (>5) CSF indirect fluorescent antibody test (IFAT) to *N. hughesi* with minimal blood contamination (Finno *et al.* 2007). There is no cross-reactivity of the IFAT for *N. hughesi* with antibodies against *S. neurona* (Packham *et al.* 2002). Furthermore, blood contamination of CSF appears to have a more detrimental effect on Western blot testing than on IFAT testing. Either Western blot or IFAT on an uncontaminated CSF sample is appropriate if high sensitivity (and therefore high negative predictive value) is desired, whereas if high specificity (and therefore high positive predictive value) is desired, the IFAT may be the better choice (Johnson 2008). Random amplified polymorphic DNA assay differentiated *S. neurona* from *S. cruzi* and *S. campestris*, as well as *T. gondii* and five *Eimeria* spp. (Granstrom *et al.* 1994).

Pathology

Gross lesions in protozoal myelo(meningo)-encephalitis consist of multifocal haemorrhages possibly in conjunction with malacia within the brainstem, pons, and spinal cord usually visible on cross-sections. Microscopically, multifocal necro-haemorrhagic areas are seen with gliosis and inflammatory infiltrates composed of gitter cells, lymphocytes, histiocytes, plasma cells, and fewer eosinophilic and neutrophilic granulocytes. The meninges are usually involved. Perivascular mononuclear cuffs admixed with eosinophils are present. The spinal cord white matter may show demyelinating features such as axonal swelling, spheroid formation, and digestion chambers (Jubb *et al.* 2007).

Management/Treatment

Clinical improvement has been shown following treatment of cases of EPM due to *N. hughesi* with ponazuril (5 mg/kg BW PO sid for 30–60 days), an antiprotozoal drug (Finno *et al.* 2007). Other antiprotozoal drugs available to treat EPM are nitazoxanide (25 mg/kg BW PO sid for days 1–5 and 50 mg/kg BW PO sid for days 6–28), and the combination of pyrimethamine (1 mg/kg BW PO sid) and sulfadiazine (20 mg/kg BW PO sid). It should be realized that serum antibody titres with reference to *N. hughesi* are not a reliable indicator of disease progression (Finno *et al.* 2007). Vaccination is used to control EPM, as vaccination with rSnSAG-1 produced antibodies in horses that neutralized *S. neurona* merozoites and significantly reduced clinical signs (Ellison & Witonsky 2009). Furthermore, intermittent administration of ponazuril (at 20 mg/kg BW PO sid every 7 days, but not every 14 days, for 12 weeks) may have application in the prevention of EPM due to *S. neurona* (MacKay *et al.* 2008). Eradication of the sporocysts shed in the faeces of opossums from the environment is an important but difficult part of EPM control.

Public health significance

Not convincing yet.

Cryptosporidium parvum: CRYPTOSPORIDIOSIS

Definition/Overview
Cryptosporidium species are protozoan parasites able to cross host species barriers that cause diarrhoeic disease (cryptosporidiosis) in humans and neonatal animals (Chalmers *et al.* 2005).

Aetiology
Among the enteric equine protozoan parasites (besides *Eimeria leuckarti*, *Giardia*, and *Tritrichomonas* spp.) *Cryptosporidium parvum* is associated with cryptosporidiosis. *C. parvum* is a potentially important pathogen in immunologically normal and normoglobulinaemic equids (Chalmers & Grinberg 2005). While the host range of *C. parvum* genotype 1 (synonymous with *C. hominis*) is largely restricted to humans, genotype 2 has a broad host range including farm animals and man (Fayer *et al.* 2000). The domestic horse was established as a further host of *C. parvum* genotype 2 (Chalmers & Grinberg 2005) subtype VIaA14G2 (Burton *et al.* 2010). In addition, foal *C. parvum* isolates were genetically diverse, markedly similar to human and bovine isolates, and carried GP60 IIaA18G3R1 alleles, indicating a zoonotic potential (Grinberg *et al.* 2008).

Epidemiology
Asymptomatic carriage can occur, but even small numbers of oocysts shed in faeces can pose a health risk to humans and animals alike, since the infectious dose is low and the organism can survive in the environment (Dupont *et al.* 1995). *Cryptosporidium* infection rates of 15–31% have been reported in foals in Ohio and Kentucky, USA. Chronological study of infection in 35 healthy foals showed that foals started to excrete *Cryptosporidium* oocysts between 4 and 19 weeks of age. The cumulative infection rate of *Cryptosporidium* in foals was 71%. Some foals were concurrently infected with both *Cryptosporidium* and *Giardia* and excretion of oocysts or cysts was intermittent and long lasting.

The longest duration of excretion was 14 weeks for *Cryptosporidium*. Excretion of *Cryptosporidium* oocysts stopped before weaning and infected foals were deemed the major source of *Giardia* infection in foals (Xiao & Herd 1994). Furthermore, the prevalence of *Cryptosporidium* species in mid-Wales was higher in foals (6% positive symptomless foals) compared with older horses (0%) (Chalmers *et al.* 2005). In comparison, the estimated maximum true prevalence of faecal shedding of *C. parvum* was 2.3% in horses used in the backcountry, USA (Atwill *et al.* 2000), 18% of faecal specimens from foals in New Zealand (Grinberg *et al.* 2009), and 8% for *Cryptosporidium* in Italy. Distribution of *Cryptosporidium* prevalence was statistically related to farms and age of animals, but was unrelated to the presence of diarrhoea. Risk factors for shedding included residence farms and age older than 8 weeks (Veronesi *et al.* 2010).

Pathophysiology
The oocysts of *Cryptosporidia* spp. sporulate within the enteric host cell thereby causing maldigestion and malabsorption leading to diarrhoea.

Incubation period
Not established in the equine species yet.

Clinical presentation
Cryptosporidium-positive foals were significantly older (13–40 days, median age of 28 days) than negative foals (4–67 days, median 18 days). The number of foals with diarrhoea or soft faeces was not significantly different between positive and negative foals (Burton *et al.* 2010). It should be realized that *C. parvum* oocysts can be found in the faeces of foals without clinical signs. On the other hand, the protozoan parasite is associated with self-limiting diarrhoea in foals ranging in age from 5 days to 6 weeks (Gajadhar *et al.* 1985).

Differential diagnosis
The differential diagnosis includes various causes of diarrhoea in foals (see p. 262). Overall, *C. perfringens*, rotavirus, and large numbers of *Cryptosporidium* spp. or *S. westeri* were isolated from 80% of foals with diarrhoea without statistical interactions between any of the pathogens associated with diarrhoea (Netherwood *et al.* 1996).

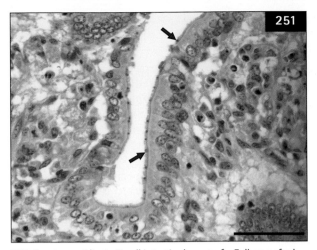

251 Cryptosporidiosis. Small intestinal crypt of a Fell pony foal (suffering from the congenital immunocompromising Fell pony syndrome rendering it susceptible to opportunistic infections) contains several small pale basophilic dot-like apicomplexan coccidian organisms attached to the enterocyte microvillous brush border (arrows). *Cryptosporidium parvum*. (H&E stain. Bar 50 μm.)

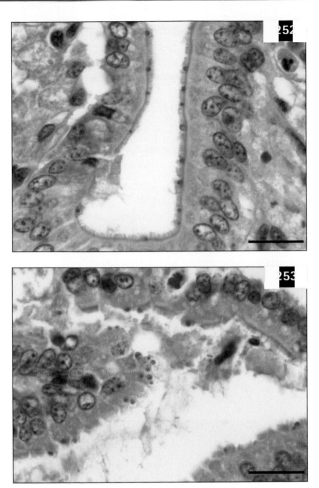

252, 253 Cryptosporidiosis. Higher magnifications of the small intestine crypt with several developing stages of cryptosporidia embedded in the microvillous border. These protozoa are located extracytoplasmically yet are intracellular, enclosed by a host's parasitophorous vacuole. Slight differences in diameter (ranging from 2–6 μm) and internal structures can only just be observed in these light microscopic photographs. *Cryptosporidium parvum*. (H&E stain. Bar 20 μm.)

Diagnosis

The oocysts can be detected in the faeces by microscopic examination following Ziehl–Neelsen staining. However, the use of microscopy on faecal samples during diagnosis permits identification only to the genus level, since many species are morphologically similar. The application of molecular tools (mainly investigation of polymorphisms within various genes by PCR and restriction enzyme digestion, and DNA sequence analysis) has enabled identification of the infecting species/genotype (Chalmers & Grinberg 2005). Furthermore, use of loop-mediated isothermal DNS amplification (LAMP) is proposed as an efficient and effective tool for epidemiological survey studies including screening of healthy animals in which *Cryptosporidium* oocyst shedding is characteristically low and probably below the detection limit of PCR in conventional sample concentrates (Bakheit *et al.* 2008).

In comparison, on direct immunofluorescence assay, 7.4% of foal samples and 1.7% of mare samples were designated positive for *Cryptosporidium* spp., whereas on small-subunit rRNA-based PCR 5.1% of foal samples were positive (Burton *et al.* 2010).

Pathology

On histological examination organisms are generally encountered in the distal portion of the small intestine, where they are associated with villous atrophy (villous blunting and fusion) and compensatory crypt hyperplasia. Mild mixed inflammatory hypercellularity can be observed in the associated mucosal lamina propria (**251–253**).

Management/Treatment

Treatment of diseased horses (254) is supportive, as the efficacy of nitazoxanide as a therapeutic agent against *Cryptosporidium* spp. in foals is unknown.

Public health significance

C. parvum has a wide mammalian host range, including humans, for whom exposure to farmed animals is a known risk factor for acquisition of cryptosporidiosis (Hunter *et al.* 2004, Smith *et al.* 2010, Burton *et al.* 2010, Veronesi *et al.* 2010). The average sample prevalence of *Cryptosporidium* infection on farms was highest in cattle, sheep, and pigs (approximately 40–50%), in the mid-range in goats and horses (20–25%), and lowest in rabbits/guinea pigs, chickens, and other birds (approximately 4–7%) (Smith *et al.* 2010).

    C. parvum shed by infected foals may therefore be infectious for man, based on anecdotal data according to which veterinary students acquired cryptosporidiosis following exposure to infected foals (Cohen & Snowden 1997).

254 A lethargic dehydrated diarrhoeic foal due to cryptosporidiosis.

Eimeria leuckarti

Definition/Overview

The equine species is regarded as a natural host of *Eimeria leuckarti*, which predominantly develops in the cytoplasm of hypertrophic host cells in the lamina propria of the small intestine. *E. leuckarti* is considered to be nonpathogenic.

Aetiology

Infection with *Eimeria* species (*E. leuckarti*, *E. solipedum*, and *E. uniungulsti*) is seen worldwide in horses (Barker & Remmer 1972, Hirayama *et al.* 2002). *E. leuckarti* occurs in the small intestine of horses and asses (Soulsby 1968, Barker & Remmer 1972, Hirayama *et al.* 2002). Its oocysts are some of the largest in the genus *Eimeria*, at 80–87.5 × 55–59 μm oval, flattened at the narrower end, the oocyst wall 6.5–7 μm thick, dark brown with distinct micropyle. Sporulation time is 20–22 days at 20°C (Soulsby 1968).

Epidemiology

The prevalence of oocysts of *E. leuckarti* in faeces of foals in central Kentucky ranged from 36 to 100% (Lyons & Tolliver 2004, Lyons *et al.* 2007) compared to 0.5% in adult horses in Brazil (De Souza *et al.* 2009).

Pathophysiology

The gametocytes develop in the cytoplasm of hypertrophic host cells in the lamina propria of the small intestine. It has been suggested that the host cell of *Eimeria* species is possibly derived from intestinal epithelial cells and then displaced into the lamina propria of the small intestine (Hirayama *et al.* 2002). However, *E. leuckarti* is considered to be nonpathogenic.

    Early gametocytes are found in host cells in the lamina propria of villi in the small intestine at 14 days post-inoculation. By 23 days post-inoculation, macrogametes and microgametes can be distinguished microscopically in the host cells. At 28 days post-inoculation, macrogametes start to develop an oocyst wall in the cytoplasm of host cells. As a consequence, the lifespan of host cells parasitized by *E. leuckarti* is at least 28 days, even though the lifespan of normal intestinal epithelial cells may be 2–3 days (Barker & Remmer 1972).

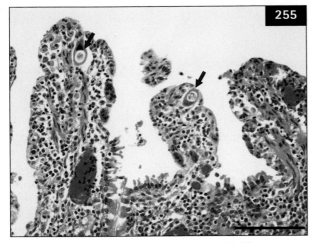

255 Intestinal coccidiosis. Subacute enteritis with villous blunting and enterocyte exfoliation. Intraepithelial protozoal coccidian parasites are present within the superficial lamina propria of the villous tips (arrows). *Eimeria leuckarti*. (H&E stain. Bar 100 μm.)

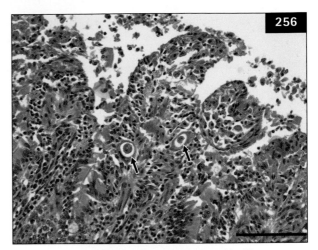

256 Intestinal coccidiosis. Subacute enteritis with villous blunting and enterocyte exfoliation. Two large protozoal coccidian parasites are present within the superficial lamina propria located at the base of the villi (arrows). *Eimeria leuckarti*. (H&E stain. Bar 100 μm.)

Clinical presentation

The true clinical significance of this parasite is poorly understood. The equine species is regarded as the natural host of *E. leuckarti*.

Differential diagnosis

Not appropriate.

Diagnosis

Diagnosis of infection is routinely based on finding the oocysts of *E. leuckarti* in faeces by coprological examination. Furthermore, various stages of *E. leuckarti* can be found in the tips of villi of the duodenum following endoscopically-guided biopsy.

Pathology

Although *Eimeria* organisms at various stages (mainly microgametes and macrogametes) can be found in the cytoplasm of hypertrophied host cells in the lamina propria at the tips of villi of the jejunum and ileum (Hirayama *et al.* 2002), their presence is merely found incidentally during post-mortem examination (**255–259**).

Management/Treatment

Not appropriate yet.

Public health significance

Not convincing yet.

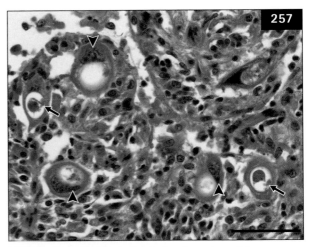

257 Intestinal coccidiosis. Several protozoal coccidian developmental stages present within hypertrophied host cells in the superficial lamina propria. Two medium swollen infected host cells each contain a macrogamete surrounded by a pale parasitophorous vacuole (arrows). Large single vacuoles are present in hypertrophic host enterocytes with swollen crescent-shaped nuclei (arrowheads). *Eimeria leuckarti*. (H&E stain. Bar 50 μm.)

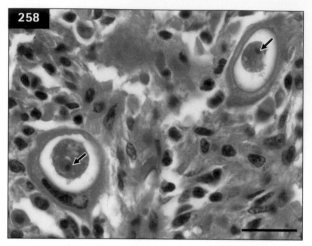

258 Intestinal coccidiosis. Higher magnification depicting two large macrogametes surrounded by a pale parasitophorous vacuole. Note the single basophilic protozoan nuclei (arrows) and a swollen nucleus of the hypertrophic host cell (bottom left). *Eimeria leuckarti.* (H&E stain. Bar 20 μm.)

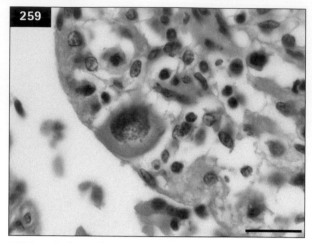

259 Intestinal coccidiosis. Higher magnification of a relatively small intraepithelial schizont containing numerous small basophilic elongated merozoites. *Eimeria leuckarti.* (H&E stain. Bar 20 μm.)

Babesia caballi/Theileria equi: BABESIOSIS/PIROPLASMOSIS

Definition/Overview

Babesiosis is a tick-transmitted intraerythrocytic parasitic disease of horses associated with fever, haemolytic anaemia, and haemoglobinuria caused by either *Babesia caballi* or *Theileria equi* (formerly *Babesia equi*).

Aetiology

Piroplasms of the genus *Babesia*, along with their relatives in the Theileriidae, comprise a genetically and antigenetically diverse group of tick-transmitted intraerythrocytic pathogens (Persing & Conrad 1995). The small piroplasm of horses, long known as *Babesia equi*, is already commonly designated *Theileria equi*. The classical differences between the main genera of nonpigment-forming haemoparasites are the absence or presence of extra-erythrocytic multiplication (schizogony) and in the cycle in the vector tick, which includes transovarial transmission in *Babesia*, but only transstadial transmission in *Theileria*. Also, the multiplication in the red cell of *Babesia*, by budding, most often results in two daughter cells (merozoites), while that of *Theileria* gives four merozoites, often as a 'Maltese cross'. However, on molecular grounds, it may be necessary to create a new genus for *T. equi* and similar parasites (Uilenberg 2006). The name 'piroplasm' originally comes from the fact that the parasites after multiplication are often pear-shaped. The old name

Piroplasma still survives in this way, and also in the fact that both babesiosis and theileriosis are commonly grouped together under the designation 'piroplasmoses'. It is now generally accepted that formerly used genus names are synonyms of *Babesia* or *Theileria* (Uilenberg 2006). It has been shown that twelve distinct *T. equi* 18S rRNA sequences and six *B. caballi* 18S rRNA sequences occur in South Africa, which form three and two phylogenetic clades, respectively (Bhoora *et al.* 2009).

B. caballi and *T. equi* are present in temperate as well as in tropical regions. Fourteen species of ixodid ticks of the genera *Dermacentor*, *Hyalomma*, and *Rhipicephalus* have been identified worldwide as vectors of either *T. equi* or *B. caballi*.

T. equi was identified in 80% of horses suffering from piroplasmosis in France and *B. caballi* in only 1.2%. Of interest, *T. equi* was also detected in 19% of dogs suffering from piroplasmosis and *B. caballi* in 0.6%, whereas *B. canis canis* was identified in 10% of horses suffering from piroplasmosis as well as *B. canis rossi* in 0.9% of horses (Fritz 2010).

Epidemiology

Piroplasmosis, a disease endemic to most tropical and subtropical areas, appears to be spreading to more temperate zones (Butler *et al.* 2005). A seroprevalence of 68% was found with reference to piroplasmosis in Italy; 12% of the horses had anti-*T. equi* antibodies, 18% anti-*B. caballi* antibodies, and 38% had antibodies against both species (Moretti *et al.* 2010). The overall seroprevalence in Switzerland was 7.3%,

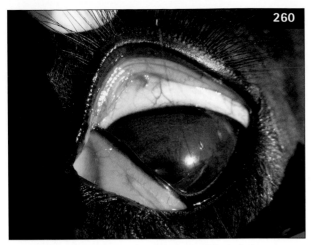

260 Clinical signs associated with babesiosis include icterus.

261–263 The differential diagnosis of various causes of fever and anaemia includes pemphigus foliaceus as seen in a 2-year-old Warmblood gelding.

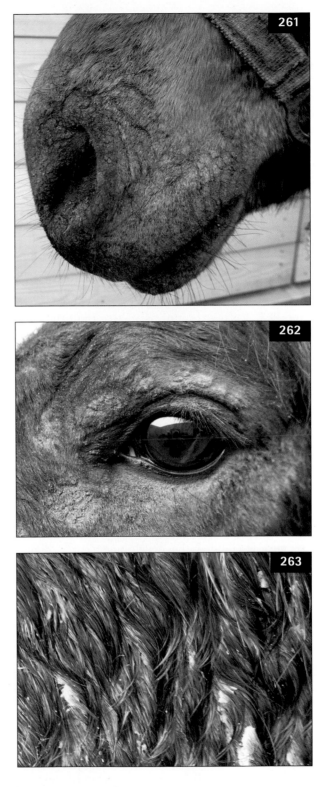

T. equi being the most important pathogen (Sigg *et al.* 2010), whereas a higher overall prevalence of *B. caballi* (54%) than of *T. equi* (22%) was found in Brazil (Kerber *et al.* 2009).

Pathophysiology

Natural transmission occurs via ticks that become infected by ingesting infected host erythrocytes. However, the pathogen can be transmitted mechanically. Ticks may also act as vectors of co-infections such as *A. phagocytophilum*.

Incubation period

About 12–19 days for *T. equi* and 10–30 days for *B. caballi* (Butler *et al.* 2005).

Clinical presentation

Equine piroplasmosis occurs in acute, subacute, and chronic forms. Clinical signs include fever, depression, anorexia, weakness, icterus (**260**), anaemia, mucosal petechiae, ventral oedema, and haemoglobinuria. Horses surviving clinical infection may remain inapparent carriers. Disease due to *B. caballi* is less severe than that caused by *T. equi* and mortality rate is lower. Death may occur within 24–48 hours after onset, preceded by lateral recumbency. It is not possible to differentiate between *B. caballi* and *T. equi* infections based solely on clinical signs (de Waal 1992, Brüning 1996, Butler *et al.* 2005).

Differential diagnosis

The differential diagnosis includes various causes of fever and anaemia (**261–263**) (see p. 263).

Diagnosis

Identification of parasites in blood smears is the diagnostic mainstay (**264–267**), but this has certain limitations, particularly when parasitaemia is low (Krause *et al.* 1996). *B. caballi* infections especially tend to be associated with extremely low parasitaemias, often due to the early elimination of most parasites after a short period of infection, thus making diagnosis almost impossible (Frerichs *et al.* 1969). Serodiagnosis by use of the CF test alone may give false-negative test results, especially in horses that are parasite carriers, and has been shown to be less sensitive than the IFAT (Weiland 1986). PCR proved very useful for the detection of haemoparasites (Caccio *et al.* 2000), and combined with reverse line blot (RLB) offers the possibility of simultaneous detection and identification of different species infecting horses (Nagore *et al.* 2004). However, it has been shown that quantitative real-time PCR assays are more sensitive than the RLB assay for the detection of *T. equi* and *B. caballi* infections in field samples (Bhoora *et al.* 2010). TaqMan real-time PCR detected DNA of piroplasms in 31% of samples, while serological methods found antibodies in 36% of horses (Jaffer *et al.* 2010).

Although the CF test has been recommended for detecting the presence of antibodies to *Babesia* spp., it has been shown to have several disadvantages, including false-positive results and low sensitivity for detecting latent infections (false-negative results). The CF test may therefore not be a suitable test for pre-import testing (Butler *et al.* 2008).

In vitro cultivation of both parasite species and the identification of parasite proteins for diagnostic use have facilitated the development of a highly sensitive and specific ELISA (Brüning 1996). Recently, a highly sensitive and specific quantitative TaqMan real-time PCR assay, based on the 18S rRNA gene, was developed for the detection of *T. equi* infections in horses (Kim *et al.* 2008).

It has also been shown that even high-dose treatment with imidocarb may not be capable of eliminating *B. caballi* and *T. equi* infections from healthy carriers (Butler *et al.* 2008).

Pathology

Pathology might reveal jaundice, splenomegaly, haemorrhagic fluid within the pericardium, kidney degeneration, haemorrhages, and haemoglobinuria. Bone marrow should not be excluded as a potential reservoir site for *T. equi* and *B. caballi* in infected asymptomatic horses (Pitel *et al.* 2010).

Management/Treatment

Management of tick-transmitted parasitic diseases relies on eradicating the vector tick and the development of effective vaccines. Treatment of diseased horses should include supportive treatment, especially with regard to anaemia.

There are a number of effective babesiacides: imidocarb dipropionate, which is often the only available drug on the market, and diminazene aceturate are the most widely used (Vial & Gorenflot 2006). For instance, diminazene aceturate has been mentioned to be effective in the chemosterilization of *B. caballi* and in the elimination of clinical signs in *T. equi* infections. Antitheilerial drugs such as buparvaquone have been shown to be effective in combatting disease due to *T. equi* (Brüning 1996).

Imidocarb dipropionate (a carbanilide derivate) should be administered at a dosage of 2 mg/kg BW IM sid for 2 days in cases of *B. caballi* infection, and at a dosage of 4 mg/kg BW IM four times with a 72-hour interval in cases of *T. equi* infection (Meyer *et al.* 2005, Butler *et al.* 2005). However, treatment with five consecutive doses of imidocarb dipropionate (4.7 mg/kg BW IM q 72 h) turned out to be unable to eliminate spontaneous *B. caballi* and *T. equi* infections from healthy carriers (Butler *et al.* 2008). Nevertheless, a high-dose regimen (4.0 mg/kg BW IM four times at 72-h intervals) of imidocarb dipropionate cleared *B. caballi* infection following inoculation with $10^{5.2}$ *B. caballi* parasites (Schwint *et al.* 2009). It should be mentioned that imidocarb dipropionate crosses the equine placenta (Lewis *et al.* 1999). Cholinergic side effects of imidocarb may be alleviated by treatment with atropine.

Public health significance

Some *Babesia* spp. can infect humans, particularly *B. microti*, *B. divergens*, and related species; human babesiosis is a significant emerging tick-borne zoonotic disease. Clinical manifestations differ markedly between European and North American diseases. In clinical cases, a combination of clindamycin and quinine is administered as the standard treatment, but also administration of atovaquone–azithromycin is successful (Vial & Gorenflot 2006).

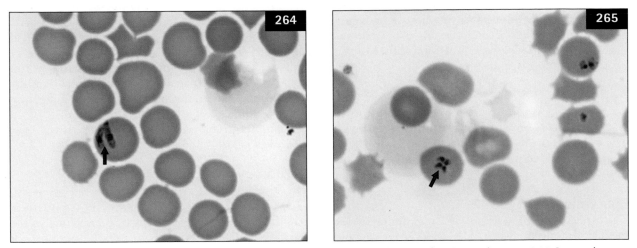

264, 265 Equine piroplasmosis. Cytology specimens of blood smears depicting a close-up of equine erythrocytes. **264**: One erythrocyte in the centre contains two relatively large paired elongated 'pear-shaped' bluish intracytoplasmic merozoites or daughter cells (arrow), typical for *Babesia caballi*; **265**: few erythrocytes contain small bluish intracytoplasmic merozoites of *Theileria equi*, positioned in a typical 'Maltese cross' formation by four clustered merozoites (arrow). (May–Grünwald–Giemsa stains.) (Courtesy of Dr C.M. Butler.)

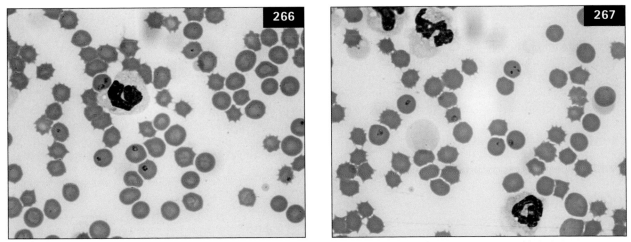

266, 267 Micrographs of equine blood smears with numerous intraerythrocytic irregular dark bluish merozoites of *Theileria equi*. (May–Grünwald–Giemsa stains.)

Giardia duodenalis

Definition/Overview
Although *Giardia duodenalis* (previously known as *Giardia lamblia*) has been incriminated as a cause of diarrhoea, the true pathological significance of this protozoan is poorly understood.

Aetiology
G. duodenalis is a protozoan parasite with a two-stage life cycle consisting of trophozoite and cyst. The cysts are ovoid and refractile, 8–14 × 6–10 μm in size. Reproduction is by binary fission (Soulsby 1968).

Epidemiology
The prevalence of *Giardia* sp. was found to be highest among foals of 5–8 weeks of age and lactating mares in Ohio and Kentucky. *Giardia* infection was found in all age groups, although the infection rates for foals were higher (17–35%). Chronological study of infection in 35 foals showed that foals started to excrete *Giardia* cysts between 2 and 22 weeks of age. The cumulative infection rate of *Giardia* in foals was 71%. Some foals were concurrently infected with both *Cryptosporidium* and *Giardia* and excretion of oocysts or cysts was intermittent and long lasting. The longest duration of excretion was 16 weeks for *Giardia*. Excretion of *Giardia* cysts continued after weaning and infected mares were deemed to be the major source of *Giardia* infection in foals. The high infection rate of *Giardia* in nursing mares suggests a periparturient relaxation of immunity (Xiao & Herd 1994). Furthermore, 4.6% of packstock was found to be shedding *G. duodenalis* cysts in their faeces, with herd-level prevalences of 0–22% (Atwill *et al.* 2000).

Incubation period
Not established in the equine species yet.

Clinical presentation
Although the presence of *Giardia* spp. in horses with diarrhoea has been reported (Kirkpatrick & Skand 1985), horses infected with *Giardia* spp. rarely show any associated clinical signs of diarrhoea, colic, lethargy, and anorexia (**268**) (Bemrick 1968, Manahan 1970). However, *Giardia* infection was associated with chronic diarrhoea, weight loss, lethargy, inappetence, and dermatitis in a 4-year-old Thoroughbred (Kirkpatrick & Skand 1985).

Differential diagnosis
The differential diagnosis includes various causes of acute diarrhoea (**269, 270**) (see p. 263).

Diagnosis
The diagnosis should be based on the demonstration of faecal cysts combined with the presence of diarrhoea and response to treatment. Faecal cysts can be detected by the zinc sulphate centrifugal flotation method (Soulsby 1968, Kirkpatrick & Skand 1985). Usually only cysts are passed but in some cases the free flagellates may be found (Soulsby 1968). In addition, detection of *Giardia* antigen in stool samples is possible by means of a semiquantitative enzyme immunoassay test (Wienecka *et al.* 1989).

Pathology
On histological sections the flattened pyriform *Giardia* trophozoites are usually seen with their concave ventral surface facing and attaching to the enterocyte brush border. Increased amounts of intraepithelial lymphocytes are common, without other considerable histopathology. The archetypal binucleated 'face-like' or 'owl-like' appearance of trophozoites is more commonly encountered in mucosal smears.

Management/Treatment
Clinical signs resolved following treatment with metronidazole suspension (5 mg/kg BW PO tid for 10 days) in a 4-year-old Thoroughbred (Kirkpatrick & Skand 1985).

Public health significance
It has been shown that horses can be infected with assemblage AI and AII genotypes of *G. duodenalis*. They therefore constitute a potential zoonotic risk to humans, as genotypes in assemblage AI and AII provide the greatest zoonotic risk to humans either directly or via watersheds (Traub *et al.* 2005).

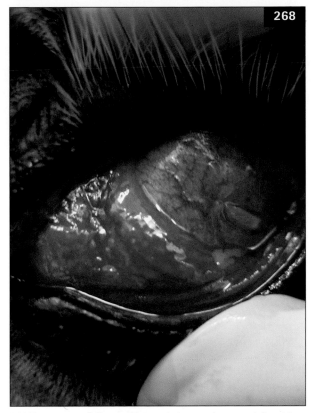

268 Treatment of diseased horses is supportive especially with regard to dehydration as reflected by red mucous membranes.

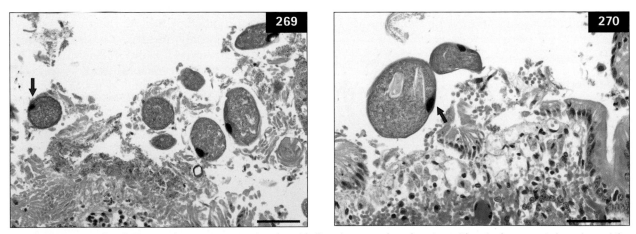

269, 270 Micrographs of ciliates: colon mucosa-associated ovoid ciliated protozoal trophozoites with a single excentric large basophilic macronucleus (arrows). *Balantidium coli*. (H&E stain. Bar 50 μm.)

Trypanosoma brucei evansi/T. b. equiperdum: TRYPANOSOMOSIS

Definition/Overview

Trypanosomosis is caused by *Trypanosoma brucei evansi*, a salivarian trypanosomatid ('surra') or *T. b. equiperdum* ('dourine'). These trypanosomes are not monophyletic clades and do not qualify for species status. They should be considered two subspecies strains of *T. brucei*, which spontaneously arose recently (Lai *et al.* 2008). Dourine is a venereal reportable disease in horses and donkeys found only in Africa, South and Central America, and the Middle East. Serological testing using CF is recommended for diagnosis (Metcalf 2001, Menezes *et al.* 2004, Gillingwater *et al.* 2007). However, no definitive diagnosis of dourine can be made at the serological or molecular level yet, whereas oedematous cutaneous plaques are regarded as pathognomonic (Claes *et al.* 2005). Surra (or mal de Cadeiras) is mainly a (wasting) disease affecting equids, camels, and cattle as well as other domestic and wild animal species (in total eight mammal orders spread over America, Europe, and Asia) (Menezes *et al.* 2004). In horses, infection may cause severe neurological abnormalities (Berlin *et al.* 2009). Chemotherapy appears to be the most effective form of control for *T. b. evansi*, whereas infections caused by *T. b. equiperdum* are considered incurable (Gillingwater *et al.* 2007). Furthermore, in horses as well as in donkeys, trypanosome infections may be due to *T. congolense* and *T. vivax*. *T. brucei* is rare and often found in mixed infections with *T. congolense* or *T. vivax* (Faye *et al.* 2001).

Aetiology

T. brucei is a kinetoplastid flagellate, the agent of human sleeping sickness and ruminant nagana in Africa. Kinetoplastid flagellates contain their eponym kinetoplast DNA, consisting of two types of interlocked circular DNA molecules: scores of maxicircles and thousands of minicircles. Maxicircles have typical mitochondrial genes, most of which are translatable only after RNA editing. Minicircles encode guide RNAs, required for decrypting the maxicircle transcripts. The life cycle of *T. brucei* involves a bloodstream stage in vertebrates and a procyclic stage in the tsetse fly vector. *T. equiperdum* and *T. evansi* are actually strains of *T. brucei*, which lost part or all of their kinetoplast DNA. *T. b. equiperdum* is the only trypanosome not transmitted by an invertebrate vector and it is primarily a tissue parasite that rarely invades the blood (Claes *et al.* 2005, Lai *et al.* 2008). *T. b. evansi* and *T. vivax* exhibit a very high immunological cross-reactivity, and antigens from *T. b. evansi* responsible for this phenomenon are three cross-reacting antigens with molecular masses of approximately 51, 64, and 68 kDa (Uzcanga *et al.* 2002, Camargo *et al.* 2004).

Epidemiology

In Venezuela, two non-tsetse transmitted trypanosomes, *T. b. evansi* and *T. vivax*, are the major aetiological agents of animal trypanosomosis (Camargo *et al.* 2004). Donkeys when exposed to a similar tsetse challenge are significantly less infected with trypanosomes than horses. The prevalence and the average monthly incidence of trypanosome infections in horses (45.5 and 16%, respectively) were significantly higher than in donkeys (6.2 and 9%, respectively) in the Gambia (Faye *et al.* 2001). The trypanosome prevalence was 18% and *T. congolense* was the most common species, accounting for 66% of the overall infections in donkey populations naturally infected with trypanosomes in southern Ethiopia (Assefa & Abebe 2001). The average apparent prevalence of dourine was 8.3% in Namibia (Kumba *et al.* 2002). An outbreak of animal trypanosomosis (*T. b. evansi*) has been reported in the Aveyron department of France (Watier-Grillot 2008). There is no known natural reservoir of *T. b. equiperdum* other than infected equids and transmission is via semen. Carriers are an important source of infection (Metcalf 2001, Menezes *et al.* 2004, Gillingwater *et al.* 2007).

T. b. evansi outbreaks in mainland Spain occurred after the introduction of dromedary camels (Tamarit *et al.* 2010).

Pathophysiology

The outcome of the infection is defined by both host genetic background and peculiarities (virulence factors) of the distinct *T. b. evansi* isolates (Menezes *et al.* 2004).

Incubation period

Equines inoculated intravenously with 10^6 trypomastigotes of *T. b. evansi* developed motor incoordination of the pelvic limbs 67–124 days after inoculation (Lemos *et al.* 2008). *T. b. evansi* was detected in blood smears of a susceptible stallion 13 days after infection with the parasite via the CSF of the subarachnoid space by lumbosacral puncture, demonstrating the ability of *T. b. evansi* to cross the blood–brain barrier (Barrowman 1976). The incubation period of *T. b. equiperdum* is 1–2 weeks, and starts with oedema, tumefaction, and damage to the genitalia including paraphimosis (Brun *et al.* 1998, Claes *et al.* 2005).

Clinical presentation

The clinical course of surra ranges from 2 to 20 days with clinical signs including marked progressive ataxia, nystagmus, cranial nerve deficits including blindness, head tilt and circling, hyperexcitability, obtundity, proprioceptive deficits, head pressing, and paddling movements (Berlin *et al.* 2009, Rodrigues *et al.* 2009). Dourine in horses is chronic, persists for 1–2 years and is generally divided into three phases, although the clinical course can vary considerably under different conditions. The first period is characterized by oedema, tumefaction, and damage to the genitalia including paraphimosis, and begins 1–2 weeks after infection. The second stage is pathognomonic for dourine. In this period, typical cutaneous plaques (5–8 cm in diameter and 1 cm thick) or skin thickness can occur. The third phase is characterized by progressive anaemia, disorders of the nervous system, mainly paralysis of the hindlimbs and paraplegia, and finally death (Brun *et al.* 1998, Claes *et al.* 2005).

Differential diagnosis

The differential diagnosis predominantly includes various causes of acute neurological disease (see p. 262).

Diagnosis

No definitive diagnosis of dourine can be made at the serological or molecular level. Only clinical signs are pathognomonic (typical cutaneous plaques), and international screening relies on an outdated cross-reactive serological test (the CF test) from 1915, resulting in serious consequences at the practical level (Watson 1915, Claes *et al.* 2005).

A competitive ELISA method has been developed for the serodiagnosis of dourine infection in horses. Apparent test specificity for the cELISA was 98.9%. Concordance and kappa value between the CF test and the cELISA in experimentally exposed horses were 97% and 0.95, respectively (Katz *et al.* 2000). Furthermore, the protozoa might be demonstrated in exudate and oedematous fluid. Incidentally, the causative protozoan is found in the blood.

Examination of Giemsa-stained blood smears detected 41% of surra infections; the mouse inoculation test detected 47% infections, whereas an in-house ELISA detected antitrypanosomal antibodies in 66% of infections in clinically ill horses suffering from the salivarian trypanosomatid *T. b. evansi* (Laha & Sasmal 2009). Using PCR, the number of detected cases was seven times higher than using the buffy coat method for the detection of trypanosomes in the blood, confirming the superiority of the PCR technique for the diagnosis of trypanosomosis (Faye *et al.* 2001).

The IFAT detected antibodies 15.7 days post-inoculation with 3×10^6 *T. b. evansi* parasites intravenously. The microhaematocrit centrifugation test was the most sensitive, first detecting parasites between 1 and 3 days post-inoculation (Wernery *et al.* 2001). Ante-mortem detection of *T. b. evansi* in the CSF of a horse using PCR identification of the parasite DNA has been reported (Berlin *et al.* 2009).

Pathology

Histopathology showed that the brain, spinal cord, and kidneys are the main affected tissues (Berlin *et al.* 2009). Lesions in the CNS of experimentally induced surra were those of a widespread nonsuppurative encephalomyelitis and meningomyelitis (Lemos *et al.* 2007, Berlin *et al.* 2009). Asymmetric leuco-encephalomalacia with yellowish discoloration of white matter and flattening of the gyri were observed in the brain of horses suffering from surra. Histologically, a necrotizing encephalitis was most severe in the white matter, with oedema, demyelination, and lymphoplasmacytic perivascular cuffs. Mild to moderate meningitis or meningomyelitis was observed in the spinal cord. *T. b. evansi* was detected immunohistochemically in the perivascular spaces and neuropil (Rodrigues *et al.* 2009). Lymphoid perivascular cuffs and meningeal infiltrations were predominantly composed of T and B cells (Lemos *et al.* 2007). Furthermore, histopathology might reveal a membrano-proliferative glomerulonephritis. PCR analysis has indicated the presence of parasite DNA in the cerebellum, brainstem, spinal cord, and bone marrow but not in other organs (Berlin *et al.* 2009). The characteristic gliosis observed suggests the ability of these cells as mediators of immune response (Lemos *et al.* 2008).

Management/Treatment

Because dourine is considered to be incurable, the disease is reportable and seropositive horses should be eradicated. Treatment of surra diseased horses is supportive and diminazene aceturate at 3.5 mg/kg BW IM appears to be effective in the first treatment of horses and mules infected with *T. b. evansi*. One study showed that parasites were cleared from the peripheral blood of horses on days 1 and 7 and from mules on days 1 and 14. Thereafter the number of positive animals increased. After the second treatment, 50% of horses and 25% of mules were still positive to surra 24 h after treatment, demonstrating that diminazene had no protective effect (Tuntasuvan *et al.* 2003). Treatment with diminazene (3.5–7 mg/kg BW IM) has been suggested to have a prophylactic effect (about 18 days of protection) in horses (Faye *et al.* 2001). However, bis (aminoethylthio) 4-melamino-phenylarsine dihydrochloride was found to be quite effective in curing horses with acute as well as chronic forms of dourine due to *T. b. equiperdum* at a dose rate of 0.25–0.5 mg/kg BW IM. Parasitaemia was cleared within 24 hours post-treatment and without relapse throughout the 320 days of observation (Hagos *et al.* 2010).

Relapse/breakthrough infections due to *T. congolense* were reported following a prophylactic dose of 1.0 mg/kg BW of isometamidium chloride (Assefa & Abebe 2001).

Public health significance

Non-tsetse transmitted trypanosomosis (*T. b. evansi* and *T. lewisi*) has zoonotic potential (Kaur *et al.* 2007, Watier-Grillot 2008). *T. brucei* is the agent of human sleeping sickness and ruminant nagana in Africa (Lai *et al.* 2008).

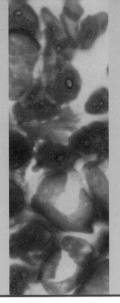

Chapter 4
Fungal diseases

INVASIVE MYCOSES

Definition/Overview

Opportunistic fungi are most commonly seen in immunocompromised hosts affecting predominantly the skin (Chaffin *et al*. 1995) and the respiratory tract, especially the guttural pouches (**271**) and the lungs (**272–275**) (King *et al*. 1962, Thirion-Delalande *et al*. 2005) and rarely other systems such as the digestive tract (**276–285**) (de Bruijn & Wijnberg 2004). Of importance, guttural pouch mycosis can lead to fatal haemorrhage. In addition, a wide variety of dermatophytes have been isolated from animals, but a few zoophilic species are responsible for the majority of cases: *Microsporum canis, Trichophyton mentagrophytes, Trichophyton equinum*, and *Trichophyton verrucosum*, as also the geophilic species *Microsporum gypseum* (Chermette *et al*. 2008) with *T. equinum* being the most prevalent. Equine dermatophytosis ('ringworm') has public health significance.

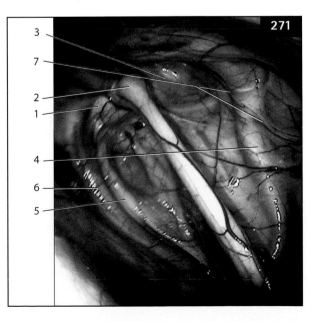

271 Endoscopic photograph of the normal right guttural pouch with the tympanic bulla (1), the stylohyoid bone (2), the occipital condyle (3), the internal carotid artery (4), the maxillary artery (5), the maxillary vein (6), and the hypoglossal nerve (7).

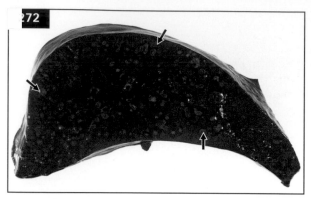

272 Multifocal mycotic granulomatous pneumonia. Note the pale miliary granulomatous foci (arrows) within the hyperaemic lung. *Aspergillus fumigatus*.

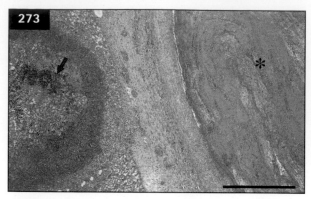

273 Mycotic pyogranulomatous pneumonia. On the left is a pyogranuloma centred on intense PAS-positive staining fungal organisms (arrow), on the right is a large intravascular thrombus (asterisk) also containing fungal hyphae (not discernible at this magnification). *Aspergillus fumigatus*. (PAS stain. Bar 1 mm.)

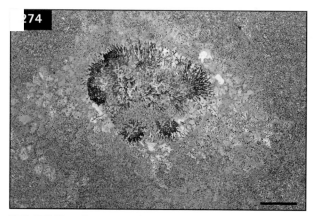

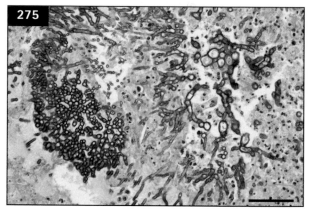

274, 275 Mycotic pyogranulomatous pneumonia. **274**: Fungal pulmonary pyogranuloma at higher magnification shows the central fungal hyphae within necrotic tissue remnants surrounded by neutrophils, macrophages, lymphocytes, and plasma cells; **275**: close-up of the pyogranuloma centre containing the branching fungal hyphae that focally exhibit larger bulbous swellings in their otherwise long slender hyphae. *Aspergillus fumigatus*. (PAS stain. Bars 200/50 μm, respectively.)

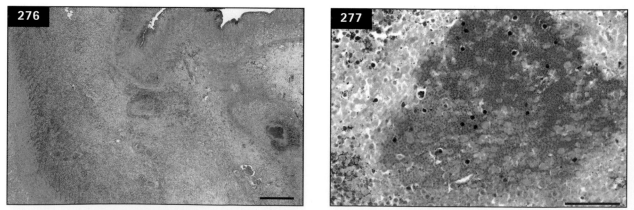

276, 277 Mycotic colitis. Necrosuppurative and histiocytic colitis (**276**). The ulcerated mucosa (top right) and submucosa are distended due to a severe diffuse pyogranulomatous inflammation, oedema, and haemorrhage. Note the intense PAS-positive staining foci of fungal spores demarcated by neutrophils at higher magnification (**277**). *Aspergillus* sp. (PAS stain. Bars 1 mm/50 μm, respectively.)

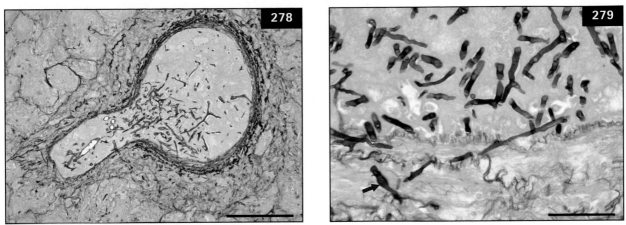

278, 279 Mycotic colitis. Black-stained fungal hyphae exhibit extensive invasion of a medium sized submucosal artery (angioinvasiveness). Higher magnification (**279**) clearly depicts the black-stained fungal hyphae within the vessel wall (arrow) and lumen (top half). *Aspergillus* sp. (Grocott–Gomori's methanamine silver stain. Bars 200/50 μm, respectively.)

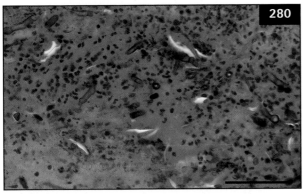

280 Mycotic rhinitis. Biopsy specimen from a nasal passageway containing several septate and branching pigmented hyphae amid a suppurative exudate. (H&E stain. Bar 50 μm.)

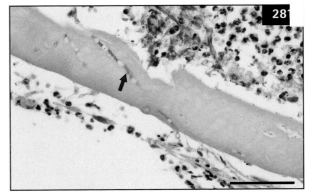

281 Keratomycosis. Fungal hyphae infiltrate the corneal stroma and destructively penetrate Descemet´s membrane (arrow). The anterior eye chamber also contains fungal hyphae amid a suppurative exudate (top right). Most commonly this represents an opportunistic infection of a corneal laceration. *Aspergillus* sp. (H&E stain. Bar 50 μm.)

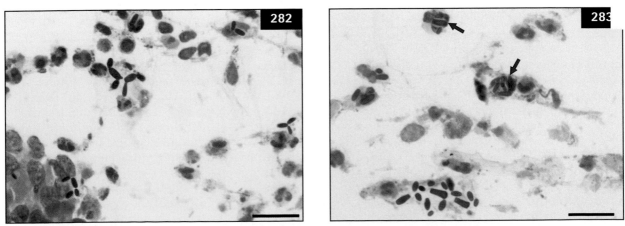

282, 283 Uterine candidiasis. Smear from uterine exudate contains large numbers of round to ovoid yeast forms which occasionally display budding amid mucus, degenerate neutrophils, macrophages, and fragments of endometrial mucosa. Note that few yeasts are phagocytosed by inflammatory cells (arrows). *Candida* sp. (May–Grünwald–Giemsa stain. Bar 10 μm.)

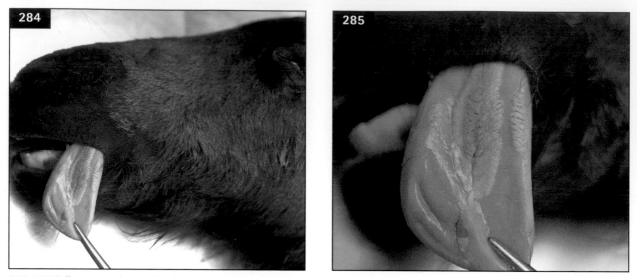

284, 285 Fell pony syndrome. Focal extensive lingual hyperkeratosis (thrush). A thick light greenish hyperkeratotic plaque or pseudomembrane on the dorsal aspect of the tongue in a young Fell pony. This lesion is frequently encountered in the Fell pony syndrome in which a hereditary congenital immunodeficiency can give rise to opportunistic infections of several organ systems (especially pneumonias) including a hyperkeratotic glossitis due to yeast infection. *Candida albicans*.

Aetiology

Aspergillus species are globally ubiquitous saprophytes found in a variety of ecological niches. Almost 200 species of aspergilli have been identified, fewer than 20 of which are known to cause human disease. Among them, *A. fumigatus* is the most prevalent and is largely responsible for the increased incidence of invasive aspergillosis in the immunocompromised patient population (Dagenais & Keller 2009). *A. fumigatus* is also the major organism found in the guttural pouch (auditory tube diverticulum) of horses affected with mycosis (Lepage *et al.* 2004, Ludwig *et al.* 2005) besides *A. versicolor, A. nidulans*, and *A. niger* (Ludwig *et al.* 2005). In comparison, in ocular flora of clinically normal horses fungi included *A. nidulans* (56%), *Cladosporium* spp. (32%), and *A. fumigatus* (22%) (Gemensky-Metzler *et al.* 2005). There were no significant differences between the number or type of organisms cultured during the sampling seasons in ocular flora of clinically normal horses in Florida, whereas the likelihood of detecting an organism depended on the horse's age (Andrew *et al.* 2003).

Epidemiology

Emericella nidulans from bedding materials in the equine environment has been associated with guttural pouch mycosis (Kosuge *et al.* 2000).

Pathophysiology

Invasive mycoses pose a major diagnostic and therapeutic challenge. Many fungal pathogens occur almost exclusively in opportunistic settings such as in the immunocompromised host (Patterson 2005).

Incubation period

Not established in the equine species yet.

Clinical presentation

The presenting signs of guttural pouch mycosis were, in order of frequency, epistaxis at rest, nasal catarrh, pharyngeal paralysis, ipsilateral laryngeal hemiplegia, swelling of the submandibular/parotid region, extension of the head and neck, and dyspnoea; cases that presented with pharyngeal paralysis were usually fatal (**286–296**) (Church *et al.* 1986). A 6-month-old filly suffering from the condition was presented with unilateral epistaxis (Millar 2006). Of horses with guttural pouch mycosis, 31 horses were identified with unilateral (n = 25) or bilateral (n = 6) guttural pouch mycosis. The 37 guttural pouches had lesions on the left (n = 20) and right (n = 17) sides. Circumscribed or diffuse mycotic lesions affected the medial compartment alone (n = 28), lateral compartment alone (n = 2), or both compartments (n = 7) (Lepage & Piccot-Crézollet 2005). Sequelae included acquired unilateral laryngeal paralysis (Dixon *et al.* 2001), lingual hemiplegia (Kipar & Frese 1993), atlanto-occipital arthropathy (Walmsley 1988), headshaking (Lane & Mair 1987), visual disturbances leading to blindness (Hatziolos *et al.* 1975), mycotic encephalitis (McLaughlin & O'Brien 1986), and sudden death due to excessive blood loss. Some cases of pharyngeal hemiplegia can make a complete recovery although it may take 12–18 months (Greet 1987).

Differential diagnosis
The differential diagnosis includes causes of (unilateral) epistaxis without fever such as trauma, e.g. haemorrhage into the guttural pouch associated with rupture of the longus capitis muscle (Sweeney *et al.* 1993), and progressive ethmoidal haematoma.

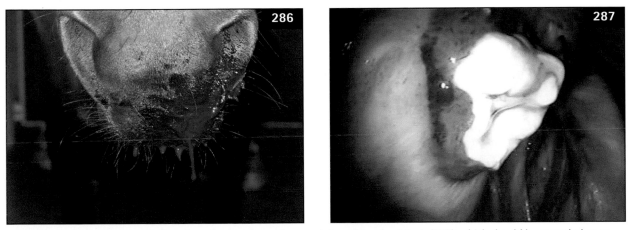

286, 287 A predominant presenting sign of guttural pouch mycosis is unilateral epistaxis (**286**), which should be regarded as an emergency given the fact that sudden death due to excessive blood loss is not unusual. *Aspergillus fumigatus* is the major organism found in the guttural pouch of horses affected by mycosis (**287**).

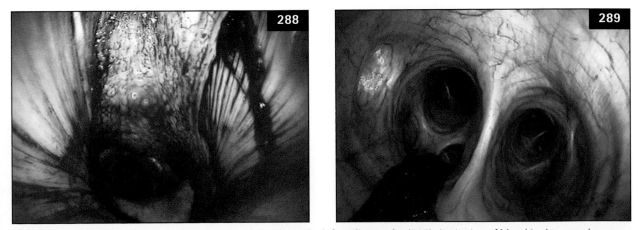

288, 289 Fresh blood oozing from the left guttural pouch via the left auditory tube (**288**). Aspiration of blood in the same horse as visualized in the trachea (**289**).

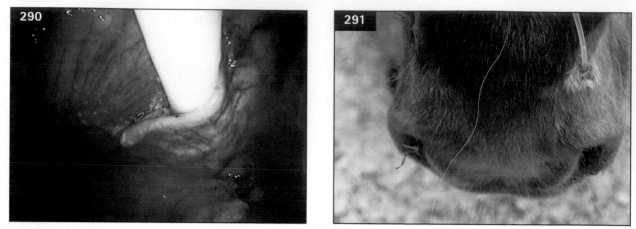

290, 291 Specific treatment options of guttural pouch mycosis include medical treatment involving local administration of antifungal preparations such as enilconazole via a specially designed catheter as seen via the auditory tube (**290**) and percutaneously (**291**).

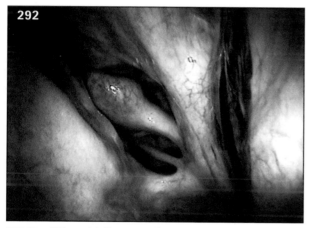

292 The differential diagnosis of guttural pouch mycosis includes trauma as illustrated here by fresh blood oozing from the apertura naso-maxillaris following sinus trauma.

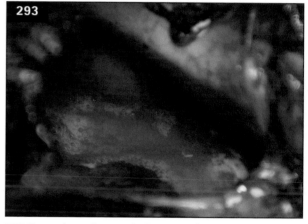

293 Guttural pouch mycosis. A seropurulent exudate occupies the guttural pouch. *Aspergillus fumigatus.*

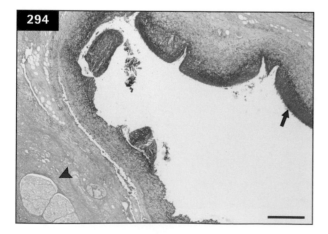

294 Guttural pouch mycosis. Intensely bright purple-staining fungal organisms lining the guttural pouch mucosa (arrow). Multifocal extensive neutrophilic infiltrates surround the guttural pouch and embed the facial nerve (arrowhead). *Aspergillus fumigatus.* (PAS stain. Bar 200 μm.)

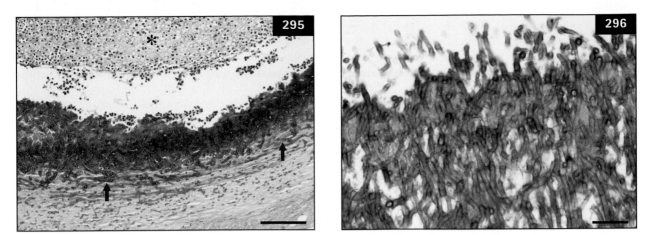

295, 296 Guttural pouch mycosis. **295**: Close-up of fungal hyphae (arrows) invading and destroying the pouch mucosa. On the top half the purulent exudate (asterisk) is noticeably present (empyema); **296**: higher magnification of the fungal septated and sharp-angled dichotomatously (i.e. into two evenly sized daughter hyphae) branching hyphae. *Aspergillus fumigatus*. (PAS stain. Bars 100/20 μm, respectively.)

Diagnosis

Guttural pouch mycosis can be visualized by means of endoscopy. Furthermore, reactivity to 22 and 26 kD *A. fumigatus* antigens, as measured by immunoblot analysis, seems to be diagnostic for guttural pouch mycosis in horses (Guillot *et al*. 1997).

Pathology

Microscopic examination is necessary to identify the intralesional fungal organisms. Typically fungi-induced inflammations are suppurative and histiocytic or granulomatous with epithelioid and/or multinucleated macrophages; lymphoplasmacellular infiltrates are variable. In many cases fungi induce tissue necrosis, and fungal angioinvasion may be present in various systemic infections. Cleistothecia and/or Hulle cells have been observed in guttural pouch mycosis (Ludwig *et al*. 2005).

Management/Treatment

Treatment of horses with guttural pouch mycosis is initially supportive, aimed at possible haemorrhagic shock. Specific treatment options include: medical treatment involving local administration of various antifungal preparations via a specially designed catheter and/or the oral administration of benzimidazole drugs (Church *et al*. 1986, van Nieuwstadt & Kalsbeek 1994, Davis & Legendre 1994); inserting a transarterial coil into the internal carotid, external carotid, and maxillary arteries (transarterial coil embolization or TCE), which is effective in occluding the arteries and in inducing regression of the mycotic lesions without adjunctive medical treatment (Lepage *et al*. 2004, Freeman 2006); and ligation of the internal carotid artery on the cardiac side of the lesion, also an effective means of reducing the chance of fatal epistaxis in cases of guttural pouch mycosis (Greet 1987).

Dermatophytosis (**297–305**) is usually self-limiting, but topical fungicidal administration might be considered. Furthermore, an inactivated vaccine against 'ringworm' is available. However, the scientific literature is sparse, making it difficult to conclude on efficacy and appropriate use (Lund & Deboer 2008).

Public health significance

The aetiology of human invasive mycoses has shown a shift from *Candida albicans* to *Aspergillus* spp. and other moulds, perhaps due in part to effective control of *C. albicans* with azole prophylaxis, particularly with fluconazole (Patterson 2005).

Invasive aspergillosis is rare in immunocompetent people (Brooks *et al.* 2011) and is regarded as a devastating human illness, with mortality rates in some patient groups reaching as high as 90% (Dagenais & Keller 2009). In comparison, the zoophilic dermatophyte species *Microsporum canis* belonging to the *Arthroderma otae* complex is associated with moderately inflammatory tinea corporis and tinea capitis, but highly inflammatory 'ringworm' as well in humans. Human infections are likely to be acquired from the fur of cats, dogs, and horses with isolates from horses not showing a monophyletic clustering (Sharma *et al.* 2007).

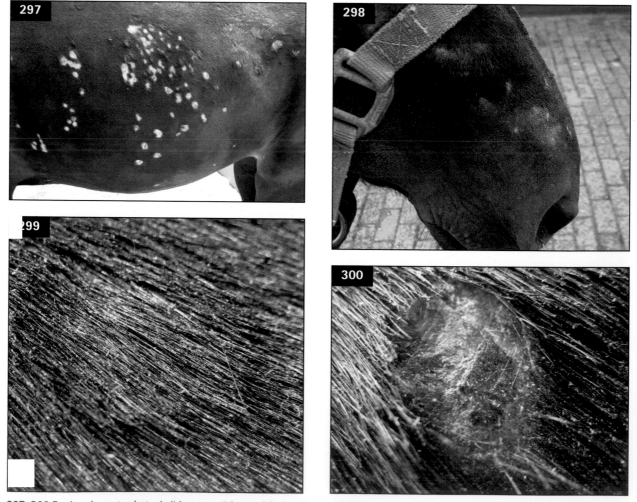

297–300 Equine dermatophytosis ('ringworm') has public health significance.

301 Dermatophytosis. Chronic mild dermatitis with epidermal hyperplasia and hyperkeratosis. The epidermis is thickened with superficial crusting and scaling. The superficial dermis contains mild to moderate amounts of perivascular to interstitial mixed cellular inflammatory infiltrates. *Trichophyton* sp. (H&E stain. Bar 200 μm.)

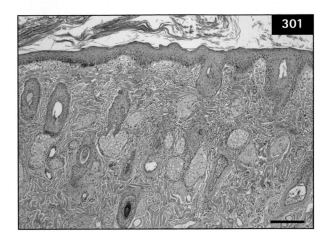

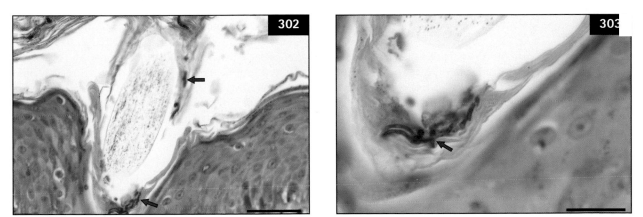

302, 303 Dermatophytosis. Close-up micrograph of an infundibular orifice containing a hair and surrounding keratin invaded by several fungal hyphae (arrows). *Trichophyton* sp. (PAS stain. Bars 50/20 μm, respectively.)

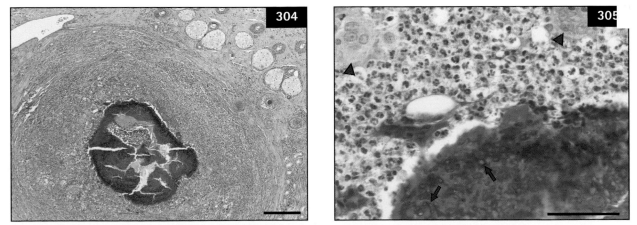

304, 305 Dermal eumycotic mycetoma. Focal pyogranulomatous panniculitis. Within the subcutis is an inflammatory nodule centred on compacted intense staining fungal hyphae surrounded by neutrophils, large epithelioid macrophages, and multinucleated giant cells. At higher magnification (**305**) numerous individual hyphae (small arrows) are discernible as well as multinucleated giant cells (arrowheads). Most commonly involved are *Curvularia* spp. and *Scedosporium* spp. (PAS stain. Bars 500/50 μm.)

Histoplasma capsulatum var. *farciminosum*: EQUINE EPIZOOTIC LYMPHANGITIS/ HISTOPLASMOSIS/PSEUDOFARCY

Definition/Overview

Equine epizootic lymphangitis (EL) (also called equine histoplasmosis or pseudofarcy) is a relatively common infectious disease of horses and other equids in certain parts of the world, and histoplasmosis is the most common endemic mycosis causing human infection. The disease is characterized by a cord-like appearance of the subcutaneous lymphatic and cutaneous pyogranulomas, the discharge from which contains spherical or pear-shaped bodies of the causal agent, *Histoplasma capsulatum* var. *farciminosum* (Al-Ani 1999).

Aetiology

H. capsulatum var. *farciminosum* is a dimorphic fungus. Genetically distinct geographical populations or phylogenetic species should be recognized, with phylogeny suggesting that the radiation of *Histoplasma* started between 3 and 13 million years ago in Latin America (Kasuga *et al.* 2003).

Epidemiology

An overall prevalence of 18.8% was recorded in Ethiopia. EL was prevalent in hot and humid towns with an altitude ranging from 1500–2300 m above sea level, but was nil or low in cold and in dry and windy towns (Ameni 2006*a*). The organism can be found in apparently healthy horses (Randall *et al.* 1951).

Pathophysiology

Similar to the other fungi in this category, initial exposure to *H. capsulatum* is by way of the respiratory tract, but once inhaled into the alveoli, the organism readily spreads in macrophages throughout the reticuloendothelial system (Kauffman 2009). Furthermore, the pathogen disseminates via the lymphatic vessels producing nodules with a characteristic corded appearance (Scantlebury 2008).

Incubation period

In one study of EL, two horses were experimentally infected. Following injection into the pre-scapular and pre-femoral lymph nodes, with scarification of the skin of the left hindlimb, conjunctiva of the right eye, and the nasal membrane of the right nostril, nodular lesions of EL appeared during the fourth week of infection at all sites in the horse infected with the yeast form, whereas lesions only appeared in the

lymph nodes and skin scratches of the horse infected with the mycelial form after 3 months. Both forms were recovered from the lesions of infected horses (Ameni 2006*b*).

Clinical presentation

Four disease presentations have been described, although combinations of these may occur within the same host. The cutaneous form is characterized by pyogranulomatous nodules occurring on any part of the body. The other forms of the disease are ocular (keratitis), respiratory, and asymptomatic carriers (Richter *et al.* 2003, Scantlebury 2008). Newborn foals died from severe granulomatous pneumonia within a few days of birth, and a weanling Thoroughbred developed granulomatous pneumonia and lymphadenitis at 5 months of age. EL also caused granulomatous placentitis and abortion in the 7–10th months of gestation (Hall 1979, Rezabek *et al.* 1993). Clinical signs in a 2-year-old Trakehner filly with pulmonary histoplasmosis included weight loss, intermittent fever, dyspnoea, and depression (Cornick 1990). Abdominal histoplasmosis was reported in Thoroughbred mares (Katayama *et al.* 2001, Nunes *et al.* 2006).

Differential diagnosis

Differentials include glanders/cutaneous farcy, ulcerative lymphangitis associated with *C. pseudotuberculosis* and *M. hemolytica* (Miller & Dresher 1981), sporothricosis, strangles (Scantlebury 2008), *R. equi* (associated with skin penetration by *S. westeri*), melioidosis, and botryomycosis.

Diagnosis

The diagnosis is based on clinical signs, a positive reaction to the skin hypersensitivity (histofarcin skin) test, combined with demonstration of typical organisms in stained smears of aspirated pus from unruptured nodules, culture, and tissue sections. Serological tests have been described (Al-Ani 1999, Ameni *et al.* 2006) such as an IFAT (Fawi 1969) and ELISA (Gabal & Mohammed 1985). The concentration of histofarcin that caused an optimum skin hypersensitivity reaction was 0.2–0.4 mg/ml in a 0.1 ml dose and this was attained 24–48 h post-injection. The sensitivity and specificity of the histofarcin test were 90.3% (95% CI = 73.1, 97.5%) and 69% (95% CI = 48.1, 84.9%) in disease-endemic districts. On the other hand, specificity was 100% (95% CI = 94.8, 100%) in disease-free districts. Positive and negative predictive values of the histofarcin test were 77.8% (95% CI = 60.4, 89.3%) and 85.7% (95% CI = 62.6, 96.2%), respectively. However, a large proportion (31%) of 'false positives' was recorded in endemic districts, which could be due to the pre-clinical stage of the disease (Ameni *et al.* 2006).

Diagnosis in a 2-year-old Trakehner filly with pulmonary histoplasmosis was based on thoracic radiography, transtracheal wash cytology, and lung aspirate cytology (Cornick 1990).

Pathology

Cutaneous lesions begin as papules or nodules that later ulcerate into crateriform lesions. In the lung and other tissues multiple granulomas or pyogranulomas are found. The fungal yeast form is abundantly found intralesionally and in exudates. Freely present or within macrophages it is round to ovoid and measures 2–3 μm in diameter (Jubb *et al.* 2007). Abdominal histoplasmosis in a 4-year-old female Thoroughbred race horse suffering from acute peritonitis was considered secondary to granulomas formed in the duodenum, lung, liver, and abdominal lymph nodes primarily caused by *Yersinia enterocolitica* (Katayama *et al.* 2001).

Management/Treatment

Preference should be given to eradication, although amphotericin B is the drug of choice for the treatment of clinical cases (Al-Ani 1999). A 5-week regimen of amphotericin B administered intravenously to a 2-year-old Trakehner filly with pulmonary histoplasmosis resulted in clinical recovery and return of the animal to normal activity (Cornick 1990).

An attenuated vaccine and a killed formalized vaccine are available and can be used in endemic areas to control the disease (Al-Ani 1999).

Public health significance

Histoplasmosis is the most common endemic mycosis causing human infection. Large outbreaks have been ascribed to histoplasmosis, but most infections are sporadic. Improvements in diagnostic tests have made it feasible to establish a diagnosis of histoplasmosis more quickly, thus allowing appropriate antifungal therapy to be started promptly (Kauffman 2009). Classical histoplasmosis caused by *H. capsulatum* var. *capsulatum*, and African histoplasmosis caused by *H. capsulatum* var. *duboisii* are both endemic in Africa. *H. capsulatum* var. *capsulatum* is known to occur naturally in caves inhabited by bats. Outbreaks of histoplasmosis have been reported in cave explorers. Surveys of histoplasmin skin sensitivity carried out in Africa have shown the rate of positive reactors to be 0–28% (Gugnani 2000).

Chapter 5
Ectoparasitical diseases

Gasterophilus spp.

Definition/Overview

Bot flies (*Gasterophilus* spp.) commonly infect horses with second- and third-stage larvae found attached to the mucosa of the stomach and duodenum. Sometimes larvae are noticed in the oral cavity.

Aetiology

The two species predominantly involved are *G. intestinalis* (two rows of spines on each segment) and *G. nasalis* (onc row of spines on each segment) (Soulsby 1968). *G. pecorum* has been reported in the soft palate of a 4-year-old British pony (Smith *et al.* 2005). The latter has complete rows of spines only on segments two to five (Soulsby 1968). *G. nasalis* specimens from different geographical areas display a level of genetic diversity (Pawlas-Opiela *et al.* 2010). Abundant microorganisms are observed in the endoperitrophic space of the anterior midgut in *G. intestinalis* instars (Roelfstra *et al.* 2010).

Epidemiology

The infection rate in equids 1-year-old or older at necropsy in central Kentucky was 12% for second instars and 14% for third instars for *G. intestinalis*, and for *G. nasalis* it was 2% for second instars and 14% for third instars (Lyons *et al.* 2000). In comparison, a low prevalence of *G. intestinalis* infection was detected (1.4%) in the Czech Republic (Bezdekova *et al.* 2007).

Pathophysiology

It has been shown that the stage L_2 is more immunogenic than the stage L_3, most probably as an effect of the higher enzymatic production of L_2 while migrating through the host tissues (Roelfstra *et al.* 2009).

The life cycle usually involves one generation per year in temperate regions. Adult *G. intestinalis* botflies lay their yellow eggs predominantly on the hairs of the forelimbs of the horse in autumn and they are licked off the hair during grooming. The eggs are ready to hatch in 5–10 days. After hatching, the larvae spend about 4 weeks in the oral cavity followed by migration to the stomach/duodenum, where they attach to the mucosa for about 10–12 months and then pass out through the intestine. *G. intestinalis* is usually found attached to the gastric squamous mucosa (306–309), whereas *G. nasalis* is found attached to the glandular mucosa of the stomach, pylorus, and duodenum. When mature in spring or early summer they are passed out in faeces to pupate and develop to the adult bot fly 4–5 weeks later (Soulsby 1968).

Clinical presentation

The clinical significance of bot larvae in the stomach is not well understood, but they have been associated with gastric ulceration, peritonitis secondary to gastroduodenal perforation, gastroesophageal reflux (310), splenitis (Dart *et al.* 1987) and pleuritis (van der Kolk *et al.* 1989). Furthermore, colonic perforation has been associated with aberrant migration of a *G. intestinalis* larva (Lapointe *et al.* 2003).

306 Third-stage *Gasterophilus intestinalis* larvae attached to the gastric squamous mucosa, as visualized by endoscopy.

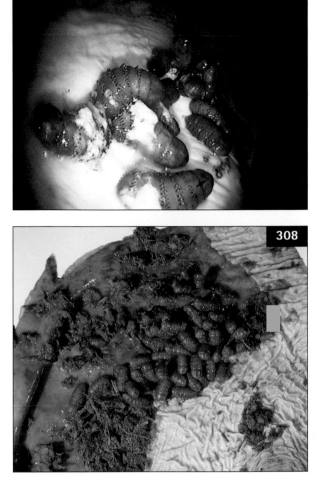

307, 308 Gastric gasterophilosis. Numerous fly larvae (bots) firmly attached to the stomach mucosa. *Gasterophilus intestinalis* is preferentially located on the pale squamous nonglandular fundus of the stomach (**307**). *Gasterophilus nasalis* is typically located at the pinkish glandular fundus part of the stomach (**308**). Although severe infestations with these bots can lead to gastric ulcerations, it usually is a coincidental necropsy finding.

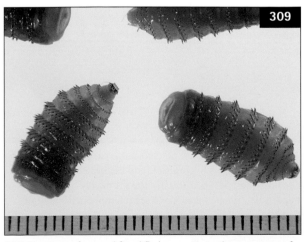

309 Close-up of several fixed fly larvae. Note the two rows of backward oriented cuticular spines per circumferential band. *Gasterophilus intestinalis*. (Scale in mm.)

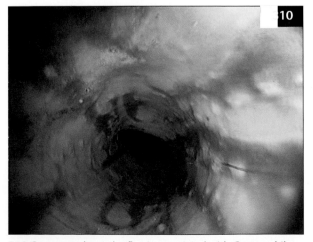

310 Gastroesophageal reflux is associated with *Gasterophilus intestinalis* infestation, as visualized by endoscopy of the oesophagus.

Diagnosis

The eggs can be found by examining the sites in which they are deposited, and larvae in the oral cavity can be seen on direct inspection (Soulsby 1968). Botfly larvae attached to the mucosa of the digestive tract can be visualized by means of endoscopy. Furthermore, an ELISA based on excretory/secretory antigens of second instar *Gasterophilus* for the diagnosis of gasterophilosis in grazing horses has been developed (Sánchez-Andrade *et al.* 2010).

Pathology

Predominantly associated with gastric mucosal erosion and ulceration (**311–316**). Additional pathology depends on sequelae.

Management/Treatment

Avermectin anthelmintics preferably administered in late autumn are highly effective against botfly larvae. In addition, treatment with 0.4 mg/kg BW moxidectin orally also had a very high activity against both *G. intestinalis* and *G. nasalis* up to 34 days after treatment of ponies (Coles *et al.* 1998). Furthermore, removing the eggs from the hairs of the forelimbs should be considered as a preventive measure.

Public health significance

Botflies have public health significance and their zoonotic risk should be minimized. Although it rarely infests man, larvae may cause a cutaneous swelling at the point at which the first larva penetrates the skin. More rarely the larvae reach the human stomach and cause irritation there (Soulsby 1968).

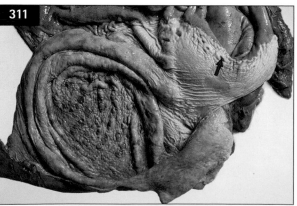

311 Chronic multifocal gastritis. Multiple grey-blue slightly prominent foci composed of chronic haemorrhage, fibrosis, and scant mononuclear infiltrates within the squamous nonglandular fundus. Scars probably due to a former fly larvae *Gasterophilus intestinalis* infection are seen. Note the several small crateriform ulcerations near the margo plicatus (arrow), consistent also with fly larvae scars.

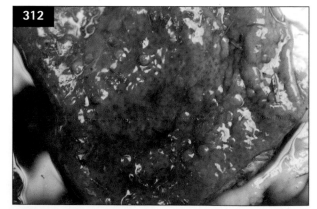

312 Multifocal to coalescing chronic hyperplastic gastritis. The glandular fundus is hyperplastic and thickened due to poorly circumscribed pale proliferative lesions mainly composed of hyperplastic gastric glands and scant lymphocytic infiltrates. For gasterophiliasis differential diagnoses include infection with the nematodes *Trichostrongylus axei* and *Draschia megastoma*.

313, 314 Chronic catarrhal gastritis in a donkey. **313**: Contrary to the chronic multifocal ulcerative gastritis in gasterophiliasis, this glandular fundus is diffusely thickened and hyperaemic due to a nematode infection; **314**: the corresponding micrograph depicts the hyperaemic inflamed gastric mucosa with intralesional nematodes (arrows). *Trichostrongylus axei*. (H&E stain. Bar 200 μm.)

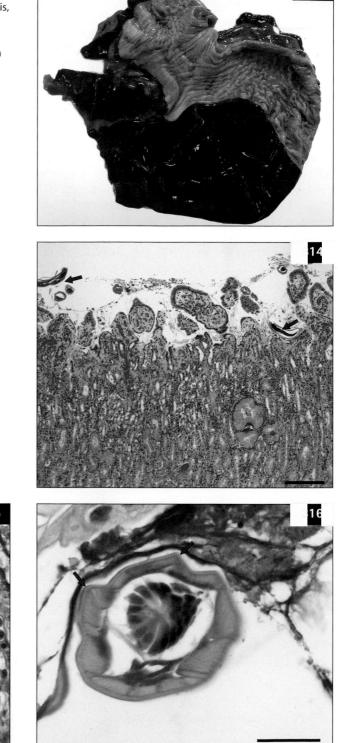

315, 316 Chronic catarrhal gastritis in a donkey. Close-up micrographs of *T. axei* embedded within the gastric mucosa on partial longitudinal section (**315**) with accompanying lymphoplasmacytic infiltrates. On cross section (**316**) note the multiple longitudinal cuticular ridges (arrows). *Trichostrongylus axei*. (PAS stain. Bars 50 μm.)

MITES

Definition/Overview
In equids, chorioptic mange is a common dermatitis (Rendle *et al.* 2007) and in horses, *Chorioptes bovis* mites were mainly found in the Belgian and Friesian breeds (40% and 62% infected, respectively) (Cremers 1985).

Aetiology
Chorioptes (**317**) resembles *Psoroptes*, but the tarsal suckers have unjointed pedicles. The life history is completed in 3 weeks and resembles that of *Psoroptes*. *Psoroptes* eggs are laid on the skin at the edges of the lesion and hatch normally in 1–3 days. The larvae feed and, 2–3 days after hatching, moult to the nymphal stage, passing the last 12 hours in a state of lethargy. The nymphal stage lasts 3–4 days, including a lethargic period of 36 hours before the moult occurs. The smaller nymphs usually become males. As a rule the pubescent females appear before the males, sometimes as soon as 5.5 days after hatching, while the males do not appear before the 6th day. As a rule the proportion of males to females is 1–2:4. The pubescent female moults 2 days after commencement of copulation and the ovigerous female begins to lay 1 day later, or 9 days after hatching from the egg. The shortest period observed is 8 days. The female lives 30–40 days and lays about five eggs daily and a total of 90 or more. In *Sarcoptes* mites development from the time the eggs are laid lasts about 17 days.

Unlike the species of the Sarcoptidae and Chorioptidae, Psoroptidae (genus *Psoroptes* (Acari: Psoroptidae)) are specific to their hosts (Soulsby 1968) and are believed to have a central African origin (Fain 1975). Furthermore, it is suggested that the ear mite, *P. cuniculi*, and the sheep scab mite, *P. ovis*, are variants of the same species (Bates 1999). Within the genus *Chorioptes* two phenotypes can be distinguished, designated as *C. bovis* and *C. texanus*.

Epidemiology
The apparent lack of host specificity of both species suggests that mites are dispersed freely in a wide range of hosts, and this might have contributed to the wide geographic distribution of these species (Essig *et al.* 1999).

Clinical presentation
Distribution of lesions varies according to the type of mite. Chorioptic mange has been detected in para-anal fold, distal portion of legs (**318–320**) and tail lesions. Psoroptic mange has been detected in withers, mane, shoulder, and flank lesions, whereas sarcoptic mange has been isolated mainly from lesions on the head and neck (Osman *et al.* 2006).

Differential diagnosis
The differential diagnosis includes various causes of pruritus (see p. 263).

Diagnosis
Adult mites and eventually smaller nymphs or larvae and eggs can be found by microscopic examination of skin scrapings.

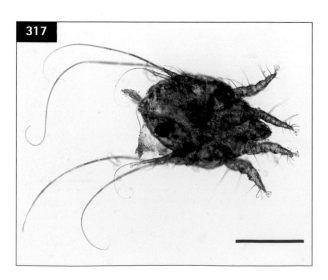

317 Chorioptic mange. Micrograph of adult *Chorioptes bovis* (*C. equi*) mite (itchy leg mite) measuring approximately 0.4 mm in length. As an arachnid it is composed of a relative large abdomen and a smaller fused head and thorax. Note the four pairs of jointed legs covered with small chitinized hairs or setae, whilst in addition the backward-facing hind legs harbour lengthy curved hairs. No antennae are present. Psoroptidae, *Chorioptes bovis* (*C. equi*). (Bar 200 μm.)

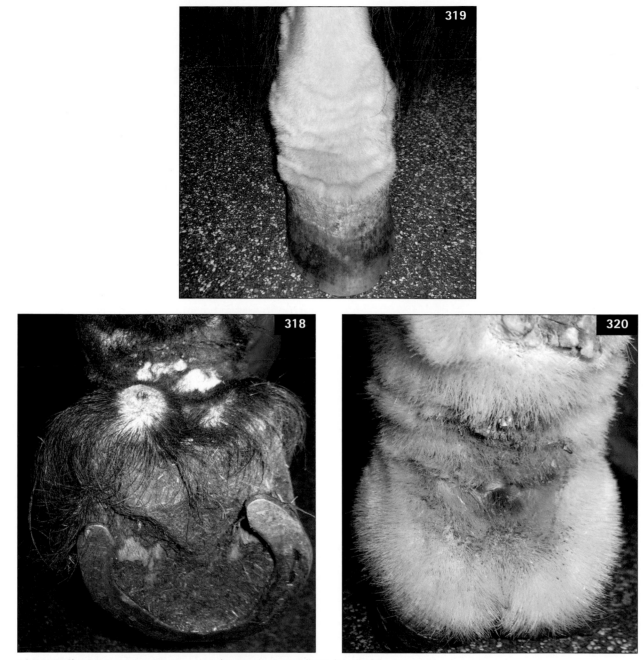

318–320 Chorioptic mange is a common dermatitis, especially in draught horses.

Pathology

Predominantly associated with chronic superficial dermatitis and epidermal hyperplasia and hyperkeratosis (**321–323**).

Management/Treatment

The treatment of the superficial *Chorioptes* mite is challenging as treatment failure and relapse are very common. Oral moxidectin (0.4 mg/kg BW given twice with a 3 week interval) in combination with environmental insecticide treatment (4-chloro-3-methylphenol and propoxur) was ineffective in the treatment of *C. bovis* in feathered horses (Rüfenacht *et al.* 2011). Treatment with sulphurated lime dip as a 5% solution four times at 7-day intervals with most horses clipped and/or shampooed prior to

treatment resulted in elimination of chorioptic infection (Paterson & Coumbe 2009).

There was no significant difference between the effectiveness of doramectin (0.3 mg/kg BW SC on two occasions 14 days apart) or fipronil (all limbs of the horses sprayed with fipronil 0.25% solution) in the treatment of equine chorioptic mange (Rendle *et al.* 2007). However, topical eprinomectin pour-on solution treatment (at a dose of 500 µg/kg BW once weekly for four applications) was effective and safe therapy against natural infestations of psoroptic mange (Ural *et al.* 2008). It has been suggested that moxidectin oral gel is an effective and good alternative for the treatment of chorioptic mange in horses to avoid drug resistance that may develop as a result of the intensive use of ivermectin alone for long periods (Osman *et al.* 2006).

Public health significance

Sarcoptic mange has public health significance, and is a reportable disease.

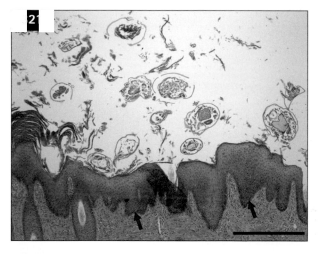

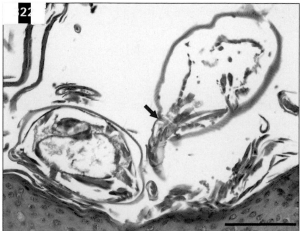

322 Chorioptic mange, leg mange. Close-up of two cross-sectioned mites embedded within the scaling stratum corneum. Histologically, mites are characterized by an eosinophilic ridged chitinous exoskeleton and striated muscles attached to jointed appendages (arrow). *Chorioptes bovis* (*C. equi*). (H&E stain. Bar 100 µm.)

321 Chorioptic mange, leg mange. Chronic superficial lymphohistiocytic and eosinophilic dermatitis with epidermal hyperplasia and hyperkeratosis. Numerous chorioptic adult mites, including smaller nymphs or larvae and eggs, on the skin surface interspersed within the scaling and crusting stratum corneum incite a superficial dermal mixed inflammatory infiltrate, as well as a hyperplastic thickening of the epidermis with formation of epidermal papillae or rete ridges (arrows). *Chorioptes bovis* (*C. equi*). (H&E stain. Bar 500 µm.)

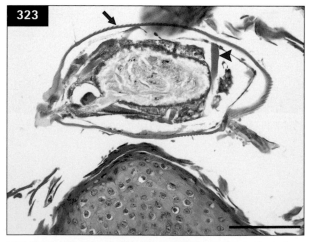

323 Chorioptic mange, leg mange. Close-up of a sectioned mite. Note the small spines or ridges (arrow) on the chitinous cuticle, which shows birefringence when viewed under polarized light, and striated musculature (arrowhead). *Chorioptes bovis* (*C. equi*). (H&E stain. Bar 100 µm.)

LICE

Definition/Overview

Pediculosis in equids is associated with either *Werneckiella* (chewing louse, formerly *Damalinia*) *equi* (**324**), or blood sucking lice *Haematopinus equi* or *H. asini*. Both types of louse can cause skin irritation and pruritic automutilated alopecic areas. Pediculosis is usually an indication of underlying predisposing factors such as overcrowding, poor hygiene, and possibly debilitating disease.

Aetiology

The operculated eggs are cemented, without stalks, to the hairs of the host. There is no metamorphosis. The egg hatches into a form which resembles the adult and is called the first nymph. There are three ecdyses, the first nymph becoming the second nymph, which becomes the third nymph and this becomes the adult. As a consequence, the whole life history is passed on the host.

Epidemiology

Uninfected hosts are infected by close contact with infected ones, but lice may also be spread by equipment and personnel (Soulsby 1968).

Clinical presentation

Clinical signs present in the head and the neck/mane area were found to be an indication of lice infestation in horses. Focal alopecia was the main clinical sign in Icelandic horses (84%) on lice-positive horses, while scaling and crusts occurred in 11% and 10% of cases, respectively (Larsen *et al.* 2005). In another report no correlation between lice burden and clinical signs was detected (Mencke *et al.* 2005). However, it should be realized that in clinically healthy horses pediculosis is very rare, consequently signs of the primary disease might predominate and obscure the clinical presentation of pediculosis.

Differential diagnosis

The differential diagnosis includes various causes of pruritus (see p. 263).

Diagnosis

Pediculosis can be assessed by visual inspection of the hair coat (**325**).

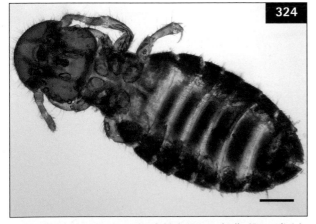

324 Pediculosis. Micrograph of adult *Werneckiella* (*Damalinia*) *equi* louse dorsoventrally flattened measuring approximately 2 mm in length. Note the three pairs of jointed legs with terminal clinging hooks set on the mid section (thorax) and two antennae sprouting from the broad head; small hairs or setae cover most of the body. *Werneckiella* (*Damalinia*) *equi*. (Bar 200 μm.)

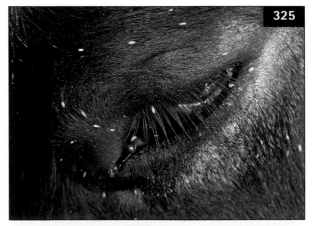

325 Pediculosis. The peri-ocular haired skin is infested with numerous small light brown lice. This biting louse *Werneckiella* (*Damalinia*) *equi* can be found in areas such as the head, neck, flanks, and tail base, as the females prefer to lay their eggs in finer hair. It feeds on skin debris.

Pathology

Especially associated with secondary skin lesions due to pruritus.

Management/Treatment

A double application of 4 ml and 8 ml 10% imidacloprid spot-on on days 0 and 28 induced a drop in lice counts 2 days after either treatment, with all animals free of live lice on day 56 with dermatological lesions decreased significantly (Mencke *et al.* 2005).

Public health significance

As species-specific ectoparasites, lice from horses may cause a minimal transient pruritus.

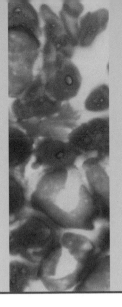

Chapter 6
Helmintic diseases

Fasciola hepatica

Phylum Platyhelminthes/Class Trematoda/Order Echinostomida/Suborder Fasciolata/Family Fasciolidae/Genus *Fasciola*

Definition/Overview

Fasciola hepatica is the most common liver fluke, with worldwide distribution. It is of economic importance in sheep and cattle, but horses are infrequently infected. Prenatal infections are reported in foals. Chronic fascioliasis is the most common form of the infection in sheep, cattle, and other animals (including man) (Soulsby 1968, Owen 1977).

Aetiology

Although fluke disease can be caused by species from three different groups (liver, lung, and intestinal) *F. hepatica* is the most important fluke parasite in domesticated animals, along with *F. gigantica* (Soulsby 1968, Keiser & Utzinger 2009). The bodies of trematodes or flukes are dorso-ventrally flattened and, unlike those of tapeworms, they consist of one piece only. Their reproductive system is hermaphroditic. *F. hepatica* may reach a size of 30 × 13 mm. The eggs measure 130–150 × 63–90 μm. The *Fasciola* egg (**326A, B**) has a yellow shell with an indistinct operculum (Soulsby 1968). Sequence-related amplified polymorphism (SRAP) revealed four major clusters indicating the existence of genetic variability within the examined *F. hepatica* samples from Spain. These four clusters were not related to particular host species and/or geographical origins of the samples (Alasaad *et al.* 2008).

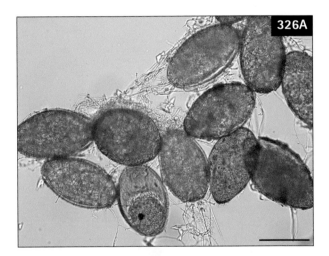

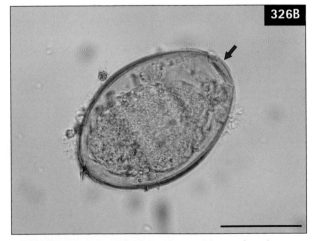

326 A, B *Fasciola hepatica* eggs obtained from a faecal sample. The ovoid thin-shelled uni-poled operculated eggs measure approximately 130 × 70 μm and are typically filled with granular yellowish-brown contents. The operculum is indicated by an arrow. (Bars 100/50 μm, respectively.)

The life cycle of Echinostomida usually requires one, two, or more than two, intermediate hosts (**327**). Important host snails for *F. hepatica* are *Galba* (formerly *Lymnaea*) *truncatula* in Europe and *Galba bulimoides* in the USA. The term metacercaria is given to the cercaria after it has encysted either inside the second intermediate host or on herbage or elsewhere (Soulsby 1968, Owen 1977).

F. hepatica develops to the adult stage in the bile ducts of the host. Their eggs pass through the bile ducts (**328–331**) and are excreted via the faeces.

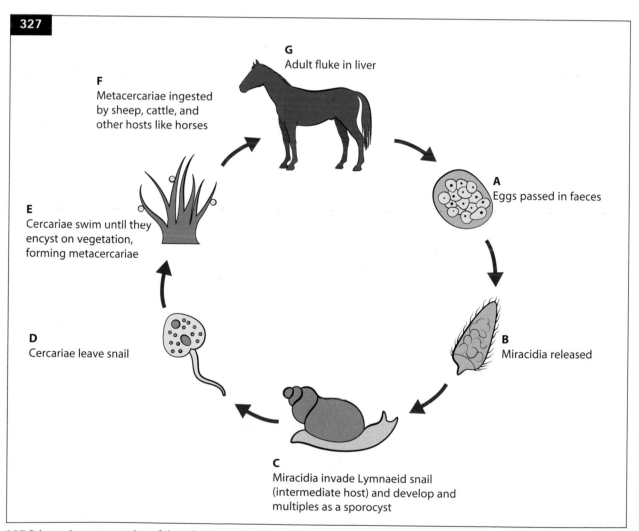

327

G
Adult fluke in liver

F
Metacercariae ingested by sheep, cattle, and other hosts like horses

A
Eggs passed in faeces

E
Cercariae swim until they encyst on vegetation, forming metacercariae

B
Miracidia released

D
Cercariae leave snail

C
Miracidia invade Lymnaeid snail (intermediate host) and develop and multiples as a sporocyst

327 Schematic representation of the infection cycle of *Fasciola hepatica*. *F. hepatica* develops to the adult stage in the bile-ducts of the host. Their eggs pass the bile ducts and are excreted via the faeces. Development of the eggs generates miracidia, which actively invade the host snail either via penetration of its skin or via ingestion by the snail, where they hatch in its gut, leaving the host as cercariae. The cercariae encyst into metacercariae on plants and are ingested by the final host. Following ingestion by the final host the metacercariae penetrate the intestinal wall and migrate through the peritoneal cavity to the liver. After invasion of the liver the cycle ends in the bile ducts.

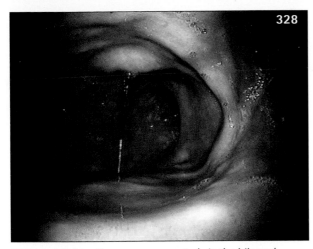

328 *Fasciola hepatica* eggs are excreted via the bile and subsequently in the faeces. Shown (dorsally) is the major duodenal papilla on which both the common hepatic duct and the pancreatic duct open into the duodenum. Opposite to the major duodenal papilla is the minor duodenal papilla, on which the accessory pancreatic duct opens into the duodenum.

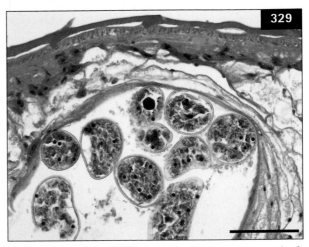

329 Hepatic fascioliasis, distomatosis. Close-up micrograph of intrauterine ovoid thin-shelled eggs of *Fasciola hepatica*. Being trematodes, adult flukes are hermaphroditic and can produce up to several thousands of eggs each day. The unipoled operculated eggs measure approximately 130 × 70 μm. *Galba truncatula*, an aquatic snail, serves as intermediate host in the development of the cercariae. Note also the fluke's spined tegument. (H&E stain. Bar 100 μm.)

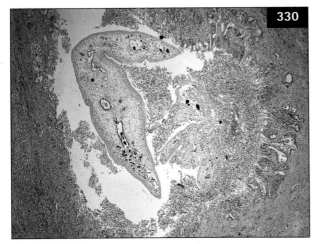

330 Hepatic fascioliasis, distomatosis. Photomicrograph of an inflamed bile duct containing a fluke embedded in cellular debris and brownish bile pigments. Note the hyperplasia of the ductal epithelium on the right and erosion of the epithelium on the left. (H&E stain.)

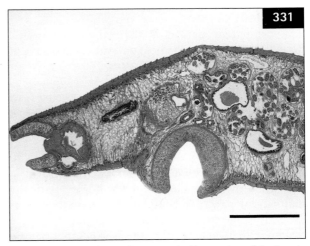

331 Hepatic fascioliasis, distomatosis. Cut section of the head of a *Fasciola hepatica* fluke. Note the two (oral and ventral) inverted cup-shaped suckers with which the fluke adheres to the inside of bile ducts. (H&E stain. Bar 1 mm.)

Development of the eggs generates miracidia, which actively invade the host snail (332) either via penetration of its skin or via ingestion by the snail, where they hatch in its gut and leave the host snail as cercariae. The cercariae encyst into metacercariae on plants and are ingested by the final host. Following ingestion by the final host the metacercariae penetrate the intestinal wall and migrate through the peritoneal cavity to the liver. After invasion of the liver the cycle ends in the bile ducts (Soulsby 1968, Owen 1977). The flukes usually live about 9 months in sheep and in one case a survival time of 11 years has been recorded (Soulsby 1968). In unusual hosts, such as man and the horse, the fluke *F. hepatica* may be found in the lungs, under the skin, or in other locations (Soulsby 1968).

Epidemiology

In 4,399 faecal samples from horses, coprological examination revealed 0.04% positive samples for *F. hepatica* (Epe *et al.* 2004). In Egypt, zoonotic fascioliasis in donkeys is increasing and post-mortem examination revealed hepatic fascioliasis in 17% of cases (Haridy *et al.* 2007).

Pre-patent period

The pre-patent period is defined as the period between infection of the host and the earliest time at which the parasite can be recovered from either faeces or urine as eggs or larvae.

Eggs of *Fasciola hepatica* can be observed 14–15 weeks post-infection in horses (Soulé *et al.* 1989). Experimental data show that the horse exhibits a pronounced resistance to the establishment of a liver fluke infection. With oral doses of up to 800 metacercariae a patent infection was established in one study in only one out of ten horses, with the majority of parasites eliminated or immobilized at an early stage of the infection, presumably before reaching the liver. This hypothesis was supported by the finding that about 15% of excysted larvae implanted intraperitoneally in two horses, succeeded in reaching maturity in the bile ducts (Nansen *et al.* 1975).

Clinical presentation

Although subclinical infection is quite common, clinical signs include fever, icterus, photodermatitis (333–335), coagulation disorders, hepatoen-cephalopathy, and weight loss. Infections may go undetected (Alves *et al.* 1988, Gorman *et al.* 1997), as horses have a high level of resistance to both *F. hepatica* and *F. gigantica* (Nansen *et al.* 1975, Alves *et al.* 1988).

Differential diagnosis

The differential diagnosis comprises various causes of icterus and fever (see p. 262).

Diagnosis

Diagnosis of infection is routinely based on finding the fluke eggs in faeces by coprological examination. However, this method is not sensitive, and infections where the parasite burden is low or when the host is harbouring immature flukes in the liver parenchyma or the bile ducts during the pre-patent phase of the infection may go undetected (Gorman *et al.* 1997). Moreover, in some species such as horses, an intermittent fluke egg elimination has been described (Owen 1977). Furthermore, some of the hepatocellular enzymes may be increased in activity like sorbitol dehydrogenase (SDH), aspartate aminotransferase (AST), alkaline phosphatase (AF), lactate dehydrogenase (LDH), and γ-glutamyl-transferase (γ-GT) associated with increased concentration of conjugated (or direct) bilirubin. Plasma glutamate dehydrogenase and γ-GT levels increased 3–5 months post-infection (Soulé *et al* 1989). Horses infected by 1,000 metacercariae and more showed 18% of positive samples by counter-electrophoresis, 49% by ELISA, and 76% by passive haemagglutination (Soulé *et al.* 1989). Against the criteria of high sensitivity and specificity, the 22–30 kDa polypeptides would appear to be the most suitable candidate antigens for use in the immunodiagnosis of fascioliasis in horses, as they were recognized by sera from all infected horses, but not by sera from uninfected horses (Gorman *et al.* 1997).

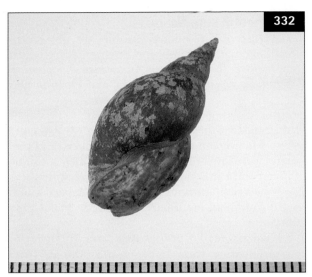

332 An empty shell of *Galba truncatula*, the important host snail for *F. hepatica* in Europe, among other freshwater snails of the family Lymnaeidae. (Scale in mm.)

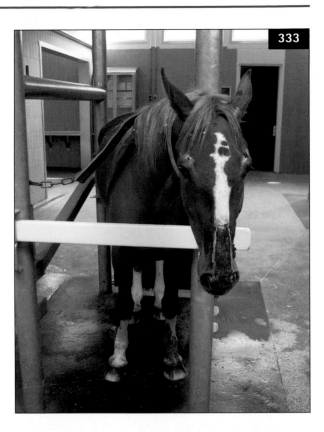

333–335 Photodermatitis in a 3-year-old Warmblood mare.

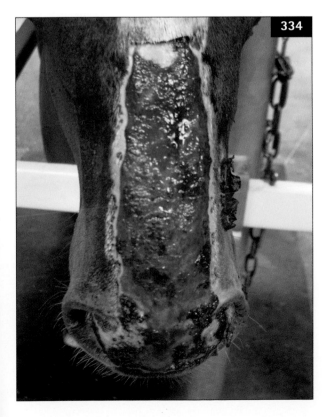

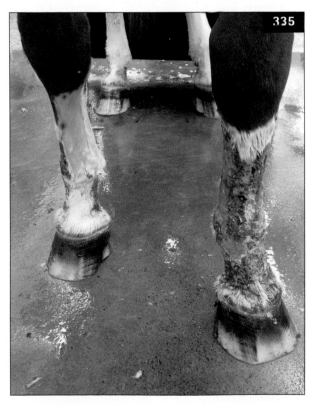

Pathology

Macroscopic evaluation of affected livers can reveal dark red necrohaemorrhagic tortuous migration tracts due to peripatetic larvae. These acute lesions of hepatocellular necrosis develop into pale, possibly contracted, streaks and foci due to infiltrating eosinophils and scarring fibrosis. Mature flukes (336) reside in bile ducts and incite a chronic cholangitis with inherent (peri)ductular fibrosis and cholestasis. Both acute and chronic lesions may be present concurrently. Dilation of bile ducts in horses is mainly due to obstruction of bile flow. Microscopically there may be intraluminal papillary projections of hyperplastic bile duct epithelium, an additional obstructing factor. The left liver lobe is generally more gravely affected than the right, indicated by atrophy and fibrosis potentially combined with compensatory hyperplasia of the right lobe (337). Further possible lesions include peritonitis and hepatic abscesses and in severe chronic infections a debilitating state of the animal, icterus, photosensitive dermatitis, and (rarely) bilateral laryngeal paralysis (338).

Management/Treatment

In foals with an adult infection and a presumed immature infection with *F. hepatica* 12 mg triclabendazole/kg BW orally is a treatment option. The absence of eggs from samples of faeces examined at intervals of up to 110 days after treatment showed that all the animals were cured (Rubilar *et al.* 1988). Eradication of the host snails from the environment is an important but difficult part of fluke control.

Public health significance

An estimated 750 million people are at risk of infections with food-borne trematodes, which comprise liver flukes (*Clonorchis sinensis, F. gigantica, F. hepatica, Opisthorchis felineus,* and *Opisthorchis viverrini*), lung flukes (*Paragonimus* spp.), and intestinal flukes (e.g., *Echinostoma* spp., *Fasciolopsis buski,* and the heterophyids) (Keiser & Utzinger 2009). Metacercarial viabilities of donkey (and pig) isolates were similar to the viabilities of metacercariae of sheep and cattle isolates, suggesting that donkeys also have a high transmission potential capacity with regard to human fascioliasis (Valero & Mas-Coma 2000).

Measurements of *F. hepatica* and *F. gigantica* eggs originating from humans and animals from sympatric areas overlap, and, therefore, they do not allow differential diagnosis when within this overlapping range. In this sense, the classic egg size range in human samples may lead to erroneous conclusions (Valero *et al.* 2009).

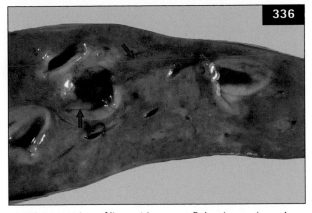

336 Cross-section of liver with mature flukes (arrows) causing chronic cholangitis. (Courtesy of Dr G. C. M. Grinwis.)

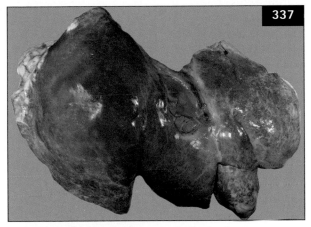

337 Hepatic fascioliasis, distomatosis. Equine liver, diaphragmatic surface, chronic cholangitis and hepatitis due to a severe infection with the common liver fluke, *Fasciola hepatica*. As a result the left lobe (right side of photograph) has diminished in size and is pale and firm because of atrophy and replacement fibrosis. The right lobes show compensatory hyperplasia. (courtesy of Dr G.C.M. Grinwis.)

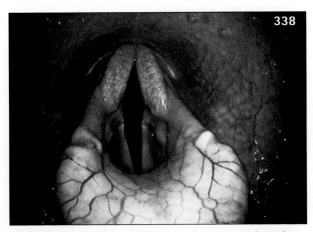

338 Bilateral laryngeal paralysis as a very rare neurological sequela of liver failure in a 9-year-old Warmblood gelding.

Anoplocephala spp.

Phylum Platyhelminthes/Class Cestoda/Subclass
Eucestoda/Order Cyclophyllidea/Suborder
Anoplocephalata/Family Anoplocephalidae/Genus
Anoplocephala

Definition/Overview

Tapeworm (genera *Anoplocephala*) of horses are
found near the ileocaecal valve and are associated
with spasmodic colic and various intussusceptions.

Aetiology

Anoplocephala perfoliata, A. magna, and
Anoplocephaloides mamillana (formerly
Paranoplocephala mamillana) (339, 340) are the
common tapeworm species of horses, with infection
following ingestion of grass mites containing the
intermediate cysticercoid stage. All equine tapeworms
require grass mites as an intermediate host in which
the intermediate cysticercoid stage is produced. *A.
perfoliata* is regarded as the most important species.
Tapeworms are hermaphrodite, endoparasitic worms
with an elongate, flat body and without a body cavity
or an alimentary canal. The body consists of a head
or scolex, usually provided with suckers and hooks,
and a strobilum, which consists of a number of
segments or proglottides. Each proglottid usually
contains one or two sets of male and female
reproductive organs. The life cycle is indirect,
requiring one or more intermediate hosts. The eggs
have a pyriform apparatus and measure 50–60 µm
(341). *A. magna* occurs in the small intestine and
occasionally in the stomach of equines. It measures
up to 80 cm in length and 2 cm wide. *A. perfoliata*
occurs in the small and large intestine of equines. *A.
perfoliata* frequently localizes near the ileo-caecal
valve, which may show ulceration, oedema, and
occasionally a marked excess of granulation tissue
(342, 343). It measures up to 8 × 1.2 cm (344–346).
The eggs measure 65–80 µm. *A. mamillana* occurs in
the small intestine and occasionally the stomach of
the horse. It measures only 6–50 × 4–6 mm. The eggs
measure about 51 × 37 µm (Soulsby 1968).

Epidemiology

In one study, *A. perfoliata* prevalence was 52%,
whereas *A. magna* was seldom found in weanlings
(Lyons *et al.* 2000). Frequent use of ivermectin might
induce tapeworm superinfestation.

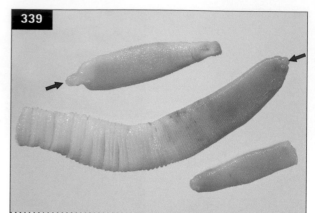

339 Cestodiasis, equine tapeworms. *Anoplocephala magna*
(middle), *A. perfoliata* (top and bottom). *Anoplocephaloides
mamillana* (not shown) is the third and smallest tapeworm in
the horse, like *A. magna* it usually inhabits the small intestines.
A. perfoliata is preferentially found at the ileocaecal junction or
proximal caecum. Note the small round scolices (arrows) and
short neck from which the proglottid segmented body or
strobilum starts. (Formalin fixed specimens. Scale in mm.)

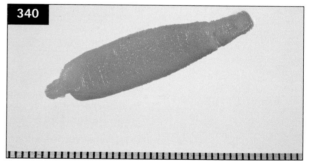

340 Cestodiasis, *Anoplocephala perfoliata* tapeworm. It can
grow up to 8 cm in length and 1.5 cm in width. (Formalin fixed
specimen. Scale in mm.)

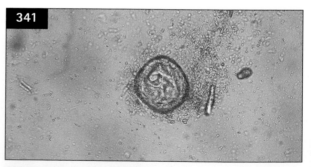

341 Cestodiasis, *Anoplocephala perfoliata* tapeworm. Eggs
mature in the proglottides, which are shed with the faeces.
Once in the environment oribatid mites (grass or soil mites)
ingest the ova and serve as intermediate hosts in which larvae
(cysticercoids) develop. These infective mites are arbitrarily
taken up by foraging horses.

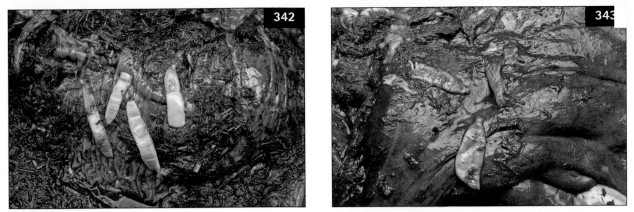

342, 343 Cestodiasis. Several typical ribbon-like tapeworms attached to the intestinal mucosa of the ileocaecal junction by means of their suckers located on the head or scolex. Mucosal erosions and ulcerations can occur in severe infections. *Anoplocephala perfoliata*.

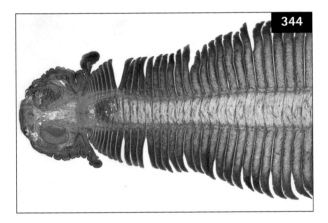

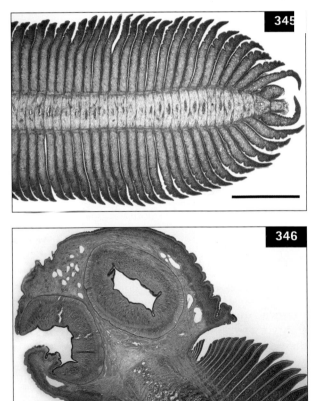

344, 345 Cestodiasis, micrograph of *Anoplocephala perfoliata*. Note the extensive segmented body. The segments or proglottides are each a fully functional element and contain a digestive system and both male and female reproductive organs with developing eggs. New proglottides grow continuously and when fully mature they break off at the posterior end and are shed in the faeces. No single central gastrointestinal tract is present; nutrients are taken up directly from the host's gut. (PAS stain. Bar 1 mm.)

346 Cestodiasis, close-up micrograph of *Anoplocephala perfoliata*. Note the round scolex with two oval suckers visible (four in total). From the short neck down the proglottides are generated. (PAS stain. Bar 500 μm.)

Pathophysiology

As adult equine tapeworms are found near the ileocaecal valve it is suggested that they may interfere with the motility of the region, thereby inducing intussusceptions (347–349).

Pre-patent period

Adult tapeworms are found 4–6 weeks after ingestion of infected mites with herbage (Soulsby 1968).

Clinical presentation

The majority of tapeworm infestations do not cause clinical signs. However, A. perfoliata is considered a likely risk factor in horses with colic and ileal impaction (Proudman et al. 1998, Proudman & Holdstock 2000). A. perfoliata has also been found in association with other intestinal disorders, especially those affecting the ileocaecal region, including peritonitis and caecal abscessation (Beroza et al. 1983), caecal rupture (Cosgrove et al. 1986), and ileocaecal, caecocolic, and caecocaecal intussusceptions (Edwards 1986).

Differential diagnosis

The differential diagnosis includes various causes of colic. Only three common parasitisms of horses are likely to be manifested as colic: Strongylus vulgaris, Parascaris equorum, and A. perfoliata (Reinemeyer & Nielsen 2009).

Diagnosis

Tapeworm proglottides may be visible macroscopically in the faeces. The detection of eggs of A. perfoliata in faeces is hampered by the necessity for there to be a ruptured proglottides in the faeces (French et al. 1994). The tapeworm eggs are characterized by the presence of a hexacanth embryo. The sensitivity of the faecal identification of the eggs of A. perfoliata in horses is therefore low and allows only a qualitative assessment of the infection. A combination of centrifugation and flotation can improve the sensitivity of the method (Beroza et al. 1983, Rehbein et al. 2011), but it has been shown to have a sensitivity of only 61% (Proudman & Edwards 1992). A serum ELISA for the diagnosis of A. perfoliata is commercially available measuring the concentration of a serum antibody that is specific for a 12/13 kDa excretory/secretory antigen, and its concentration has been shown to be correlated with the intensity of the infection (Proudman et al. 1998). Diagnosis based upon faecal egg counts of horses with known numbers of worms was least accurate in detecting worm presence.

Detection of circulating antibodies to the cestode was most sensitive using Western blot analysis (100%), but had lower specificity (87%). A serum-based ELISA had a lower sensitivity (70%) for the detection of antibodies. A coproantigen ELISA had 74% sensitivity and 92% specificity, and there was a positive correlation between antigen concentration and tapeworm intensity (Skotarek et al. 2010). Furthermore, a nested PCR assay represents a valid method for the specific molecular detection of A. perfoliata in faecal samples collected from naturally infected horses and may have advantages over coprological and serological approaches for diagnosing A. perfoliata infection (Traversa et al. 2008).

Pathology

Injury to intestinal nervous elements at the ileocaecal junction in horses with moderate to high parasitism supports a correlation between colic and A. perfoliata infestation in the horse (Pavone et al. 2010), possibly leading to obstructions and intussusceptions.

Management/Treatment

It is recommended to dose less frequently than every 6 months to remove tapeworm infections with either 1.5 mg/kg BW praziquantel or pyrantel. The optimal time for blood sampling to monitor for effective tapeworm treatment using a serum ELISA appears to be 5 months after treatment (Abbott et al. 2008). Pyrantel at twice the normal dose rate (for normal strongyles) is regarded as effective.

Public health significance

Not convincing yet.

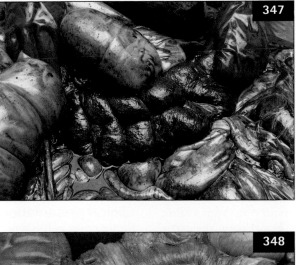

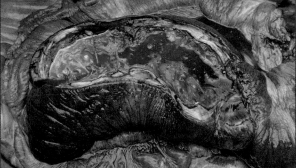

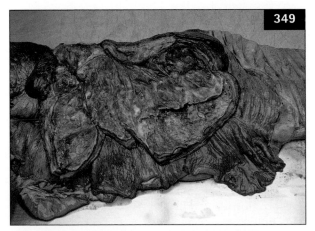

347–349 Caecocolic intussusception, cestodiasis. The opened colon (intussuscipiens) reveals the darkened incarcerated necrotic caecum (intussusceptum), which shows a thickened congested wall on the cut surface with extensive yellowish fibrinous depositions on the serosa. This is a lesion attributed to intestinal dysperistalsis due to either massive tapeworm or cyathostome infections.

Echinococcus equinus

Phylum Platyhelminthes/Class Cestoda/Subclass Eucestoda/Order Cyclophyllidea/Suborder Taeniata/Family Taeniidae/Genus *Echinococcus*

Definition/Overview

Equine cystic echinococcosis can be caused by various *Echinococcus* taxa, but only *Echinococcus equinus* (the 'horse strain') is known to produce fertile cysts.

Aetiology

E. granulosus consists of the following groups: *E. granulosus* sensu stricto (the sheep strain), *E. equinus* (the horse strain), *E. ortleppi* (the cattle strain), and *E. canadensis* (the human strain), with *E. granulosus* sensu strico having the widest global distribution (Nakao *et al.* 2007).

E. equinus infects dogs, red foxes, arctic foxes (experimentally), cats (experimentally), humans, sheep, goats, horses, donkeys, pigs, cattle, roe deer, and reindeer (in Scotland). Attempts to transmit *E. equinus* to badgers and domestic ferrets were unsuccessful. Of 123 cats infected with protoscolices of horse origin, one gravid adult parasite was recovered from one animal. *E. granulosus* sensu stricto does not mature either in foxes or in horses, *E. equinus* will mature in either (Cook 1989).

After the eggs have been ingested by the intermediate host they hatch in the intestine and the embryos migrate to the bloodstream, which carries them to various organs. The embryo grows into a large vesicle, 5–10 cm or more in diameter, known as an echinococcus or 'hydatid' cyst. The hydatid cyst (**350, 351**) has an internal germinal layer which produces numerous small vesicles or brood capsules about 5–6 months after infection. Each brood capsule may contain up to 40 scolices. The final host acquires the infection by ingesting fertile hydatids.

E. granulosus sensu stricto is 2.1–5.0 µm long and usually has only three proglottides. The sexually mature segment is the penultimate one and the gravid one is the last segment. The scolex has two rows of hooklets varying from 30 to 60 in number (**352–354**). The eggs are the typical *Taenia* eggs and they measure 32–36 × 25–30 µm (Soulsby 1968).

Epidemiology

In Europe, *E. equinus* appears to be endemic in Great Britain, Ireland, Spain, and Italy and has sporadically been reported in Belgium, Germany, and Switzerland (Blutke *et al.* 2010). Equine cyst echinococcosis in Italy had a prevalence rate of 0.3% (Varcasia *et al.* 2008).

Pre-patent period

The pre-patent period of *E. granulosus* sensu stricto in the definitive host is about 42 days while that of *E. equinus* is about 70 days (Cook 1989).

Clinical presentation

Equine cyst echinococcosis is usually an accidental finding and clinical presentation largely depends on localization of cyst(s).

Diagnosis

Ultrasonographic examination can be helpful in the (accidental) detection of cyst echinococcosis.

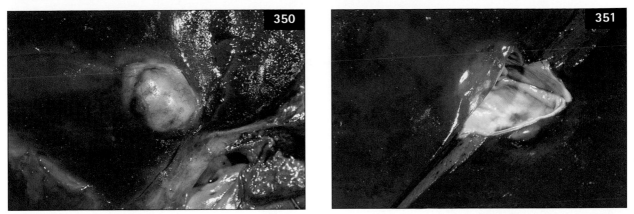

350, 351 Hepatic echinococcosis. Intact (**350**) and incised (**351**) unilocular hydatid cyst of *Echinococcus granulosus*, the intermediate stage of the cestode *E. equinus* in dogs and foxes.

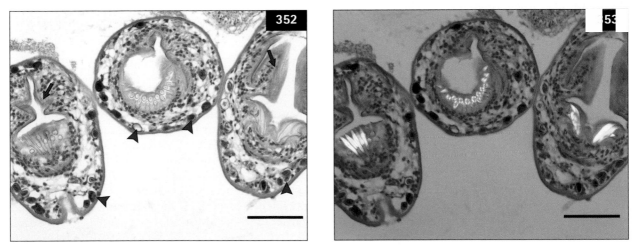

352, 353 Close-up micrographs of three protoscolices that each harbours the typical rostellar keratinized hooklets especially discernible because of their birefringence when viewed under polarized light (**353**). Note also the pale to dark basophilic calcareous corpuscles (arrowheads) and inverted suckers (arrows). *Echinococcus equinus*. (H&E stain. Bars 50 μm.)

354 Fresh unstained wet mount of a hydatid cyst's contents depicting two typically invaginated protoscolices with a central rostellar pad set with a double crown of hooks and lining calcareous corpuscles (arrows). Note the presence of several free-lying hooklets (arrowheads). *Echinococcus equinus*. (Bar 50 μm.)

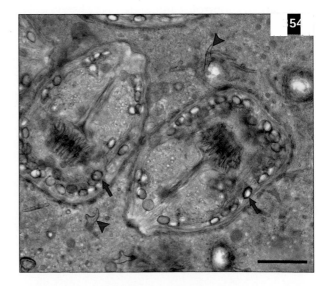

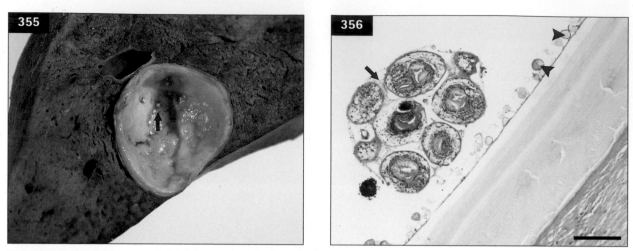

355, 356 Hepatic echinococcosis. **355**: Cut section of a formalin-fixed liver sample with a thick-walled hydatid cyst containing several small white brood capsules (arrow); **356**: corresponding micrograph depicting several protoscolices clustered in a brood capsule (arrow). Note the smaller spherical pale basophilic calcareous corpuscles (arrowheads) lining the germinal membrane of the thick hyaline laminary layer of the hydatid cyst wall. *Echinococcus equinus*. (H&E stain. Bar 100 µm.)

Pathology

Macroscopic evaluation might reveal a thick-walled hydatid cyst containing several small white brood capsules (355–358).

Management/Treatment

If necessary, therapy should be directed towards (ultrasound-guided) surgical removal of the cyst(s).

Public health significance

E. granulosus sensu stricto (the former 'sheep strain') is still common and a public health problem in many parts of the Mediterranean region, and re-emergence after failed control campaigns is observed or suspected in Bulgaria and Wales. No recent data on the cattle-transmitted *E. ortleppi* are available, but their relevance for human health seems to be minor (Romig *et al.* 2006). Cyst echinococcosis is one of the most important zoonoses in Chile. The surgical incidence of cyst echinococcosis in humans ranged between 2.3 and 8.5 cases per 10^5 people. Highest prevalence of cyst echinococcosis was detected in cattle (24%), followed by swine (14%), sheep (11%), equines (9%), and goats (6%) (Acosta-Jamett *et al.* 2010). In comparison, human cyst echinococcosis incidence rates in the range of 1.1–3.4 cases per 10^5 inhabitants coexist with ovine/bovine cyst echinococcosis prevalence rates of up to 23% in Spain (Carmena *et al.* 2008).

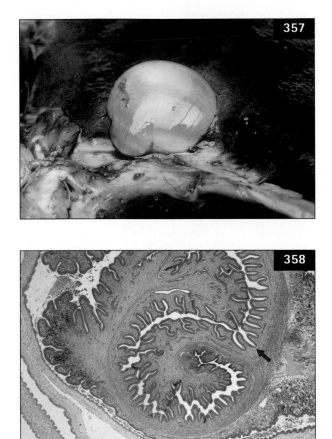

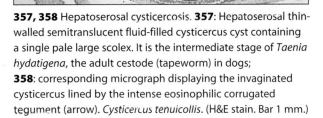

357, 358 Hepatoserosal cysticercosis. **357**: Hepatoserosal thin-walled semitranslucent fluid-filled cysticercus cyst containing a single pale large scolex. It is the intermediate stage of *Taenia hydatigena*, the adult cestode (tapeworm) in dogs;
358: corresponding micrograph displaying the invaginated cysticercus lined by the intense eosinophilic corrugated tegument (arrow). *Cysticercus tenuicollis*. (H&E stain. Bar 1 mm.)

Strongyloides westeri

Phylum Nemathelminthes/Class Nematoda/Order Rhabditida/Suborder Rhabditata/Superfamily Rhabditoidea/Family Strongyloididae/Genus Strongyloides

Definition/Overview

Strongyloides westeri is a small nematode found as an adult in the small intestine of foals (Lyons *et al.* 1993). Diarrhoea is the most common sign of infection with *S. westeri* in neonatal foals to 4 months of age, sometimes preceded by episodes of frenzy. The parasite has no clear relationship with so-called foal heat diarrhoea.

Aetiology

The genus *Strongyloides* contains species that are parthenogenetic and their eggs may give rise, outside the host, directly to infective larvae of another parasitic generation or to a free-living generation of minute males and females. *S. westeri* occurs in the small intestine of the horse, pig, and zebra. It is up to 9 mm long and 0.08–0.095 mm thick. The eggs measure 40–52 × 32–40 μm (**359, 360**). The first-stage larvae may develop directly to become third-stage infective larvae (homogonic cycle) or they may develop to free-living males and females that subsequently produce infective larvae (heterogonic cycle). In the homogonic cycle, the first-stage larvae metamorphose rapidly to become infective larvae, as little as 24 hours being required for this at 27°C. Infection of the vertebrate host is mainly by skin penetration (Soulsby 1968).

The main source of infection in foals is believed to be from parasitic stages (L₃) in mares' milk acquired by foals while nursing (Lyons *et al.* 1993) or by skin penetration (Soulsby 1968). As a consequence, an important source of infection appears to be larvae in the tissues of the mare. Probably, to a lesser degree, infections in foals also occur from free-living third-stage larvae that are ingested in feed (Lyons *et al.* 1993).

Epidemiology

An association had already been noted between climate, behaviour of mares and foals best described as frenzied, subsequent high faecal egg counts of *S. westeri* in foals, and the development of abscesses in peripheral lymph nodes from which *Rhodococcus equi* can be isolated (Dewes 1972). The probability of sighting episodes of frenzy increased by a factor of three when within 24 hours there was 0.2 mm or more of rain, a maximum air temperature of 16.7–26.6°C and a soil temperature of 16.3–23.9°C at 30 cm (Dewes 1989).

Eggs of *S. westeri* were found in 6% of foals (ranging in age from 7–63 days and none of them treated with an antiparasitic compound) on 78% of farms in central Kentucky, USA, considered to have overall excellent deworming programmes (Lyons *et al.* 1993). It appears that foals develop a resistance to *S. westeri* by the age of 15–23 weeks and the infection then disappears (Russell 1948).

Pathophysiology

Intraoral and percutaneous (intra-aural) administration of infective larvae resulted in suitable test infections in contrast with administration by stomach tube (Drudge *et al.* 1982). Infection causes inflammation of the proximal part of the jejunum associated with diarrhoea in some cases.

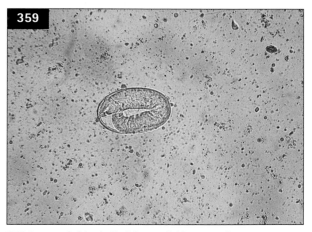

359 Larvated-thin shelled *Strongyloides westeri* egg.

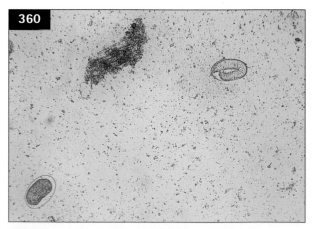

360 *Strongyloides westeri* egg (right-upper part) and *Cyathostomum* egg (left-lower part).

Pre-patent period

The pre-patent period is 5–7 days (Soulsby 1968). In accord, high egg counts of *S. westeri* appeared in faeces 4–5 days following episodes of frenzy and persisted for several days. The youngest foal in which eggs were first detected (20,000 eggs per gram [epg]) was 12 days old, the highest faecal egg count was 94,700 epg in a foal 20 days old, and the oldest foal in which eggs were detected for the first time was 104 days old (Dewes 1989). Milk may contain larvae for 47 days post-partum and the shortest pre-patent period after nursing on infected milk is given as 8 days (Lyons *et al.* 1973).

Clinical presentation

Percutaneous invasion by infectious larvae in foals was associated with the appearance of small spots of hair of darker hue on the face, neck, and limbs of subjects with light coloured coats, and occasionally a mild dermatitis (Dewes & Townsend 1990). The attack of frenzy occurred shortly after rain in warm humid conditions among mares and foals confined to yards surfaced with soil. Onset was sudden, affected every horse in the yard simultaneously and occupied about 35 minutes. Foals started by first scratching the face, ears, and neck with their hind feet, stamped, walked quickly, circled, and rolled in the mud. Mares stamped, rolled, sweated profusely, and breathed rapidly through nostrils flared by distress (Dewes 1989). Patent infection without clinical signs is not uncommon in foals. It is proposed that the percutaneous invasion of foals by third-stage larvae of *S. westeri* facilitated invasion of *R. equi*, an ubiquitous saprophytic opportunist pathogen (Dewes 1989).

Overwhelming strongyloidosis has been suggested in a 6-month-old foal evaluated because of weakness, weight loss, and inappetence of 3 weeks' duration. Strongyloidosis might have occurred when it was first exposed to other foals at 5 months of age, because it had not been naturally exposed to the organism at a younger age and was immunologically naive (Brown *et al.* 1997).

Differential diagnosis

The differential diagnosis includes various causes of diarrhoea in foals (see also p. 262) such as *Clostridium perfringens* (significantly associated with foal diarrhoea [OR = 3.0] as well as significantly associated with fatal diarrhoea [OR = 4.5]), rotavirus (OR = 5.6), *Cryptosporidium* spp. (OR = 3.2), and *Salmonella* spp. (OR = 14.2). Overall, *C. perfringens*, rotavirus, and large numbers of *Cryptosporidium* spp. or *S. westeri* were isolated from 80% of foals with diarrhoea without statistical interactions between any of the pathogens associated with diarrhoea. Thermophilic *Campylobacter* spp., *Yersinia enterocolitica*, *Escherichia coli*, and other parasites were not associated with diarrhoea. Carriage of *C. perfringens*, rotavirus and *Cryptosporidium* spp. was significantly greater in healthy foals in contact with cases of diarrhoea than in foals that were not in contact with diarrhoea (Netherwood *et al.* 1996).

Diagnosis

Diagnosis of infection is routinely based on finding *S. westeri* eggs in faeces by coprological examination combined with the occurrence of yellowish diarrhoea.

Pathology

Massive infection can cause eosinophilic enteritis with villous atrophy of the proximal part of the jejunum with intramucosal nematodes and ova.

Management/Treatment

Ivermectin at a dosage of 200 µg/kg BW IM revealed a greater than 99% reduction in *S. westeri* egg output during the 21 days following treatment of foals (Mirck & van Meurs 1982). Foals from treated mares (ivermectin at a dosage rate of 200 µg/kg BW IM on the day of parturition) had significantly fewer *S. westeri* epg faeces from 17 to 28 days post-partum. There were no differences observed in the frequencies of severity of foal heat diarrhoea between the treated and control groups (Ludwig *et al.* 1983). Feeding pyrantel tartrate daily, beginning at about 3 months of age was associated with prevalence of eggs of *Parascaris equorum* being low (0–31%), of strongyles being high (at least 80%), of *S. westeri* very low, and oocysts of *Eimeria leuckarti* medium to high (36–85%). It is uncertain whether the low ascarid prevalence was from activity of pyrantel tartrate and/or the other drugs or to a limited source of infective eggs (Lyons *et al.* 2007).

The numbers of free-living males and females and rhabditiform and filariform larvae could be reduced for at least 5 months by dressing with salt (Dewes & Townsend 1990). Interestingly, the fungi *D. flagrans* and *M. thaumasium* look promising for use in the biological control of *S. westeri* (Araujo *et al.* 2010).

Public health significance

Not convincing yet.

Halicephalobus gingivalis

Phylum Nemathelminthes/Class Nematoda/Order Rhabditida/Suborder Cephalobina/Superfamily Panagrolaimoidea/Family Panagrolaimidae/Genus *Halicephalobus*

Definition/Overview

Halicephalobus gingivalis is an ubiquitous saprophytic nematode that has been reported to infect humans and horses (Pearce *et al.* 2001), causing extensive tissue damage due to aberrant migration of the nematodes.

Aetiology

Nematodes in the genus *Halicephalobus* are free-living, saprophytic, and opportunistic parasites commonly found in organic matter (Kinde *et al.* 2000). Among these, *H. gingivalis* (formerly known as *H. deletrix* and *Micronema deletrix*) is the most important equine pathogen. Eggs in the two-cell stage embryonate to larvae in 17 hours at 28°C but do not hatch for an additional 24 hours. First-stage larvae are unusually large and variable in length (136–199 μm, average 168 μm). Inactive third-stage larvae are 180–240 μm (average 203 μm) in length (Anderson *et al.* 1998).

Epidemiology

Transmission of *H. gingivalis* from dam to foal has been suggested (Wilkins *et al.* 2001).

Pathophysiology

H. gingivalis has the ability to produce destructive lesions and extensive tissue damage because of its migratory behaviour. The ability of these nematodes to reproduce parthenogenetically within the host results in massive numbers occurring in various tissues, thereby setting up the probability of killing the host (Kinde *et al.* 2000).

Pre-patent period

Not established in the equine species yet.

Clinical presentation

The nematode may form granulomas in the integument or may disseminate to various organs with a tropism for the CNS (**361, 362**) and kidneys (**363–366**). Once clinical signs of CNS involvement develop, the disease is rapidly fatal (Pearce *et al.* 2001). Clinical signs usually depend on the organs affected.

Differential diagnosis

The differential diagnosis predominantly includes various causes of acute neurological disease (see p. 262).

Diagnosis

Diagnosis is usually made at autopsy although *H. gingivalis* has been recovered from the semen and urine of two horses (Kinde *et al.* 2000).

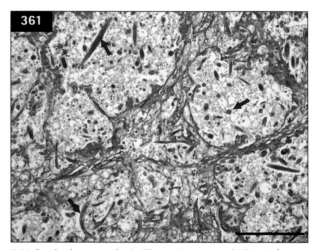

361 Cerebral nematodiasis. The optic nerve, which is in fact brain tissue and not a nerve as such, is massively infected by small thin nematode larvae and adults (arrows) that incite a mild granulomatous inflammatory reaction and severe loss of nervous tissue. *Halicephalobus gingivalis*. (PAS stain. Bar 200 μm.)

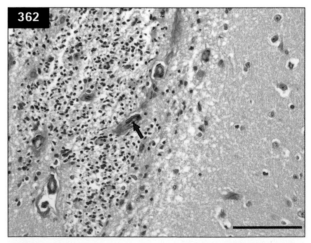

362 Cerebral nematodiasis. Focal extensive lymphohistiocytic meningoencephalitis. Within the cerebrum and adjacent meninges mononuclear inflammatory infiltrates are centred on a nematode (arrow). *Halicephalobus gingivalis*. (PAS stain. Bar 100 μm.)

Pathology

Macroscopically extensive multifocal to coalescing firm pale nodular lesions may affect typically the kidneys and other organs. Histology might reveal multiple granulomatous inflammatory foci containing huge numbers of parasites, with organs commonly affected by *H. gingivalis* in horses including brain and meninges, kidneys, lymph nodes,

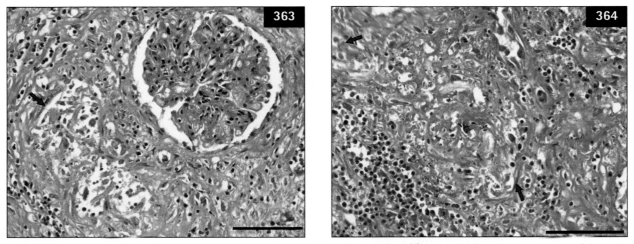

363, 364 Renal nematodiasis. Chronic lymphoplasmacytic and histiocytic nephritis with extensive fibrosis. In the centre of the right micrograph **(364)** is a pale eosinophilic necrotic and sclerotic remnant of a glomerulus surrounded by mainly lymphoplasmacytic infiltrates within a fibrotic interstitium. Multiple invading nematodes are present (arrows). *Halicephalobus gingivalis*. (H&E stain. Bars 100 μm.)

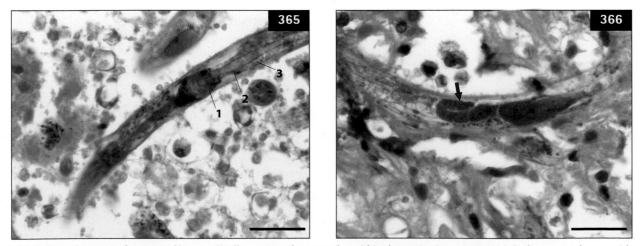

365, 366 Higher magnifications of longitudinally sectioned nematodes within the optic nerve. **365**: Rhabditiform oesophagus with bulbous (1), the adjoining narrow isthmus (2), and anterior corpus (3); **366**: typical morphologic feature of a female didelphic *Halicephalobus gingivalis*; the retroflexion of an ovarian arm is depicted (arrow). (PAS stain. Bars 20 μm.)

spinal cord, adrenal glands, and oral and nasal cavities. Additional organs reported to be affected to a lesser degree include eye (**367**), heart, stomach, liver, ganglia, and bones (Cantile *et al.* 1997, Kinde *et al.* 2000, Shibahara *et al.* 2002, Nadler *et al.* 2003, Bryant *et al.* 2006, Boswinkel *et al.* 2006, Ferguson *et al.* 2008).

Management/Treatment
Although ivermectin (1.2 mg/kg BW PO every 2 weeks for three treatments (Pearce *et al.* 2001)) might be effective, results of treatment may be variable due to the presence of enormous numbers of parasites in granulomatous tissue, even intracerebrally (Ferguson *et al.* 2008). Similarly, oral administration of moxidectin and local application of an ointment containing prednisolone and moxidectin revealed a poor clinical response in a 24-year-old Warmblood horse (Muller *et al.* 2008).

Public health significance
Halicephalobus sp. has been reported to have infected human beings (Gardiner *et al.* 1981).

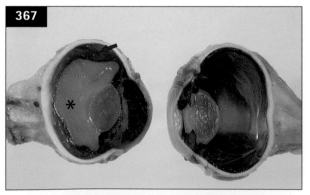

367 Granulomatous verminous endophthalmitis. On the left a cross-sectioned eye globe shows a diffuse thickening of the uvea (arrow). Note the opacity of the vitreous body (asterisk) compared with the nonaffected eye on the right. This horse suffered from an infection with the free-living rhabditiform nematode *Halicephalobus gingivalis*. It can spread systemically after penetration of nasal mucosa and skin, and has a tropism for the CNS and the kidneys in the horse.

Strongylus spp.
Phylum Nemathelminthes/Class Nematoda/Order Strongylida/Suborder Strongylata/Superfamily Strongyloidea/Genus *Strongylus*

Definition/Overview
Intermittent colic predominantly seen in young horses due to infestation with the large strongyle *Strongylus vulgaris* is regarded as uncommon nowadays due to common use of anthelmintics.

Aetiology
The strongyle nematodes have a direct life cycle. The large strongyles of the genus *Strongylus* migrate through the body of the host and are also known as redworms, associated with the presence of blood from the host in their digestive tract. Following ingestion via the intestinal tract, *S. vulgaris* larvae migrate via the arteries in the intestinal tract (**368**, **369**) to the cranial mesenteric artery. After spending several months in the cranial mesenteric artery mature larvae travel to the caecum and colon ascendens via the arterial system. The large strongyle larvae of *S. edentatus* penetrate the intestinal wall and travel via the portal vessels to the liver where they stay for about 4 weeks. Subsequently, they use the hepatorenal ligament to reach the subperitoneal tissues, where they remain, prior to the last part of their journey to the large colon and caecum. The migratory route of the large strongyle larvae of *S. equinus* differs from that of *S. edentatus* in that they migrate to the pancreas and subperitoneal tissues subsequent to penetration of the liver (Soulsby 1968).

S. vulgaris occurs in the large intestine of equines (**370**). The male is 14–16 mm long and the female 20–24 mm long and about 1.4 mm thick. This worm is distinctly smaller than the two preceding species. Embryonation commences immediately but is dependent on suitable environmental conditions such as moisture, oxygen, and a favourable temperature. At about 26°C a first-stage larva is produced in 20–24 hours; this hatches from the egg to become a free-living stage. Infective larvae penetrate the intestinal wall where, about 8 days after infection, fourth-stage larvae are produced. These penetrate the intima of the submucosal arterioles and migrate in these vessels towards the cranial mesenteric artery. They are to be found here from the 14th day after infection onwards, associated with thrombi and later (pseudo)aneurysms. Starting on about the 45th day after infection fourth-stage larvae pass back via the arterial system to the submucosa of the caecum and colon, and here become fifth-stage larvae about 3 months after infection. They then enter the lumen

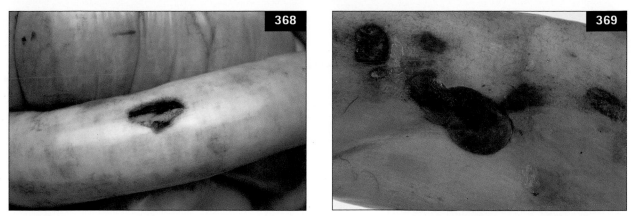

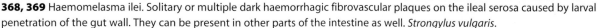

368, 369 Haemomelasma ilei. Solitary or multiple dark haemorrhagic fibrovascular plaques on the ileal serosa caused by larval penetration of the gut wall. They can be present in other parts of the intestine as well. *Strongylus vulgaris.*

and reach maturity, egg production occurring about 200 days after infection (Soulsby 1968).

S. *equinus* occurs in the caecum and colon of equines. The male is 26–35 mm long and the female 38–47 mm long and about 2 mm thick. The eggs are oval, thin-shelled, segmenting when laid, and measure 70–85 × 40–47 µm. Exsheathed infective larvae penetrate the mucosa of the caecum and colon and enter the subserosa where they cause the formation of nodules. Eleven days after infection, fourth-stage larvae occur in the nodules and these migrate to the peritoneal cavity and then to the liver in which they wander for about 4 months. There they moult to the fifth larval stage and leave the liver and return to the large intestine, but the route employed is unknown except that larvae may be found in the pancreas during this process. After entry into the lumen of the colon, they reach maturity, eggs being produced about 260 days after infection (Soulsby 1968).

S. *edentatus* also occurs in the large intestine of equines. The male is 23–28 mm long and the female 33–44 mm long and about 2 mm wide. This worm resembles S. *equinus* macroscopically, but the head is somewhat wider than the following portion of the body. The buccal capsule is wider anteriorly than at the middle and contains no teeth. Infective larvae enter the wall of the liver via the portal system. In the liver, fourth-stage larvae are produced about 11–18 days after infection. They may migrate in the liver for up to 9 weeks and then pass between the peritoneal layers of the hepatic ligaments to reach the parietal peritoneal region in the right abdominal flank.

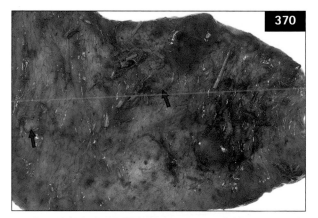

370 Strongylosis. Large intestinal mucosa with blood-stained adult *S. vulgaris* (arrows). Note the two prominent mucosal nodules containing young adult nematodes. *Strongylus vulgaris.*

Late fourth- and early fifth-stage larvae are found at this site in association with haemorrhagic nodules that vary in size from 1 to several centimetres in diameter. Larvae are found here up to about 3 months after infection, but they then migrate between the layers of the mesocolon to the walls of the caecum and colon, here again causing haemorrhagic nodules. Eventually the young adult worms pass to the lumen and become mature. Eggs are produced about 300–320 days after infection (Soulsby 1968).

Epidemiology

The epidemiology of infestation depends largely on local climatic conditions, but mares are the main source of infection for foals. Arterial lesions caused by migrating *S. vulgaris* larvae were observed in 5.8% of equids at necropsy in central Kentucky, USA (Lyons *et al.* 2000). However, several decades of intensive anthelmintic use has virtually eliminated clinical disease caused by *S. vulgaris* (Nielsen *et al.* 2008).

It is of interest to note that competitive interactions have been observed between *S. edentatus* and *S. vulgaris* in the caecum and ventral colon. When *S. edentatus* is in the caecum, the favourite site of *S. vulgaris*, the latter decreases especially in the caecum. On the other hand, when *S. edentatus* is in the ventral colon, its favourite site, there is no negative relationship with *S. vulgaris* in the ventral colon and the positive correlation observed is maintained (Stancampiano *et al.* 2010).

Pathophysiology

The significance of transglutaminase in the early growth and development of *S. vulgaris*, *S. edentatus*, and *S. equinus* has been shown (Rao *et al.* 1999). The sharply delineated but superficial attachment to the equine caecum by the mouth of *S. vulgaris* leaves behind an oval area devoid of epithelial cells. However, attachment does not extend deeply enough to reach the muscularis mucosa layer of the equine intestine (Mobarak & Ryan 1999). Despite the lack of proinflammatory cytokine induction with the apparent inflammatory response to *S. vulgaris* there is evidence of a potential role of nitric oxide (NO) (Hubert *et al.* 2004). It has been stated that *S. vulgaris* amphids, tooth core, intestine, excretory gland and ducts, and hypodermis are either antigen-producing tissues, or antigens sharing common epitopes (Mobarak & Ryan 1998). Increased caecal and colonic motility is an important host response in susceptible foals exposed to *S. vulgaris* larvae (Lester *et al.* 1989).

Pre-patent period

The pre-patent period of *S. vulgaris* is about 200 days (Soulsby 1968). Following surgical implantation peak epg values of 13–327 (*S. vulgaris*) and 363–1,284 (*S. edentatus*) generally occurred during the first 3 weeks post-implantation. Duration of infections was as long as 5 years (McClure *et al.* 1994).

Clinical presentation

Clinical signs include intermittent fever as well as recurrent colic. As an example, *S. vulgaris* migration and cranial mesenteric arterial thrombus formation resulted in fatal colic in a 3-month-old Thoroughbred foal (DeLay *et al.* 2001). In addition, crusting, exudative dermatitis of the coronary bands as well as lingual and buccal ulcerations were associated with eosinophilic gastroenteritis due to *S. edentatus* in a 3-year-old Quarter Horse gelding (Cohen *et al.* 1992).

Differential diagnosis

Only three common parasitisms of horses are likely to be manifested as colic: *Strongylus vulgaris*, *Parascaris equorum*, and *Anoplocephala perfoliata* (Reinemeyer & Nielsen 2009).

Diagnosis

The diagnosis of *S. vulgaris* infestation is based on clinical signs (including enlarged and painful cranial mesentery artery as noticed on rectal palpation and/or ultrasound) combined with increased strongyle faecal egg counts and the presence of hyperbetaglobulinaemia. Larval culture is indicated for definitive diagnosis, as small and large strongyle eggs cannot be differentiated on microscopic examination (Chapman *et al.* 1994). However, a fluorescence-based quantitative TaqMan real-time PCR assay reliably and semiquantitatively detected small numbers of *S. vulgaris* eggs in faecal samples (Nielsen *et al.* 2008). In addition, an RLB assay identified 13 common species of equine small strongyles (cyathostomins) and discriminated them from three *Strongylus* spp. (large strongyles) (Traversa *et al.* 2007).

Pathology

In cases of *S. vulgaris* infestation, necropsy reveals thrombosis and inflammation of the cranial mesenteric artery with thickening of its wall erroneously referred to as aneurysm (**371–376**).

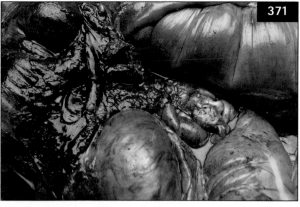

371 Verminous aneurysm. Incised saccular aneurysm with mural osseous metaplasia of the cranial mesenteric artery (arrow), the result of a chronic arteritis due to fourth-stage nematode larvae of *Strongylus vulgaris*.

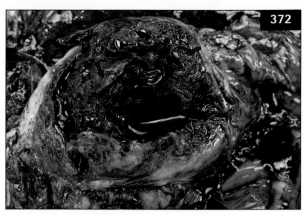

372 Verminous aneurysm. Close-up of an incised aneurysm of the cranial mesenteric artery. Note the fourth-stage larvae (arrows) of *Strongylus vulgaris*.

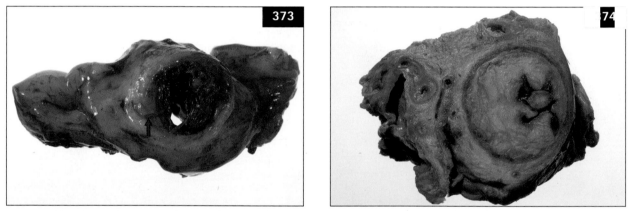

373, 374 Chronic verminous arteritis. **373**: Close-up of a cross-sectioned branch of the mesenteric artery. Note the thickened vessel wall with reddish fourth-stage larvae (arrow) embedded within a thrombus. *Strongylus vulgaris*; **374**: a similar nearly completely obstructing thrombus (formalin fixed specimen).

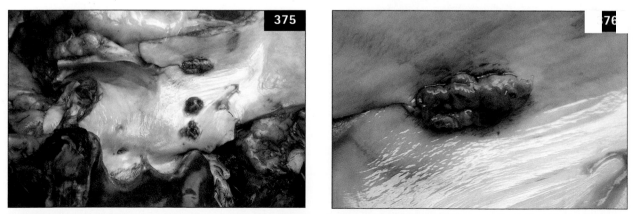

375, 376 Chronic proliferative verminous arteritis of the aorta in a donkey. Multiple intraluminal protruding inflammatory foci have resulted from migration of fourth-stage larvae in the aortic wall. This lesion can give rise to thromboemboli which may infarct the intestine with subsequent severe colic. *Strongylus vulgaris*.

Histological examination revealed that thrombosis and the severity of inflammation (377) varied on a seasonal basis and were directly associated with larval presence (378, 379). Intimal and adventitial fibrosis were generally of greater severity than medial fibrosis. Fibrosis of the vasa vasorum was less frequent than fibrosis of the artery itself. Morphometry revealed a significant increase in intimal, adventitial, and, to a lesser extent, medial areas in affected as compared with normal arteries. This change was due to the accumulation of collagen and was considered to result in decreased arterial elasticity. The luminal area varied widely among affected arteries (Morgan *et al.* 1991). Furthermore,

focal infarction in the digestive tract may also be noticed (380). In cases of *S. edentatus* infection, hepatitis and subserosal haemorrhage are seen, whereas pancreatitis is additionally seen in cases of *S. equinus* infestation. Migration of eosinophils to the equine large intestinal mucosa appears to be independent of exposure to parasites, indicating that large intestinal mucosal eosinophils may have more functions in addition to their role in defence against parasites (Rötting *et al.* 2008).

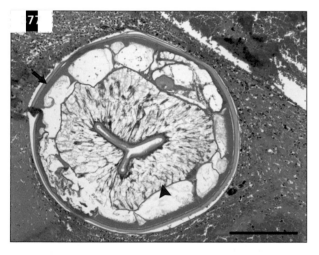

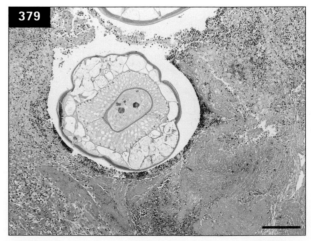

377 Verminous thromboarteritis. Cross-sectioned larva; note the thin rim of platymyarian musculature (arrow) and the prominent thick-walled intestine (arrowhead). *Strongylus vulgaris.* (H&E stain. Bar 200 μm.)

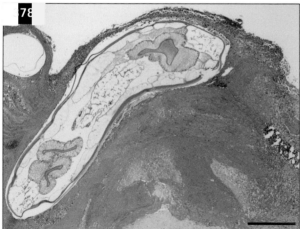

378, 379 Fibrinonecrotizing and eosinophilic thromboarteritis of a branch of the cranial mesenteric artery with a longitudinal section (**378**) and a cross-section (**379**) of an intralesional fourth-stage larval nematode. Note the irregular eroded arterial luminal surface devoid of endothelial lining. *Strongylus vulgaris.* (H&E stain. Bars 500/200 μm, respectively.)

Management/Treatment

In order to prevent anthelmintic resistance it is of importance to combine prudent use of anthelmintics with frequent monitoring of the level of herd infestation by means of strongyle faecal egg counts. The use of pasture rotation and removal of manure if possible are additional important management factors. Treatment of diseased horses is supportive, especially with regard to the verminous arteritis with TMP/S and NSAIDs.

The available oral anthelmintics that are effective against adult and migrating large strongyles are the benzimidazoles (fenbendazole at 5 mg/kg BW) and macrocyclic lactones (ivermectin at 200 µg/kg BW and moxidectin at 400 µg/kg BW) (Monahan *et al.* 1996, Bauer *et al.* 1998, Costa *et al.* 1998). A tablet formula of ivermectin–praziquantel showed 100% anthelmintic efficacies on *S. vulgaris*, *S. equinus*, and *S. edentatus* (Bonneau *et al.* 2009). There is no effective vaccine available yet for horses (Swiderski *et al.* 1999), although protection by immunization with irradiated larvae was associated with an anamnestic eosinophilia and post-immunization antibody recognition of *S. vulgaris* L_3 surface antigens (Monahan *et al.* 1994).

Public health significance

Not convincing yet.

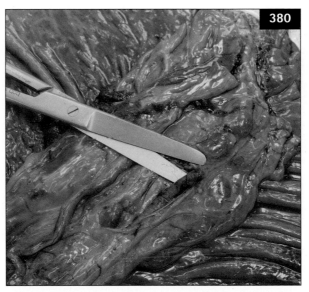

380 Arterial thromboembolus in the mesocolon, resulting in necrosis of the infarcted segment of the intestine. *Strongylus vulgaris.*

Cyathostomum spp.

Phylum Nemathelminthes/Class Nematoda/Order Strongylida/Suborder Strongylata/Superfamily Strongyloidea/Genus *Cyathostomum*

Definition/Overview

Weight loss and anaemia predominantly seen in young horses can be due to infestation with small strongyles (genera *Cyathostomum* and *Trichonema* spp.), regarded as the economically most important equine internal parasites. The term strongylosis is used to indicate infestation with either the large strongyles (genera *Strongylus* and *Triodontophorus* spp.) and/or small strongyles.

Aetiology

The nematodes are free-living or parasitic, unsegmented worms, usually cylindrical and elongate in shape. With a few exceptions the sexes are separate. The white adult nematodes (**381, 382**) belonging to the Tribe *Cyathostominea* genus *Cyathostomum* consisting of 52 species (Lichtenfels *et al.* 2002) are found in the caecum and colon ascendens. Thin-shelled oval strongyle eggs (**383, 384**) and reddish fourth-stage (L$_4$) larvae are passed with the faeces (**385, 386**). The former develop to infective third-stage larvae on pasture as their life cycle is direct. Infestation is by ingestion of the infective larvae. The small strongyles do not migrate through the body of the

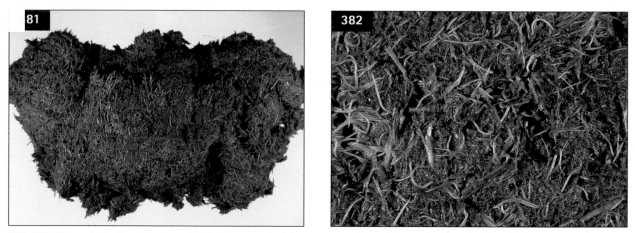

381, 382 Strongylosis. Faecal bolus extensively covered with numerous white adult small strongyles that feed on intestinal contents and are of minimal pathogenic importance. *Cyathostomum* spp.

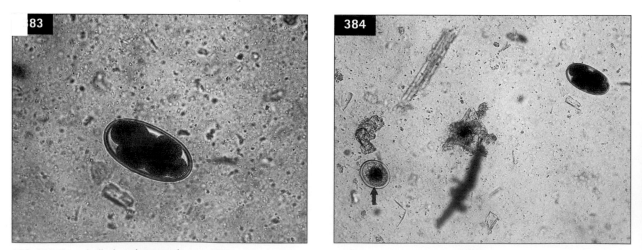

383, 384 Thin-shelled oval strongyle egg (**383**) compared to a *Parascaris equorum* egg (arrow) (**384**).

host (Soulsby 1968). With reference to individual species analysis, 28.5% of the L_4 were identified as *C. longibursatus*, 25.7% as *C. nassatus*, 15.9% as *C. ashworthi*, 7.3% as *C. goldi*, 1.7% as *C. catinatum*, and 20.9% unidentified isolated from the diarrhoeic faeces of horses. When L_4 within faeces from individual horses were compared, no sample was found to comprise parasites of one species. The least number of species identified in a single sample was two (Hodgkinson *et al.* 2003). As part of an investigation into mechanisms involved in reactivation of mucosal larval stages, a gene encoding a predicted LIM domain-containing protein (Cy-LIM-1) was identified. LIM domains are cysteine- and histidine-rich motifs that are thought to direct protein–protein interactions. Proteins that contain these domains have a wide range of functions including gene regulation, cell fate determination, and cytoskeleton organization (Matthews *et al.* 2008).

Epidemiology

The epidemiology of infestation depends largely on local climatic conditions, but mares are the main source of infection for foals. Arrested development by means of encystation within the intestinal wall is a strategy employed in areas with bad winter conditions. An unusual feature of cyathostome biology is this propensity for arrested larval development within the large intestinal mucosa for more than 2 years. From limited studies it appears that this arrested larval development is favoured by: feedback from luminal to mucosal worms; larger size of challenge dose of larvae, and trickle (versus single bolus) infection. During arrested larval development cyathostomes have minimal susceptibility to all anthelmintic compounds, thus limiting the effectiveness of therapeutic and/or control strategies (Love *et al.* 1999). Transcription of the protein cyathostomin gut-associated larval antigen-1 (Cy-GALA-1) was restricted to cyathostomin encysted larvae, and the presence of native protein was limited to developing larval stages (McWilliam *et al.* 2010).

Pathophysiology

The clinical signs are due to damage to the mucosa either from so-called plug feeding of the adult worms and/or from inflammation caused by the synchronous emergence of larval stages within the wall of the digestive tract following overwintering. As a result, fluid malabsorption in caecum and colon ascendens might occur, inducing diarrhoea. Furthermore, anaemia can be caused by chronic blood loss, malabsorption of haematopoietic nutrients, and chronic inflammation itself. It is evident that cyathostomes are pathogenic at times of both penetration into and emergence from the large intestinal mucosa (Love *et al.* 1999).

To date there are few data available on the molecular mechanisms of anthelmintic resistance in cyathostomes; beta-tubulin gene is the only anthelmintic resistance-associated gene that has been cloned (Kaplan 2002).

Pre-patent period

The pre-patent period is 6–10 weeks (Soulsby 1968).

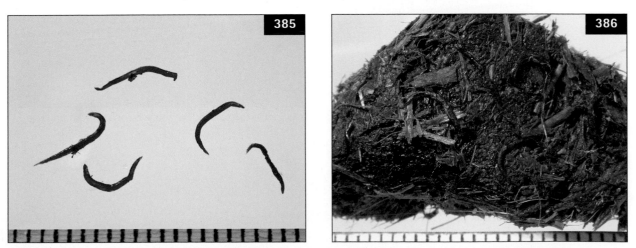

385, 386 Cyathostominae. Small reddish fourth-stage nematode larvae are passed with the faeces. *Cyathostomum* spp. (Scale in mm.)

Clinical presentation

Clinical signs include rough hair coat associated with delayed shedding, pyrexia, weight loss, poor performance, diarrhoea, and anaemia (Lyons *et al.* 2000). The occurrence of diarrhoea ranges from sudden onset to chronic debilitating concomitant with severe weight loss. Cases are most prevalent during late winter and early spring, also known as winter cyathostominosis. As a sequela, ventral oedema (**387**, **388**) might develop as well as caecocaecal and caecocolic intussusceptions (**389**) (Lyons *et al.* 2000, Mair *et al.* 2000). Larval cyathostominosis due to poor deworming during the first years of life in individual horses has a very grave prognosis. Clinical cyathostominosis occurs more commonly in young horses in late winter/early spring, but there is lifelong susceptibility to cyathostomes and they can cause clinical disease in any age of horse during any season (Love *et al.* 1999). Furthermore, clinical larval cyathostominosis is predominantly caused by mixed-species infections (Hodgkinson *et al.* 2003).

Differential diagnosis

The differential diagnosis includes various (chronic) causes of weight loss, diarrhoea, and anaemia (**390**, **391**) (see p. 262).

Diagnosis

The diagnosis is based on clinical signs combined with increased strongyle faecal egg counts, the presence of anaemia on haematological assessment, hypoalbuminaemia, and hyperbeta-globulinaemia (includes IgG(T)). Furthermore, rectal exploration sometimes reveals white adult nematodes and/or reddish fourth-stage larvae passed with the faeces. However, in individual cases the strongyle faecal egg count is not well correlated with the number of adult nematodes present, and fails to reveal the presence of larval stages. Furthermore, it is not possible to differentiate between large and small strongyles based on faecal egg morphology. However, an RLB assay enables the accurate and rapid identification of 13 common species of equine small strongyles (cyathostomins) and is able to discriminate them from three large *Strongylus* spp. (*S. edentatus*, *S. equinus*, and *S. vulgaris*) irrespective of their life-cycle stage (Traversa *et al.* 2007). Nevertheless, despite the clinical importance of these nematodes, diagnostic techniques for the pre-patent stages do not exist yet although anti-25 kDa IgG(T) levels correlated positively with mucosal and luminal burdens (Dowdall *et al.* 2004). It should be noted that for instance tetanus vaccination also induces IgG(T) production.

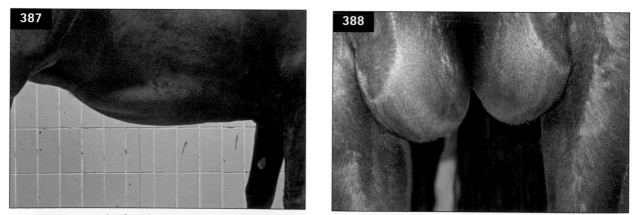

387, 388 As a sequela of cyathostominosis, ventral oedema might develop due to hypoalbuminaemia associated with protein-losing enteropathy.

389 As a sequela of cyathostominosis, rectal prolapse might develop due to hypoalbuminaemia associated with protein-losing enteropathy.

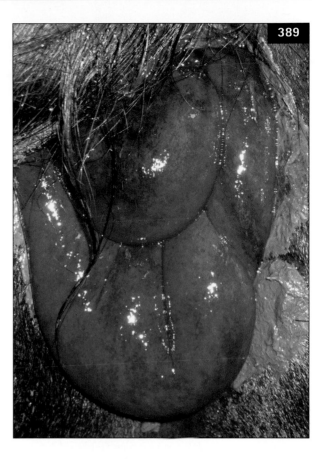

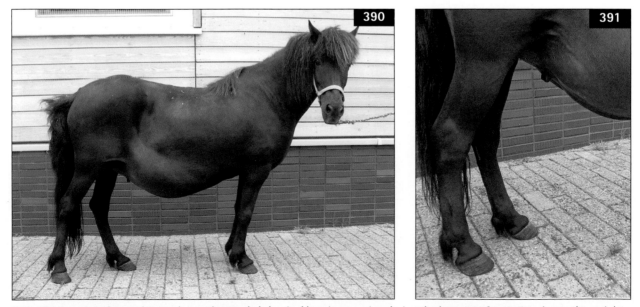

390, 391 A ruptured prepubic tendon and ventral abdominal hernia occurring during the last part of gestation due to the weight of the gravid uterus can be compared with ventral oedema due to cyathostominosis. Note the cranial dislocation of the teats.

Pathology

In massive emergence of larvae from the intestinal wall, gross necropsy findings may include a catarrhal colitis and/or typhlitis with a thickened oedematous hyperaemic mucosa (392) and ulcerations. Inhibiting or hypobiotic larvae may be seen as small mucosal grey or black dots, sometimes even the coiled dark red larvae itself may be discernible through the mucosal surface (393–397).

Management/Treatment

In order to prevent anthelmintic resistance it is of importance to combine prudent use of anthelmintics with frequent monitoring of the level of herd infestation by means of strongyle faecal egg counts. The use of pasture rotation and removal of manure if possible are important additional management factors. Treatment of diseased horses is supportive, especially with regard to diarrhoea.

The dosing interval of anthelmintics is based predominantly on the drug used. Drug resistance on individual farms can be monitored by assessment of reduction in strongyle faecal egg counts 2–3 weeks following anthelmintic treatment. A reduction rate of less than 95% might indicate anthelmintic resistance. The available oral anthelmintics which are effective against adult and nonencysted strongyles are the benzimidazoles (fenbendazole at 5 mg/kg BW and oxfendazole at 10 mg/kg BW), heterocyclic drugs (piperazine at 88 mg/kg BW), tetrahydropyrimidines (pyrantel at 6.6 mg/kg BW), and macrocyclic lactones (ivermectin at 200 µg/kg BW and moxidectin at 400 µg/kg BW). Fenbendazole at 10 mg/kg BW for 5 consecutive days and moxidectin at 400 µg/kg BW are also effective against encysted strongyles overwintering in the intestinal wall (Lyons *et al.* 2000, Deprez & Vercruysse 2003). It has been shown that treatment with either drug was efficacious against tissue larvae of cyathostomins but in contrast to moxidectin effects, killing of larvae by fenbendazole was associated with severe tissue damage, which clinically may correspond to reactions caused by synchronous mass emergence of fourth-stage larvae, i.e. may mimic larval cyathostominosis (Steinbach *et al.* 2006).

Neither ivermectin nor pyrantel anthelmintic resistance was detected on German horse farms in 2003 and 2004 with reference to cyathostomins, as based on reduction of cyathostomin egg production 14 and 21 days post-treatment (Samson-Himmelstjerna *et al.* 2007). However, the widespread incidence of resistance to certain anthelmintics is reducing treatment options (Corning 2009).

Public health significance

Not convincing yet.

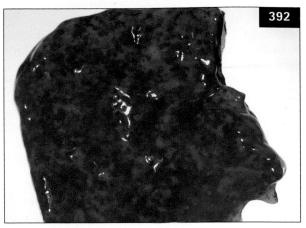

392 Cyathostominosis. Catarrhal colitis. The mucosa is hyperaemic oedematous with multiple small ulcerative lesions. *Cyathostomum* spp.

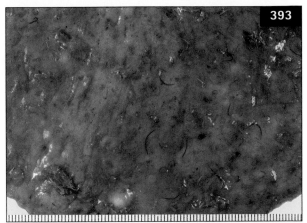

393 Cyathostominosis. Colon containing numerous small red fourth-stage nematode larvae. *Cyathostomum* spp. (Scale in mm.)

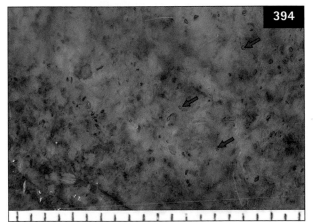

394 Cyathostominosis. Colon contains numerous red and coiled fourth-stage (L$_4$) larvae embedded within the mucosa (arrows). Note the multiple interspersed dark pinpoint haemorrhages. *Cyathostomum* spp. (Scale in mm.)

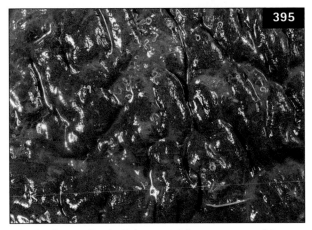

395 Cyathostominosis. Colon containing numerous white adult nematodes. *Cyathostomum* spp.

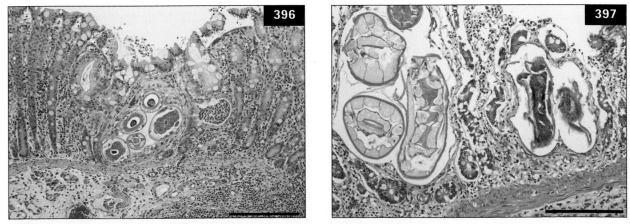

396, 397 Cyathostominosis. Large intestinal mucosa with clusters of coiled small strongyle larvae in the lamina propria inciting a mild to moderate inflammation. *Cyathostomum* spp. (H&E stain. Bars 200/100 µm, respectively.)

Dictyocaulus arnfieldi

Phylum Nemathelminthes/Class Nematoda/Order Strongylida/Suborder Strongylata/Superfamily Trichostrongyloidea/Family Dictyocaulidae/Genus *Dictyocaulus*

Definition/Overview

Dictyocaulus arnfieldi is a cause of chronic coughing in horses. The donkey is regarded as the natural host of *D. arnfieldi* and may host large numbers of lungworms without showing clinical signs. In horses, development from fifth-stage larvae to the adult stage in the bronchial tree is frequently prevented.

Aetiology

The equine lungworm is named *D. arnfieldi*. *D. arnfieldi* occurs in the bronchi of the horse, donkey, and tapir and is found worldwide. The male measures up to 36 mm and the female measures up to 60 mm long. The eggs measure 80–100 × 50–60 µm. Eggs usually do not hatch before being passed in the faeces. Following infection, the larvae penetrate into the intestinal wall and pass via the blood and lymph vessels to the lungs. The fourth-stage larvae are found in the lung parenchyma during their passage from the lymph-vessels to the bronchi. The worms grow to be adult in 39 days after infection (Soulsby 1968). Genomic DNA from the four *Dictyocaulus* species *D. viviparus*, *D. eckerti*, *D. filaria*, and *D. arnfieldi* analysed by means of random amplified polymorphic DNA (RAPD) PCR revealed that lungworms from fallow deer belong to a separate species (*D. eckerti*), whereas the similarity coefficient of *D. viviparus*, *D. eckerti*, *D. filaria*, and *D. arnfieldi* ranged from 12% to 32% (Epe *et al.* 1995).

Infection follows ingestion of third-stage larvae. These larvae travel from the digestive tract following ingestion via the lymphatic vessels and vascular system to the lungs where they develop to the adult stage in the bronchial tree. Adult females produce larvated eggs which are passed in the faeces, hatching almost immediately to first-stage larvae (Soulsby 1968).

Epidemiology

In the majority of clinical cases of lungworm infection in horses there has been previous contact with donkeys. Prevalence of natural infections of the lungworm, *D. arnfieldi*, was 54% for donkeys and mules, 2% for Thoroughbreds, 2% for Standardbreds, 0% for American Saddle Horses, 3% for other breeds or mixed breeds, and 0% for ponies in Kentucky, USA from 1983–1984 (Lyons *et al.* 1985).

Pre-patent period

Within 11 weeks of exposure both pony and donkey foals developed patent lungworm infections (Clayton & Duncan 1981).

Clinical presentation

Clinical signs in horses include chronic coughing, tachypnoea, and weight loss. However, young foals especially develop patent infection without clinical signs. In contrast, donkeys rarely show clinical signs in case of lungworm infection.

Differential diagnosis

The differential diagnosis includes various causes of chronic coughing (see p. 263).

Diagnosis

Diagnosis is based on the history, clinical signs, and the presence of first-stage lungworm larvae in the faeces as detected by means of the Baermann technique. Occasionally, adult lungworms may be visualized endoscopically in the bronchi. Furthermore, fourth- or fifth-stage larvae may be collected via transtracheal wash or bronchoalveolar lavage. Interestingly, eosinophilia proved useful in detecting lungworm infections in donkeys (Urch & Allen 1980).

Pathology

Pathological examination reveals chronic eosinophilic bronchitis containing lungworms, atelectasis, and eventually emphysema mostly evident in the caudodorsal lung regions.

Management/Treatment

Apparently normal donkeys may shed first-stage larvae frequently via the faeces. Contact with untreated donkeys should be avoided and donkeys should be regularly dewormed. Ivermectin paste is probably the drug of choice, at a dose rate of 200 µg/kg BW orally once, being highly effective against both adult and immature or inhibited stages of the horse lungworm, with no eggs present in faeces from 7 to 15 days after treatment (Britt & Preston 1985). The same was true for 0.4 mg/kg BW moxidectin orally once, with no eggs present in faeces up to 34 days after treatment in donkeys (Coles *et al.* 1998) in contrast with 7.5 mg fenbendazole/kg BW administered to donkeys (Urch & Allen 1980).

Public health significance

Not convincing yet.

Parelaphostrongylus tenuis

Phylum Nemathelminthes/Class Nematoda/ Order Strongylida/Suborder Strongylata/ Superfamily Metastrongyloidea/ Family Protostrongylidae/Genus *Parelaphostrongylus*

Definition/Overview

Neurological disease in the horse can be due to the meningeal nematode *Parelaphostrongylus tenuis* (formerly *Odocoileostrongylus tenuis*).

Aetiology

There are seven genera within the family Protostrongylidae that produce dorsal-spined larvae. Of these, species from both *Parelaphostrongylus* and *Elaphostrongylus* are known to infest the host CNS and musculature, whereas the other five genera occupy host lungs exclusively. *P. tenuis*, a member of the family Protostrongylidae within the superfamily Metastrongyloidea, also called meningeal worm or brain worm, is a common neurotropic parasitic nematode of white-tailed deer throughout eastern North America (Soulsby 1968, Anderson 2000). Mature parasites in white-tailed deer occur in the CNS and eggs are carried by the bloodstream to the lungs, where they form small emboli. Larvae hatch from such eggs, enter the alveoli, and pass out in the faeces. Terrestrial snails serve as intermediate hosts (Anderson 2000). *P. tenuis* measures 48–65 mm in length with an undivided bursa in the male. Infection of fawns with infected snails results in fourth- and fifth-stage larvae in the brain and spinal cord 25 days after infection. By 50 days immature adults are found in the dura mater of the spinal cord and cerebral hemispheres (Soulsby 1968).

Epidemiology

Protostrongylid nematode infection should be included as a differential diagnosis for instances of neurological disease in horses in endemic areas of eastern North America (Tanabe *et al.* 2007).

Pathophysiology

Parasitic migratory encephalomyelitis is a rare but important cause of neurological disease in horses. Metazoan parasites identified from the equine CNS include nematodes (*Strongylus vulgaris*, *S. equinus*, *Angiostrongylus cantonensis*, *Halicephalobus gingivalis*, *Setaria* spp., *P. tenuis*, and *Draschia megastoma*) and fly larvae (*Hypoderma* spp.) (Lester 1992, Tanabe *et al.* 2007).

Pre-patent period

Not established in the equine species yet, but perhaps 90 days as reported in white-tailed deer (Soulsby 1968).

Clinical presentation

Clinical examination in a 6-month-old Arabian colt revealed marked spastic tetraparesis and ataxia in all four limbs. The head and neck were held to the right side (Tanabe *et al.* 2007). Furthermore, a 4-year-old Hanoverian gelding was diagnosed with *P. tenuis* in the right eye. Ophthalmologic examination of the right eye upon admission revealed a white, thin, coiled, mobile nematode, located in the ventral portion of the anterior chamber of the eye with vitreal strands located temporally and inferiorly near the margin of the pupil. Results of ophthalmologic examination of the left eye were unremarkable (Reinstein *et al.* 2010).

Differential diagnosis

The differential diagnosis predominantly includes various causes of acute neurological disease (see p. 262).

Diagnosis

CSF from a 6-month-old Arabian colt contained mildly increased protein (1.2 g/l, normal range 0.05–1.0 g/l) and 1200 cells/µl (58% lymphocytes, 40% neutrophils, 2% macrophages, and a few eosinophils and erythrocytes). CT examinations were normal except for a mild atlanto-occipital joint subluxation (Tanabe *et al.* 2007).

Diagnosis of infection may be based on finding *P. tenuis* eggs (approximately 21 µm in length with a thin shell (Tanabe *et al.* 2007)) in faeces by coprological examination, combined with acute neurological disease.

Pathology

Parasitic granulomatous eosinophilic inflammation was observed in the CNS of a 6-month-old Arabian colt associated with *P. tenuis* infection. Inflammation was associated with eggs, larvae, and adult nematodes in the cerebellum (Tanabe *et al.* 2007).

Management/Treatment

It has been reported that clinical signs persisted following treatment with dexamethasone (Tanabe *et al.* 2007). In addition, surgical extraction of an intraocular infection of *P. tenuis* has been reported associated with uncomplicated recovery from the procedure and retained vision (Reinstein *et al.* 2010).

Public health significance

Not convincing yet.

Parascaris equorum

Phylum Nemathelminthes/Class Nematoda/Order
Ascaridida/Suborder Ascaridata/Superfamily
Ascaridoidea/Family Ascarididae/ Genus *Ascaris*

Definition/Overview

The roundworm *Parascaris equorum* is common in
foals and is associated with decreased weight gain.
An important sequela is death associated with
intestinal obstruction and/or rupture associated with
subsequent peritonitis due to massive numbers of
adult parasites in the small intestine.

Aetiology

P. equorum has a direct life cycle, with a free-living
and a parasitic phase (Clayton 1986). After
ingestion, embryonated eggs hatch in the host's small
intestine. The larvae penetrate the intestinal mucosa
and migrate to the liver and lungs. They then travel
up the bronchial tree, are swallowed, and develop
into mature adult ascarids in the duodenum and
proximal jejunum (**398**) (Clayton 1986, Austin *et al.*
1990). The males are 15–28 cm long and the females
up to 50 cm × 8 mm (**399**). The eggs are subglobular
with a thick, pitted albuminous layer and measure
90–100 µm in diameter (**400**). The worms reach
maturity in about 12 weeks after infection (Soulsby
1968).

Epidemiology

Specific examination for *P. equorum* indicated that
0–46% of weanlings and 10% of older horses were
infected (Lyons *et al.* 2000, Lyons *et al.* 2007).

Pathophysiology

The incidence of acute small intestinal obstruction
associated with *P. equorum* infection within 24
hours of anthelmintic treatment can be up to 72%
(Cribb *et al.* 2006). In comparison, in a previous
study 27% of horses had been administered
anthelmintics within 24 hours prior to the onset of
colic associated with ascarid impaction (Southwood
et al. 1996).

Pre-patent period

The pre-patent period of *P. equorum* is 72–110 days
(Clayton 1986, Austin *et al.* 1990).

Clinical presentation

P. equorum infection is associated with lethargy,
inappetence, unthriftiness, a rough hair coat, pot-
bellied appearance, decreased weight gain,
hypoproteinaemia, coughing, and nasal discharge in
young horses (Austin *et al.* 1990). Acute small
intestinal obstruction associated with *P. equorum*
infection is usually seen under the age of 12 months
(median age at presentation was 5 [range 3–24]
months). Horses were four times more likely to
present in autumn with colic associated with *P.
equorum* infection than in any other season (Cribb *et
al.* 2006).

Differential diagnosis

The differential diagnosis includes various causes of
chronic weight loss in elderly foals such as
strongylosis, chronic inflammation (e.g. pneumonia,
endocarditis), *Lawsonia intracellularis* infection,
cardiovascular anomalies, malocclusions, renal
hypoplasia, portal vein anomaly, and congenital
hepatic fibrosis.

Diagnosis

Diagnosis of infection is routinely based on finding
P. equorum eggs in faeces by coprological
examination combined with the occurrence of
clinical signs. Ultrasound examination of the
abdomen may visualize the parasite within the small
intestine. Remarkably, adult parasites are sometimes
collected via nasogastric reflux, thereby assisting in
diagnosis.

Pathology

Apart from the obvious presence of intraluminal
intestinal ascarid nematodes, marked white spots on
the liver capsule and firm calcified subpleural lung
nodules (chalicosis nodularis pulmonis), can be
encountered at necropsy associated with larva
migrans (**401–403**).

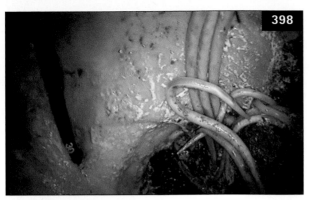

398 Several large mature roundworms encountered at endoscopy in the stomach. The endoscope enters the stomach via the cardia.

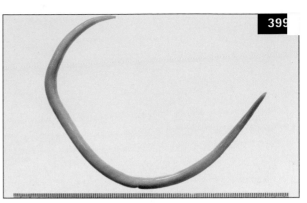

399 Parascaridiosis. Close-up of an individual mature ascarid nematode; the females can reach 50 cm in length. *Parascaris equorum*. (Scale in mm.)

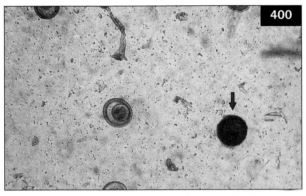

400 *Parascaris equorum* eggs are very long-lived and very resistant to usual methods of eradication: Note a dark infertile unembryonated egg on the right (arrow).

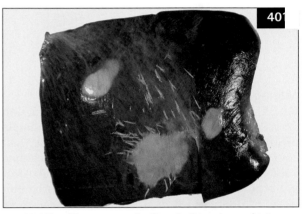

401 Multifocal hepatocapsular fibrosis. Extensive multiple white firm fibrous plaques and filaments are present on the liver capsule. Such lesions are scars attributed to parasitic migrations. Implicated are *Strongylus vulgaris* and *S. edentatus* larvae, *Parascaris equorum* larvae, and *Fasciola hepatica* metacercariae.

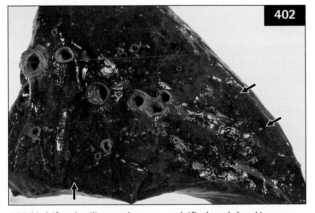

402 Multifocal miliary pulmonary calcified nodules. Numerous small (1–3 mm in diameter) firm calcified white foci (arrows) attributed to larva migrans. *Parascaris equorum*.

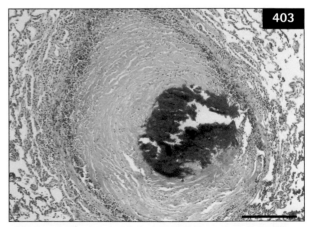

403 Chalicosis nodularis pulmonis. Micrograph of a remnant lesion in the lung of larval migration, a dark bluish-purple focus of dystrophic calcification centred on a dead larva (mostly inapparent in sections), with concentric encapsulating fibrosis and an outer rim of eosinophils and macrophages. These are coincidental findings at necropsy generally without clinical significance. *Parascaris equorum*. (H&E stain. Bar 200 μm.)

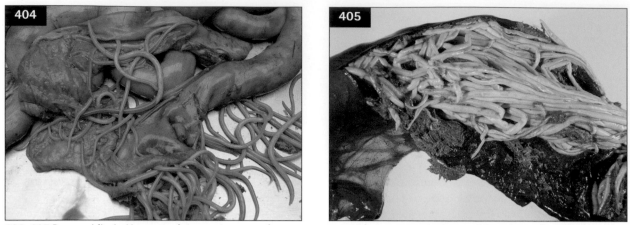

404, 405 Parascaridiosis. Numerous large mature roundworms encountered at necropsy in the small intestines of usually juvenile horses. Within a fresh necropsy the worms are frequently still alive and motile. *Parascaris equorum*.

Management/Treatment

Of 25 cases of acute small intestinal obstruction associated with *P. equorum* infection, 16 had simple obstructive ascarid impactions and nine had complicated obstructive ascarid impactions including volvulus or intussusception (**404–407**). Ascarid impactions that required surgical treatment had an overall long-term survival of 27%. Formation of adhesions was the most frequent finding associated with death in horses that did not survive more than 1 year. On the other hand, small intestinal obstruction associated with *P. equorum* infection accounted for 0.4% of colic surgery performed on horses less than 1 year of age. In cases of heavy parasite burden, anthelmintic treatment should be preceded by the administration of mineral oil via nasogastric tube in order to reduce the risk of post-treatment ascarid obstruction/intestinal rupture (Cribb *et al*. 2006).

Horses older than 6 months develop immunity to *P. equorum* (Clayton 1986). Various broad-spectrum anthelmintics (including piperazine) are effective against *P. equorum*. However, an emerging resistance of *P. equorum* to ivermectin has been reported (Boersema *et al*. 2002, Cribb *et al*. 2006,

Samson-Himmelstjerna *et al*. 2007, Schougaard & Nielsen 2007). A paste formulation of pyrantel pamoate (at a dosage of 13.2 mg/kg BW) was 97.3% effective against macrocyclic lactone-resistant *P. equorum* (Reinemeyer *et al*. 2010).

Faecal monitoring for anthelmintic efficacy should be an integral component of the anthelmintic treatment programme for all foals from 3–4 months of age (Cribb *et al*. 2006).

The infective eggs are very long-lived and very resistant to usual methods of eradication. Likewise, regular steam-cleaning of the stall environment, removal of faeces from pasture at least twice a week (**408**), and pasture rotation are additional techniques for reducing environmental burdens of *P. equorum* eggs (Cribb *et al*. 2006). At 45°C and 50°C, 2 log10 reduction of viability is reached after between 8 and 24 h of incubation, and it takes less than 2 h at 55°C and 60°C to achieve a viability reduction of 2 log10 *P. equorum* eggs. These temperatures are potentially encountered during horse manure composting (Hébert *et al*. 2010).

Public health significance
Not convincing yet.

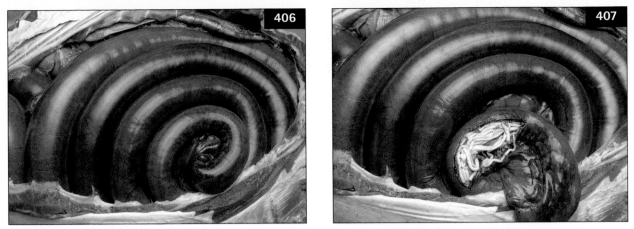

406, 407 Parascaridiosis. Intestinal volvulus (approximately 720° clockwise), an exceptional associated lesion with heavy burdens of jejunum-obstructing roundworms that most probably provokes a causative peristalsis. Other associated lesions are jejuno–jejunal intussusceptions and perforations. Note the markedly hyperaemic congested and thickened intestinal wall. *Parascaris equorum.*

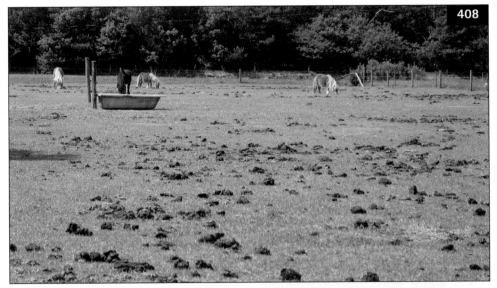

408 Removal of faeces from pasture at least twice a week is an additional method for reducing environmental burdens of *Parascaris equorum* eggs.

Oxyuris equi

Phylum Nemathelminthes/Class Nematoda/
Order Oxyurida/Suborder Oxyurata/Superfamily
Oxyuroidea/Family Oxyuridae/Genus Oxyuris

Definition/Overview

Oxyuris equi occurs in the large intestine of equines in all parts of the world, with pruritus in the perianal region as a classical clinical sign.

Aetiology

The male is 9–12 mm long and the female up to 150 mm long (**409, 410**). The mature females have a slaty-grey or brownish colour and narrow tails which may be more than three times as long as the rest of the body. The males and young females inhabit the caecum and large colon. After fertilization the mature females move down to the rectum and crawl out through the anal opening with the anterior parts of their bodies. The eggs are elongate, slightly flattened on one side, provided with a plug at one pole (so-called operculum), and measure about 90 × 42 μm. They are laid in clusters on the skin in the perineal region (**411, 412**). Development of the egg is rapid, reaching the infective stage in 3–5 days (**413**) (Soulsby 1968).

Epidemiology

Prevalences and intensities of *O. equi* adults and larvae were reduced compared with a survey conducted 20 years earlier in the same region in Louisiana, USA (Chapman *et al.* 2002).

Pre-patent period

The sexually mature adult stage is reached about 4–5 months after infection (**414, 415**) (Soulsby 1968).

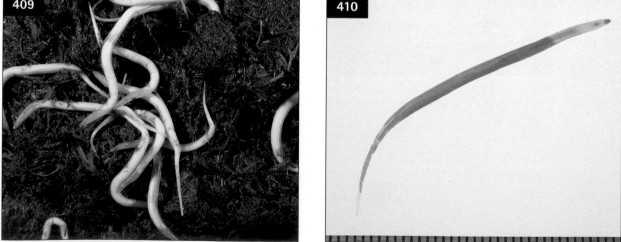

409, 410 Infection with the horse pinworm may lead to perineal irritation and pruritus due to perianal yellow-white crusty egg clutches deposited by female nematodes, which can be recognized in faecal examination because of their typical slender pointed anterior end. *Oxyuris equi.* (Scale in mm.)

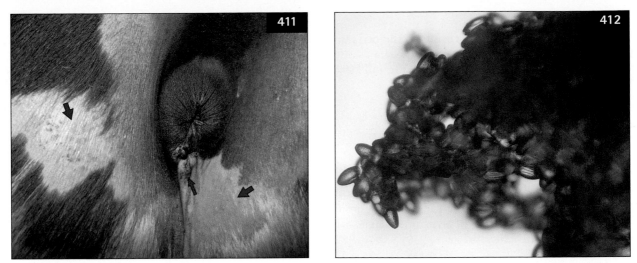

411, 412 Perineal alopecia (**411** bold arrows). The egg masses (**412**) are seen as a yellowish streak below the anus (**411**; small arrow).

413 Eggs of *Oxyuris equi.*

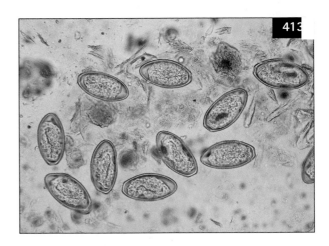

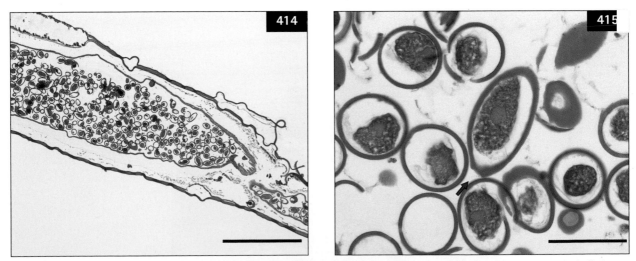

414, 415 Histological micrograph of the pointed rear end of a female pinworm harbouring many round to ovoid thick-shelled embryonated eggs, magnified in **415**. Note the plug at one pole (arrow). Application of cellophane tape to the perianal skin may recover ova and possible remnants of dried female pinworms that may be used in a diagnostic microscopic wet mount. *Oxyuris equi.* (H&E stain. Bars 500/50 µm, respectively.)

Clinical presentation

The classical clinical sign is pruritus in the perianal region ultimately leading to focal alopecia in the perineal region and broken hairs on the tail base (416–418).

Differential diagnosis

The differential diagnosis includes various causes of pruritus (see p. 263).

(see p. 263)

Diagnosis

Application of cellophane tape to the perianal skin may recover ova and possible remnants of dried female pinworms that may be used in a diagnostic microscopic wet mount.

Pathology

Pathology is associated with broken hairs on the tail base and secondary skin lesions due to pruritus. Remarkably, *O. equi* eggs were recovered from haemomelasma ilei lesions on the ileal serosa of a Thoroughbred yearling filly (Tolliver *et al.* 1999).

Management/Treatment

Ivermectin paste administered to horses orally at 200 μg/kg BW (Klei *et al.* 2001) and moxidectin at 300–400 μg/kg BW (Monahan *et al.* 1996, Bauer *et al.* 1998) were highly effective against *O. equi*.

Following anthelmintic treatment, the perineal region should be washed regularly. The lack of anthelmintic treatment appeared not to affect prevalence rates for *Anoplocephala perfoliata* and *Anoplocephala magna* in contrast to prevalence rates for *O. equi*, *Strongylus* spp., *Triodontophorus* spp., *Craterostomum acuticaudatum*, and *Parascaris equorum* (Torbert *et al.* 1986). A recent study showed that numbers of *O. equi* adults recovered post-mortem were significantly decreased by both pyrantel pamoate and ivermectin treatment, with efficacies of 91.2% and 96.0%, respectively. In addition, both products demonstrated >99% efficacy against fourth-stage *O. equi* larvae, demonstrating acceptable adulticidal and larvicidal efficacy of both pyrantel pamoate and ivermectin against *O. equi*. The existence of macrocyclic lactone or pyrimidine resistance in the pinworm populations evaluated could not be shown (Reinemeyer *et al.* 2010).

In vitro assays showed that the fungal species *Pochonia chlamydosporia* had a negative influence on eggs of *O. equi* and might be considered as a potential biological control agent of this nematode (Braga *et al.* 2010).

Public health significance

Not convincing yet.

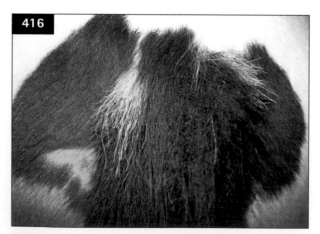

416 Perineal pruritus in chronic pinworm infestation as illustrated by broken hairs on the tail base.

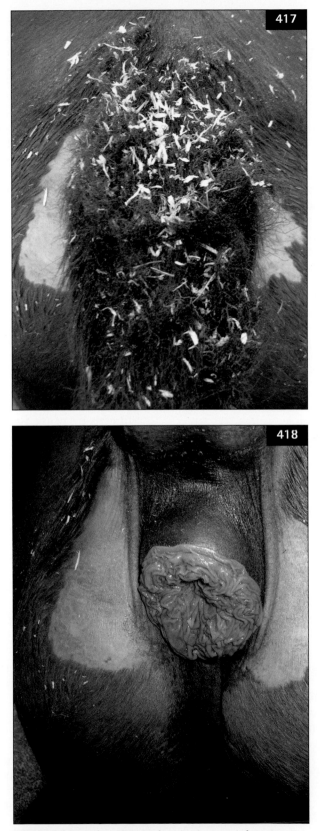

417, 418 Perineal pruritus in chronic pinworm infestation as illustrated by perineal alopecia.

Probstmayria vivipara

Phylum Nemathelminthes/Class Nematoda/Order Oxyurida/Suborder Oxyurata/Superfamily Oxyuroidea/Family Oxyuridae/Genus *Probstmayria*

Definition/Overview

Subclinical pinworm infestation with *Probstmayria vivipara* is found in the caecum and colon.

Aetiology

The adult pinworm *P. vivipara* can be found in the caecum and colon. It measures 2–2.9 mm in length. The females are viviparous, producing larvae almost as large as themselves. As a result of this almost unique method of reproduction, infections may be enormous, but the worms are not known to be pathogenic (Soulsby 1968).

Pathophysiology

The life cycle of this nematode is completely endogenous, all development taking place in the caecum and colon (Smith 1979).

Pre-patent period

Not established in the equine species yet.

Clinical presentation

Despite the large number of pinworms present, clinical signs are usually not observed.

Diagnosis

Infected animals might constantly shed pinworms in their faeces.

Epidemiology

Transfer is believed to be accomplished by contamination of food and water by larvae passed in the faeces. Prevalence ranged from 2% (Mfitilodze & Hutchinson 1989) to 12% (Tolliver *et al.* 1987).

Pathology

Insignificant findings at post-mortem examination.

Management/Treatment

A single oral dose of fenbendazole paste at 7.5 mg/kg BW was highly effective against adults of *P. vivipara* (Malan *et al.* 1981).

Public health significance

Not convincing yet.

Thelazia lacrymalis

Phylum Nemathelminthes/Class Nematoda/Order Spirurida/Suborder Spirurata/Superfamily Spiruroidea/Genus *Thelazia*

Definition/Overview

Conjunctivitis or dacryocystitis can be due to the spirurid nematode *Thelazia lacrymalis*, also known as eye worm, predominantly seen in young horses.

Aetiology

Thelazia lacrymalis is a large ovoviviparous nematode (10–25 mm in length) (**419**). The face fly, *Musca autumnalis*, is the intermediate host (Soulsby 1968, Dongus *et al.* 2003).

Epidemiology

Thelazia lacrymalis were found in 42% of the 1–4-year-old equids at necropsy in central Kentucky, USA (Lyons *et al.* 2000), and was recovered from 10% of horses examined post-mortem in Normandy, where animals aged 6 months to 2 years were most frequently infected (Collobert *et al.* 1995).

Pathophysiology

Lesions and tissue damage occur, particularly of the conjunctival sac and nasolacrimal system because of the migratory behaviour of *Thelazia lacrymalis*.

Pre-patent period

Not established in the equine species yet.

Clinical presentation

The presence of nematodes does not always induce clinical signs (Collobert *et al.* 1995). Clinical signs include blepharospasm, lacrimation, epiphora, photophobia, keratitis, corneal ulceration, abscessation of the eyelids, and conjunctivitis.

Differential diagnosis

The differential diagnosis includes conjunctivitis and keratitis especially due to *Onchocerca cervicalis* microfilaria and aberrant adult *Setaria equina* and *Parelaphostrongylus tenuis* nematodes.

Diagnosis

The diagnosis should be based on the demonstration of nematodes in the eye and adnexal structures (**419–421**) combined with the presence of characteristic lesions and response to treatment. Active serpentine movement of nematodes can be detected macroscopically. In addition, a restriction fragment length polymorphism-PCR-based assay on the first and/or second internal transcribed spacer (ITS1 and ITS2) of ribosomal DNA has been developed for the detection of *T. lacrymalis* DNA (Traversa *et al.* 2005).

Pathology

Heavy infections cause a mild conjunctivitis and adenitis of the lacrimal gland.

Management/Treatment

Levamisole 5 mg/kg BW orally or applied as a 1% eye lotion has proved to be highly efficient (Lyons *et al.* 1981). Furthermore, fly control may prevent recurrence.

Public health significance

Not convincing yet.

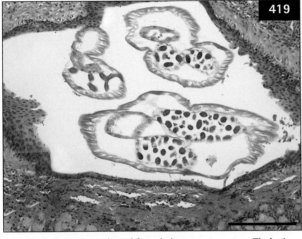

419 Thelaziasis. Intraductal female horse eye worm, *Thelazia lacrymalis*. Note numerous basophilic ovoid eggs within the paired uterus. (H&E stain. Bar 200 μm.)

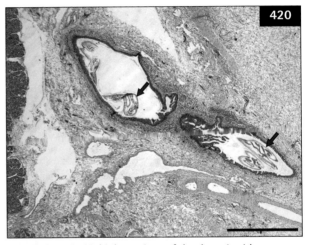

420 Thelaziasis. Multiple sections of slender spirurid nematodes within the lacrimal duct of the nictitating membrane (arrows). Nematode larvae in lacrimal secretions are transmitted by flies. Horse eye worm, *Thelazia lacrymalis*. (H&E stain. Bar 1 mm.)

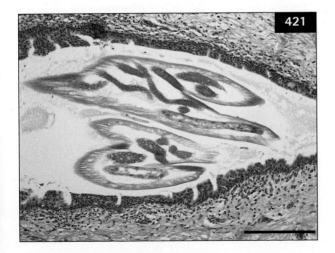

421 Thelaziasis. Mild lymphocytic periductular conjunctivitis. Usually infections are of no clinical significance, but in this case there is a moderate lymphocytic inflammatory infiltrate surrounding the infected lacrimal duct. Horse eye worm, *Thelazia lacrymalis*. (H&E stain. Bar 200 μm.)

Setaria equina
Phylum Nemathelminthes/Class Nematoda/Order Spirurida/Suborder Filariata/Superfamily Filarioidea/Family Onchocercidae/Genus Setaria

Definition/Overview
Disease of eye and adnexa is associated with aberrant *Setaria equina* nematodes, although the nematode is generally nonpathogenic (Soulsby 1968).

Aetiology
The filarioid nematode *S. equina* is a common parasite of equines in all parts of the world. The male is about 40–80 mm (**422, 423**) and the female 70–150 mm long. The tail of the female ends in a simple point. *S. equina* is a vector-borne filarial nematode that causes a relatively benign infection of equids in which the adult worms reside in the peritoneal cavity and sometimes in the scrotum (Soulsby 1968). It has also been recorded from the pleural cavity and the lungs of the horse. Microfilariae develop in the thoracic muscles of culicine mosquitoes such as *Aedes aegypti*. Infective larvae are produced in 12–16 days (Soulsby 1968).

Epidemiology
Peripheral blood samples collected randomly revealed a prevalence of 9.2% of *S. equina* in Hungary, and the level of microfilaraemia was between 1 and 1,138 larvae in 2 ml of blood. There was a significant association between the prevalence of microfilaraemia and the presence of still waters (Hornok *et al.* 2007).

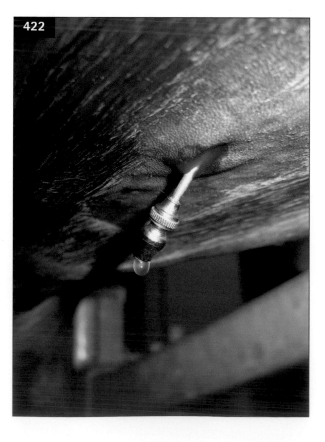

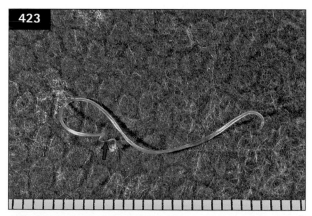

422, 423 Abdominal punctuate (**422**) yielded an adult onchocercid filarioid nematode (**423**); note the strongly coiled tail (arrow), a typical male determinant. These parasites inhabit the peritoneal cavity as end-stage in horses and generally do not cause major lesions. Here adult females produce microfilariae which, when present in the bloodstream, enter blood sucking arthropod vectors in which infectious larvae develop. Migrating larvae however can cause lesions in the CNS and eyes. *Setaria equina*. (Scale in mm.)

In Ankara, Turkey, 15% of slaughtered equines harboured adult *S. equina* (Oge *et al.* 2003). A *Setaria* sp. from the abdominal cavity and *Strongylus vulgaris*, *Strongylus edentatus*, and *Strongylus equinus* from the caecum showed recovery rates of 7%, 8%, 8%, and 1%, respectively, from Thoroughbreds in Kentucky, USA during 1981–1982. Parasites recovered from the stomach and infection rates were: immature *Habronema* spp. (24%), adult *H. muscae* (38%), immature *Draschia megastoma* (13%), adult *D. megastoma* (62%), and adult *Trichostrongylus axei* (4%). Lesions caused by *D. megastoma* were found upon gross observation in 58% of the stomachs. *Anoplocephala perfoliata* was recovered from 54% of the horses, whereas *A. magna* was not found. There was no obvious difference in infection rates of the stomach worms and tapeworms according to age or sex of the horses. Seasonal differences were apparent only for immature *Habronema* spp. and immature *D. megastoma*, for which infection rates began increasing in June, peaking in October and declining thereafter (Lyons *et al.* 1983).

Pathophysiology
S. equina might produce lesions and tissue damage because of its migratory behaviour.

Pre-patent period
In the horse adult parasites occur 8–10 months after infection (Soulsby 1968).

Clinical presentation
A slight fibrinous peritonitis may occur but this is usually of no consequence (Soulsby 1968).The presence of nematodes in the stomach usually does not induce clinical signs, although aberrant migration of the nematode is associated with disease of the eye and adnexa. Clinical signs include blepharospasm, lacrimation, epiphora, photophobia, keratitis, corneal ulceration, abscessation of the eyelids, and conjunctivitis.

Differential diagnosis
The differential diagnosis includes parasitic conjunctivitis and keratitis especially due to *Onchocerca cervicalis* microfilaria and adult *Thelazia lacrymalis* and *Parelaphostrongylus tenuis* nematodes.

Diagnosis
Blood smears may be used to detect microfilariae of *Setaria* spp. When blood samples were checked for microfilariae, using Knott's method and a combination of membrane filtration followed by histochemical staining for acid phosphatase, only

4% of the equines were found to be microfilaraemic (Oge *et al.* 2003). Interestingly, a standard method used to purify and cryopreserve peripheral blood mononuclear cells resulted in the unintended co-isolation of *Setaria equina* microfilariae (Yeargan *et al.* 2009).

Pathology
Setaria spp. adults generally cause no significant peritoneal lesions. However, migrating *Setaria* larvae within the CNS and eyes can incite localized eosinophilic granulomatous inflammation. Sheathed microfilariae can be patent in the blood (Jubb *et al.* 2007).

Management/Treatment
The avermectins are macrocyclic lactones produced by *Streptomyces avermitilis*. One of them has been chemically modified and given the generic name ivermectin. The compounds have shown efficacy against various stages of filarial parasites including *S. equina* in horses (Campbell 1982). Diethylcarbamazine citrate is a drug that is successful in eliminating human filariasis, possibly via trapping larvae in organs and killing them through cellular adherence (El-Shahawi *et al.* 2010).

The search for macrofilaricides remains a research priority in man. One of the most promising leads is treatment directed at *Wolbachia*, the intracellular bacterial symbiont of filarial parasites (Stolk *et al.* 2005). Depletion of *Wolbachia* by doxycycline kills most adult worms, without causing severe side effects. As a consequence, doxycycline indirectly kills the adult worm (Taylor *et al.* 2005). The availability of a new generation of drugs working through a different mechanism (killing the symbiont bacteria) is good news. However, using either PCR or DNA hybridization, *Wolbachia* sp. 16S rDNA was not found in *S. equina* (Chirgwin *et al.* 2002).

Public health significance
Not convincing yet.

Appendices

APPENDIX 1
Differential diagnoses

The differential diagnosis of **foal septicaemia** includes pathogens such as *A. equuli, E. coli, Clostridium* spp., *Salmonella* spp., *Klebsiella* spp., *Enterobacter* spp., and *Streptococcus* spp.

The differential diagnosis of **acute neurological disease** includes trauma, hepato-encephalopathy, Equine herpesvirus type 1, (pseudo)rabies, Louping ill virus, Western equine encephalomyelitis virus, Venezuelan equine encephalomyelitis virus, Eastern equine encephalomyelitis virus, tick-borne encephalitis, Borna disease virus, West Nile virus infection, Bunyavirus infection, Japanese encephalitis virus, Lyme disease, equine protozoal myeloencephalitis, parasitic migratory encephalomyelitis (due to *Strongylus vulgaris, S. equinus, Angiostrongylus cantonensis, Setaria* spp., *Parelaphostrongylus tenuis, Draschia megastoma*, and fly larvae *Hypoderma* spp.), *Clostridium botulinum*, bacterial meningoencephalitis, hypoglycaemia, malignant hyperthermia, acute selenium toxicity, mycotoxicosis (rye grass), various neoplasms, and neoplasia-like cholesteatoma.

The differential diagnosis of **blood clotting disorders** includes disseminated intravascular coagulation/sepsis, anthrax, rodenticide toxicity, myelophthisis, equine infectious anaemia, thrombocytopenia purpura, immune-mediated anaemia, arsenic toxicity, hepatic failure, snakebite, factor VIII deficiency, and von Willebrand's disease.

The differential diagnosis of **various (chronic) causes of weight loss, diarrhoea and anaemia** includes malnutrition, internal abscessation/peritonitis, tuberculosis, piroplasmosis, liver cirrhosis, EIA, chronic proliferative enteritis, and various neoplasms.

The differential diagnosis of **sudden death** includes lightning strike, malignant hyperthermia, ionophore toxicity, snakebite, clostridiosis, digestive tract rupture, taxus poisoning, anthrax, aortic rupture, anaphylactic drug reaction, African horse sickness, acute selenium toxicity, atypical myopathy, third degree heart block, and retentio secundinarum.

The differential diagnosis of **icterus and fever** includes piroplasmosis, Theiler's disease, neoplasms such as haemangiosarcoma, lymphosarcoma, and hepatic carcinoma, onion and red maple leaf poisoning, snakebite, sepsis, immune-mediated anaemia, gall stones, Tyzzer's disease, leptospirosis, reactive hepatitis (for instance due to duodenitis-proximal jejunutis), as well as various viral diseases including Hendra, Getah, equine infectious anaemia, and equine viral arteritis.

The differential diagnosis of **various causes of diarrhoea in foals** includes *Clostridium perfringens, C. difficile, Y. enterocolitica, S. westeri, Cryptosporidium* spp., and *Salmonella* spp.

The differential diagnosis of **various causes of internal abscessation** (without characteristic stellate scars in the nasal septum as seen in *B. mallei)* includes *S. equi* subsp. *zooepidemicus, S. equi* subsp. *equi, C. pseudotuberculosis, R. equi*, and melioidosis.

The differential diagnosis of various causes of **fever and dyspnoea** includes bacterial and mycotic pneumonia, pleuritis, thromboembolism, endo/myo/pericarditis, influenza, EHV (including 5), VSV, EIA, WNV, AHS, EVA, EAV, Hendra virus, anthrax, *C. pseudotuberculosis, Burkholderia mallei*-infection, tuberculosis, leptospirosis, *B. bronchiseptica*, piroplasmosis, histoplasmosis/EL, rhinitisvirus, adenovirus, digestive tract rupture, smoke inhalation, snakebite, strangles, pseudorabies, Hendra virus, sarcoidosis, heat stress, acute selenium toxicity, septicaemia/disseminated intravascular coagulation, and various neoplasms such as malignant lymphoma.

The differential diagnosis of **various causes of abortion and fever** includes EHV, EIA, EVA, piroplasmosis, anaphylaxis, *T. equigenitalis*, *C. pseudotuberculosis*, salmonellosis, tularaemia, brucellosis, *R. equi*, EPM, trypanosomiasis, *B. pseudomallei*, *N. risticii*, leptospirosis, histoplasmosis, *Chlamydophila*, and, anthrax.

The differential diagnosis of **various causes of acute diarrhoea** includes strongylosis, cyathostominosis, clostridiosis (*C. perfringens* and *difficile*), *C. pseudotuberculosis*, equine idiopathic colitis X syndrome, acute selenium toxicity, antibiotic-induced diarrhoea, salmonellosis, arsenic toxicity, NSAID toxicity, peritonitis, piroplasmosis, *N. risticii*, *Rhodococcus equi* infection, sand accumulation, chronic proliferative colitis, and lymphosarcoma.

The differential diagnosis of various causes of **chronic weight loss and (intermittent) fever** includes strongylosis, internal abscessation, chronic adhesions, pneumonia, pleuritis, meningoencephalitis, osteomyelitis, gastroduodenal ulcers, endo/peri/myocarditis, chronic proliferative enteritis, sinusitis, steatitis, temporohyoid osteoarthropathy, hepatitis, dermatophilosis, pemphigoid/pemphigus, piroplasmosis, glanders, tuberculosis, dourine, brucellosis, arsenic toxicity, wooden tongue, AIHA, EVA, rabies, and neoplasm.

The differential diagnosis of **various causes of fever and limb oedema** includes rhinitis virus, influenza, EIA, EHV, Getah virus, EVA, WNV, piroplasmosis, snakebite, *A. phagocytophilum*, and purpura haemorrhagica/thrombocytopenia purpura.

The differential diagnosis of **various causes of polyuria and polydipsia** includes psychogenic, sepsis/endotoxaemia, chronic renal failure, diabetes mellitus, diabetes insipidus (central or nephrogenic), iatrogenic (sedation with α2-agonists, triamcinolone administration), *Klossiella equi* infection, and vitamin D toxicity.

The differential diagnosis of **various causes of fever and anaemia** includes strongylosis, chronic inflammation, anti-coagulant toxicity, EIA, EVA, purpura haemorrhagica, anthrax, kidney disease, snakebite, guttural pouch mycosis, squamous cell carcinoma, lymphosarcoma/myelophthisis, haemangiosarcoma, Theiler's disease, leptospirosis, pemphigus foliaceus and vulgaris, piroplasmosis, trypanosomiasis, red maple leaf poisoning, *Anaplasma phagocytophilum*-(co)infection, auto-immune-mediated anaemia, chronic proliferative enteritis, gastric ulceration, and arsenic toxicity.

The differential diagnosis of **various causes of chronic coughing** includes heaves, pleuritis, diaphragmatic hernia, pneumothorax, (follicular) pharyngitis, exercise-induced pulmonary haemorrhage (EIPH), glanders, interstitial pneumonia, tracheal foreign body, ascarids, (aspiration) pneumonia, congestive heart failure, (metastatic) neoplasm, metastatic endocarditis, and laryngeal disorders (like epiglottic entrapment, epiglottitis, and dorsal displacement of the soft palate).

The differential diagnosis of **verminous conjunctivitis** includes *Thelazia lacrymalis*, *O. cervicalis* microfilaria, and (aberrant) adult *Setaria equina* and *Parelaphostrongylus tenuis* nematodes.

The differential diagnosis of various causes of **pruritus** includes shedding of hair coat, food allergy/intolerance, atopy, insect (*Culicoides*, *Dermanyssus gallinae*) bite or contact hypersensitivity, mites, pediculosis, pemphigus foliaceus, epidural drug administration (e.g. morphine), vertebral bone fracture, exercise-associated (cholinergic) pruritus and associated with terminal disorders (e.g. paraneoplastic pruritus associated with malignant lymphoma).

APPENDIX 2

(Potential) Zoonoses

Actinobacillus equuli
Actinobacillus lignieresii
Actinomyces pyogenes
Adenovirus
<u>African horse sickness virus</u>
Anaplasma phagocytophilum
<u>*Bacillus anthracis*</u>
Bartonella spp.
Bordetella bronchiseptica
Borna disease virus
Borrelia burgdorferi sensu lato complex
<u>*Brucella* spp.</u>
Burkholderia cepacia complex
<u>*Burkholderia mallei*</u>
Burkholderia pseudomallei
Campylobacter jejuni
<u>*Chlamydophila* (previously *Chlamydia*) *psittaci*</u>
Clostridium botulinum
Clostridium difficile
Clostridium perfringens
Clostridium piliforme
Corynebacterium pseudotuberculosis
<u>*Coxiella burnetii*</u>
Cryptosporidium spp.
Dermatophilus congolensis
<u>Eastern equine encephalomyelitis virus</u>
<u>*Echinococcus equinus*</u>
Erysipelothrix rhusiopathiae
Escherichia coli
Fasciola hepatica and *F. gigantica*
<u>*Francisella tularensis*</u>
Gasterophilus intestinalis and *G. nasalis*
Giardia duodenalis
Halicephalobus gingivalis
Hendra virus
Histoplasma capsulatum var. *farciminosum*
<u>Japanese encephalitis virus</u>
Leptospira interrogans

Listeria monocytogenes
Methicillin-resistant *Staphylococcus aureus*
Microsporum canis
Microsporum gypseum
<u>*Mycobacterium bovis*</u>
<u>Nipah virus</u>
Nocardia asteroides
Pasteurella multocida
Rhinitis virus
<u>Rabies</u>
Rhodococcus equi
Rotavirus
Ross River virus
Salmonellosis
<u>Sarcoptic mange</u>
Streptococcus equi subsp. *equi*
Streptococcus equi subsp. *zooepidemicus*
Trichophyton equinum
Trichophyton mentagrophytes
Trichophyton verrucosum
<u>*Trypanosoma brucei evansi*</u>
<u>Venezuelan equine encephalitis virus</u>
<u>Vesicular stomatitis virus</u>
<u>West Nile virus</u>
<u>Western equine encephalomyelitis virus</u>
Yersinia enterocolitica

Reportable (nonzoonotic) diseases

<u>Aujeszky's disease</u>
<u>*Babesia caballi*</u>
<u>Equine infectious anaemia</u>
<u>Equine influenza</u>
<u>Equine rhinopneumonitis (EHV)</u>
<u>Equine viral arteritis</u>
<u>*Taylorella equigenitalis*</u>
<u>*Theileria equi*</u>
<u>*Trypanosoma brucei equiperdum*</u>

Underlined = Office International des Epizooties (OIE) listed diseases. Note that this OIE list may not comply with national legislations fully.

APPENDIX 3
Clinical pathology
Haematology (424–436)

The morphology of erythrocytes and white blood cells is most readily observed by examination of smears. The most suitable anticoagulant for haematological investigations is ethylenediamine tetra-acetic acid (EDTA). The majority of equine lymphocytes are of the small type with a small amount of cytoplasm and a dark-staining nucleus.

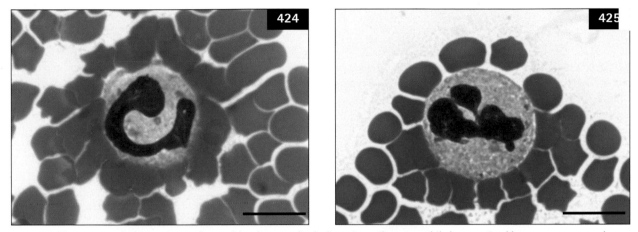

424, 425 Close-up cytology specimens from a blood smear displaying a juvenile neutrophil characterized by an unsegmented nucleus (**424**) and a mature segmented nucleus (**425**). The embedding anucleated cells are erythrocytes. (May–Grünwald–Giemsa stain. Bars 10 μm.)

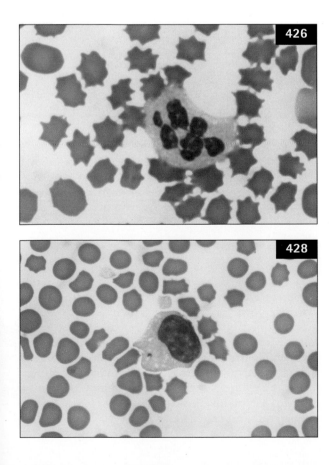

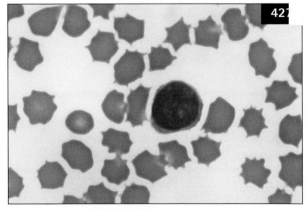

426–428 Cytology specimens from blood smears displaying a mature hypersegmented neutrophil (**426**), a lymphocyte with a dark round nucleus and scant cytoplasm (**427**), and a larger histiocytic cell with pale cytoplasm and an ovoid indented nucleus (**428**). In the background are erythrocytes. (May–Grünwald–Giemsa stain.)

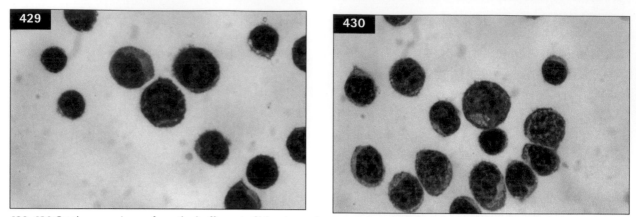

429, 430 Cytology specimens from the buffy coat of blood samples containing several smaller lymphocytes with dark round nuclei and somewhat larger monocytic cells with larger amounts of cytoplasm and less intensely stained and indented nuclei. (May–Grünwald–Giemsa stain.)

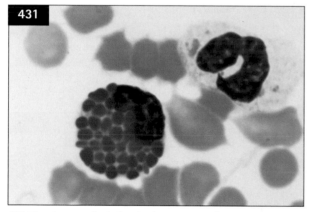

431 Blood smear depicting, in the centre, a close-up of an eosinophilic granulocyte packed with round to ovoid reddish cytoplasmic granules and an excentrically placed horseshoe-shaped nucleus, and on the right a neutrophilic granulocyte with a blunt lobed nucleus and indistinct cytoplasmic granules, amongst erythrocytes. (May–Grünwald–Giemsa stain.)

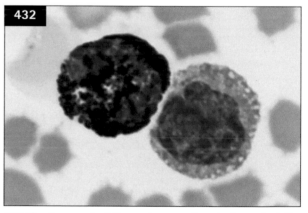

432 Blood smear depicting a close-up of, centrally on the left, a basophilic granulocyte packed with round to ovoid dark blue cytoplasmic granules and a blunt-lobed nucleus clustered on the right with a monocyte containing a central irregular nucleus and fine cytoplasmic vacuoles, surrounded by erythrocytes. (May–Grünwald–Giemsa stain.)

Occasionally larger lymphocytes may be observed. The nucleus of the equine monocyte is most commonly bean-shaped and not often folded. As with monocytes of the blood of other animal species, the nucleus has a lacy appearance and stains poorly. A **regenerative left shift** is characterized by an absolute increase in neutrophils accompanied by the appearance of immature neutrophils in the peripheral circulation. A **degenerative left shift** is one in which there is a normal, low, or falling total leukocyte count accompanied by a moderate to marked shift to the left, with the absolute number of immature neutrophils frequently exceeding the number of mature neutrophils (Coles 1986, Taylor & Hillyer 1997, Cowell & Tyler 2002). **Pancytopenia** is defined as an absolute decrease in erythrocytes, leukocytes, and platelets.

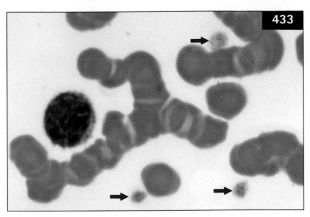

433 Blood smear depicting rouleaux formation of erythrocytes typical for equine blood, i.e. clustering of erythrocytes in a 'roof-tile' fashion thus forming cell strands of variable lengths. On the left is a small lymphocyte with a rounded compact dark nucleus and scant cytoplasm. A few scattered thrombocytes are indicated by arrows. (May–Grünwald–Giemsa stain.)

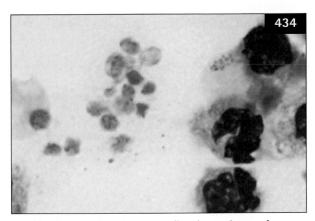

434 Blood smear depicting, centrally, a loose cluster of thrombocytes with vague cytoplasmic dark granules. On the right are several neutrophilic granulocytes and a few erythrocytes. (May–Grünwald–Giemsa stain.)

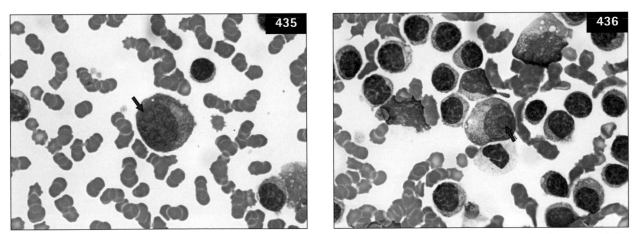

435, 436 Blood smear from a 4-year-old Friesian horse reveals several large neoplastic lymphoblasts (centre of both micrographs) with several atypical large nucleoli (arrows) consistent with a chronic lymphoid leukaemia. (May–Grünwald–Giemsa stain.)

Bronchoalveolar lavage (BAL) (437–445)

This technique samples fluid and cells from the alveoli and distal airways. BAL is undertaken in the standing, sedated horse and may be performed using an endoscope or a 'blind' technique (Taylor & Hillyer 1997).

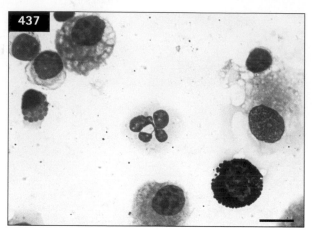

437 Cytology smear of a bronchoalveolar lavage, depicting different cell types: a neutrophilic granulocyte with a polymorphic hypersegmented nucleus (centre); an eosinophilic granulocyte with relative large reddish cytoplasmic granules (middle left); a mast cell with intense purple-staining cytoplasmic granules (bottom right); several spread large macrophages with abundant amounts of vacuolated cytoplasm; and a lymphocyte with a dark rounded nucleus and a small rim of cytoplasm (top right). (May–Grünwald–Giemsa stain. Bar 10 μm.)

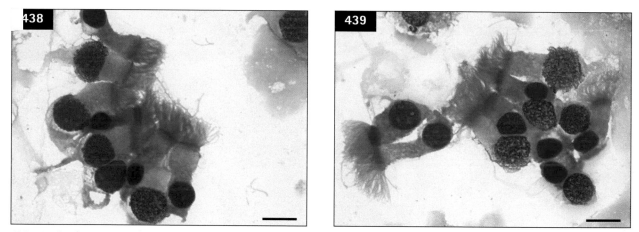

438, 439 Cytology smears of a bronchoalveolar lavage, depicting clustered high columnar ciliated epithelial cells from the respiratory tract that contain a basally located rounded nucleus and apical lining of cilia. (May–Grünwald–Giemsa stain. Bars 10 μm.)

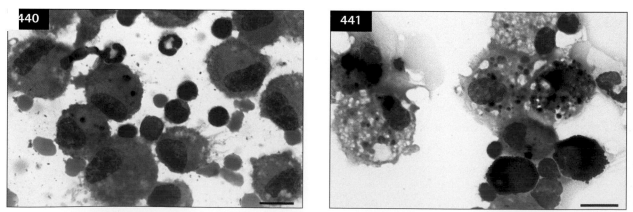

440, 441 Cytology smears of a bronchoalveolar lavage depicting several large macrophages laden with abundant amounts of variably sized haemosiderin granules. Haemosiderin is an iron metabolite of haemoglobin degradation; therefore this finding is indicative of a pulmonary haemorrhage. These granules vary in colour from light greenish (often still reminiscent of the phagocytosed erythrocytes) to dark brown respectively, inherent to the stage of iron metabolism. (May–Grünwald–Giemsa stain. Bars 10 μm.)

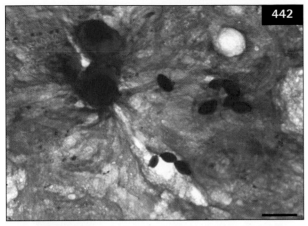

442 Cytology smear of a bronchoalveolar lavage depicting abundant mucus with several embedded yeasts (middle right). Note also a few bacteria at top left. (May–Grünwald–Giemsa stain. Bar 10 µm.)

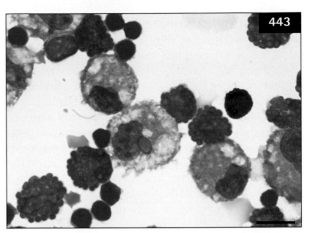

443 Cytology smear of a bronchoalveolar lavage, depicting several large macrophages with excentric nuclei and abundant cytoplasm that contains a phagocytosed ovoid yeast (centre), several accompanying eosinophils, a mast cell, and lymphocytes. (May–Grünwald–Giemsa stain. Bar 10 µm.)

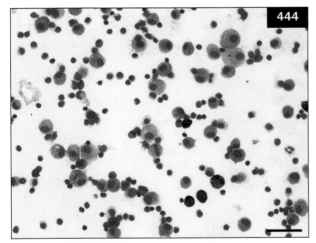

444 Cytology smear of a bronchoalveolar lavage at low magnification depicting an increased cellularity and hypereosinophilia; accompanying the readily observed bright reddish eosinophils are increased numbers of dark purple mast cells and abundant numbers of large macrophages. Hypereosinophilia can be associated with *Dermanyssus gallinae* infestations. (May–Grünwald–Giemsa stain. Bar 50 µm.)

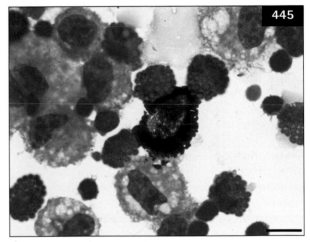

445 Cytology smear of a bronchoalveolar lavage hypereosinophilia at higher magnification depicting several eosinophils with intense reddish cytoplasmic granules, a central mast cell with intense purple cytoplasmic granules amongst larger macrophages with abundant cytoplasm, and smaller lymphocytes with rounded dark blue nuclei and scant cytoplasm. (May–Grünwald–Giemsa stain. Bar 10 µm.)

Bone marrow aspiration/biopsy (446–462)

When a peripheral blood count indicates the presence of leucopaenia, nonregenerative anaemia, or thrombocytopaenia, or if abnormal cell types appear, a bone marrow examination should be considered. Anaemias in the horse are usually not accompanied by typical peripheral blood signs of regeneration. Consequently, it may be necessary to resort to a bone marrow examination in order to evaluate erythropoietic response in this species. If the anaemia is regenerative, the myeloid:erythroid ratio is decreased, often falling below 0.5 (Coles 1986). Study of the precursor cells of lymphocytes and monocytes is difficult because these cells do not contain specific cytoplasmic granules or the nuclear lobulation that is present in the granulocytes, both of which facilitate the distinction between young and mature forms. Lymphocytes and monocytes are distinguished mainly on the basis of size, chromatin structure, and the presence of nucleoli in smear preparations. As lymphocytic cells mature, their chromatin becomes more compact, the nucleoli become less visible, and the cells decrease in size (Junqueira & Carneiro 1980).

Maturation of erythrocytes: proerythroblast → basophilic erythroblast → polychromatophilic erythroblast → normoblast → reticulocyte → erythrocyte.

Maturation of granulocytes: myeloblast → promyelocyte → myelocyte → metamyelocyte → juvenile (band-shaped nucleus) granulocyte → mature granulocyte.

Maturation of lymphocytes: lymphoblast → lymphocyte.

Maturation of platelets: megakaryoblast → megakaryocyte → platelet.

Normal myeloid:erythroid ratio has been reported as 0.71±0.11 (range 0.48–0.91) based on 24 Warmblood horses. The average bone marrow contained 28.2±7.9% intermediate normoblasts, and 23.2±5.8% orthochromatic normoblasts within the erythroid cells and 1.0±1.1% myeloblasts, 1.7±1.0% promyelocytes, 3.2±1.8% myelocytes, 5.6±3.2% metamyelocytes and 15.7±5.3% band neutrophils. In total 0.8±0.8% mitoses were noticed. It was shown that equine bone marrow contains a considerable amount of iron in the normal horse (Franken *et al.* 1982).

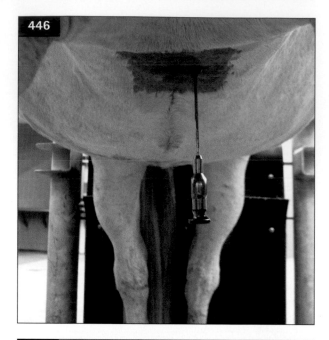

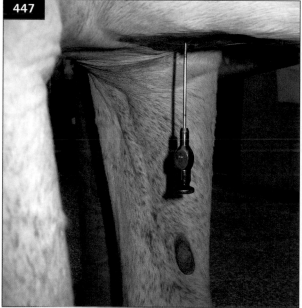

446–448 Bone marrow from the sternum can be collected from the standing horse by insertion of a special needle at the crossing point of an imaginary line drawn between the two points of the elbow (Taylor & Hillyer 1997), illustrated from the cranial (**446**) and lateral (**447**) view. The photograph (**448**) illustrates the thickness of both the deep pectoral muscle and the sternum above it in a normal Warmblood horse. (Scale in cm.)

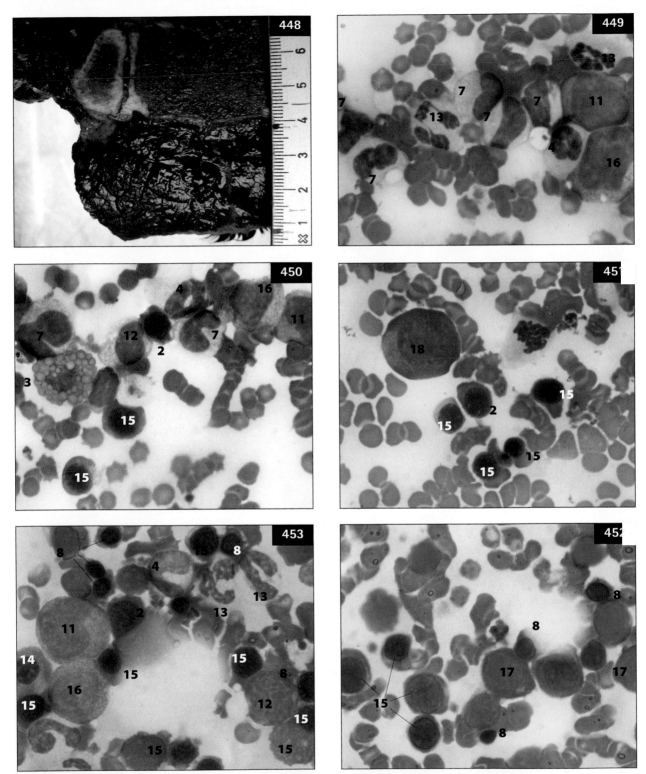

449–462 High cellular equine bone marrow aspirates from the sternum illustrating various cells. Cells shown are; basophilic granulocyte (1), basophilic rubricyte (2), eosinophilic granulocyte (3), juvenile band-shaped granulocyte (4), macrophage (5), megakaryocyte (6), metamyelocyte (7), metarubricyte (8), monoblast (9), monocyte (10), myeloblast (11), myelocyte (12), neutrophilic granulocyte (13), plasma cell (14), polychromatic rubricyte (15), promyelocyte (16), prorubricyte (17), rubriblast (18), lymphocyte (19). (May–Grünwald–Giemsa stain.) (Courtesy of Dr E. Teske.)

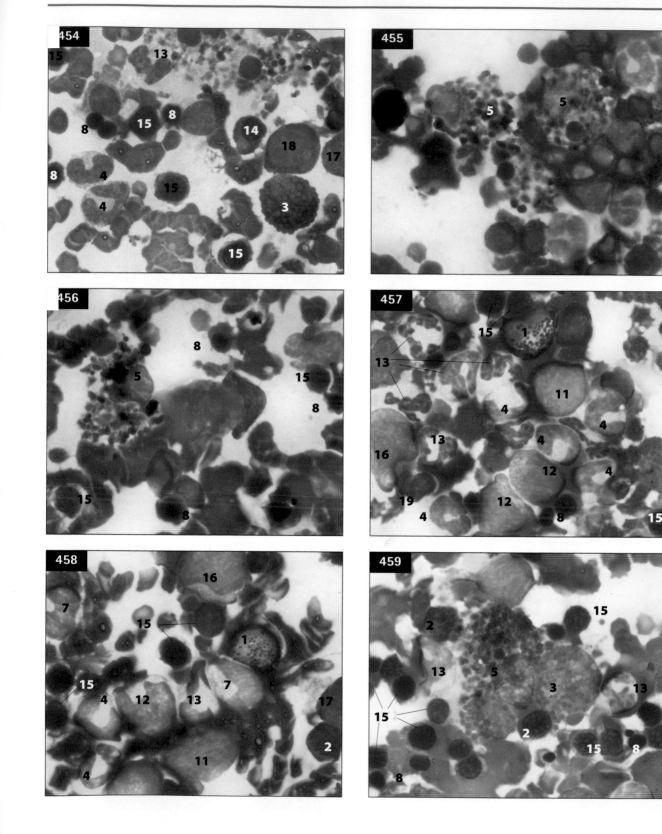

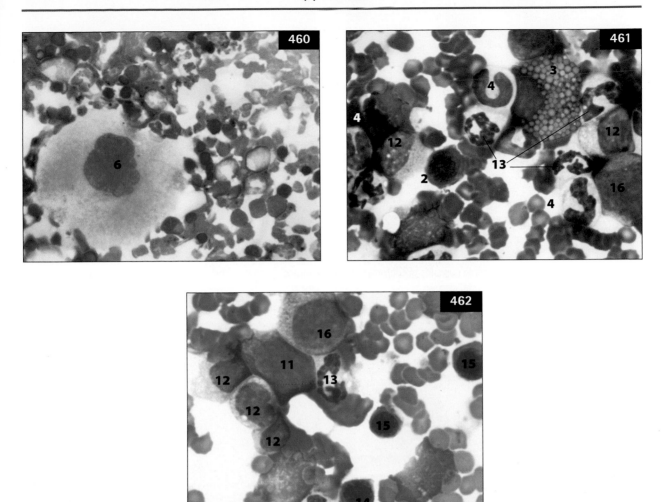

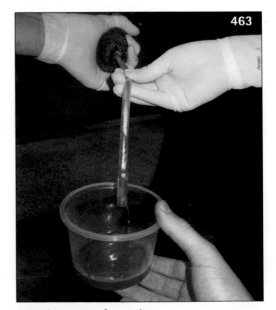

Urinalysis (463–474)

Normal equine urine is alkaline, given the vegetable diet. If the urine is alkaline, the leukocytes are usually swollen, ragged in appearance, and very granular and have a tendency to adhere in clumps (Coles 1986). It is normal to find large quantities of amorphous phosphates and calcium carbonate crystals in equine urine. Struvites are normally found in very small quantities in equine urine.

463 Urine capture for cytology.

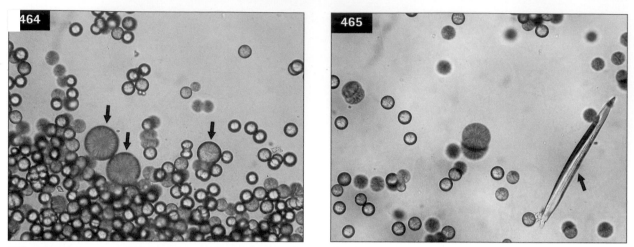

464, 465 Urine cytology. **464**: Sample contains predominantly amorphous phosphates and some round calcium carbonate crystals (arrows); **465**: a bar-like struvite crystal (arrow).

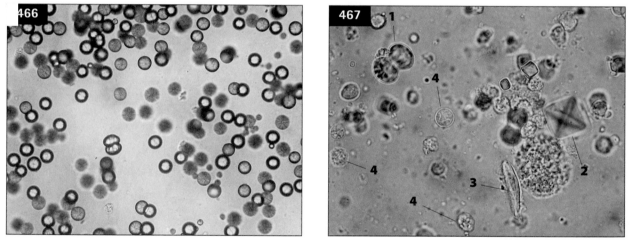

466, 467 Equine urine. The classic form of calcium carbonate crystal, being the predominant crystal in equine urine, is round in shape with radial striations and is yellow-brown (**466**); **467**: the so-called dumbbell form of the calcium carbonate crystal (1) is present, as well as a calcium oxalate crystal (2) and a bar-like struvite crystal (3). Note the leukocytes (4).

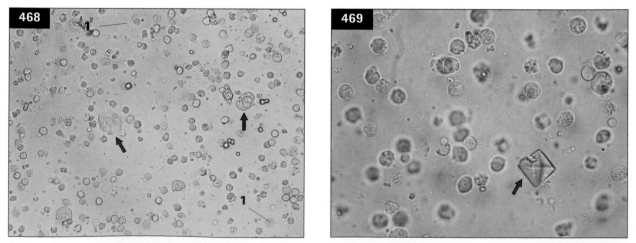

468, 469 Equine urine. Renal tubule cells (arrows) between many leukocytes (1) (**468**); **469**: a calcium oxalate crystal (arrow) is seen between many leukocytes.

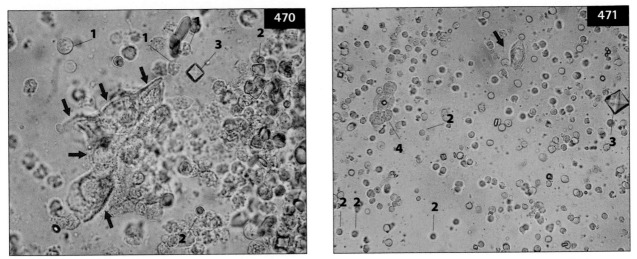

470, 471 Equine urine. **470**: Renal tubule cell cast (arrows), leukocytes (1), erythrocytes (2), and a calcium oxalate crystal (3);
471: a calcium oxalate crystal (3), a leukocyte cast (4), erythrocytes (2), and a renal tubule cell (arrow) are seen.

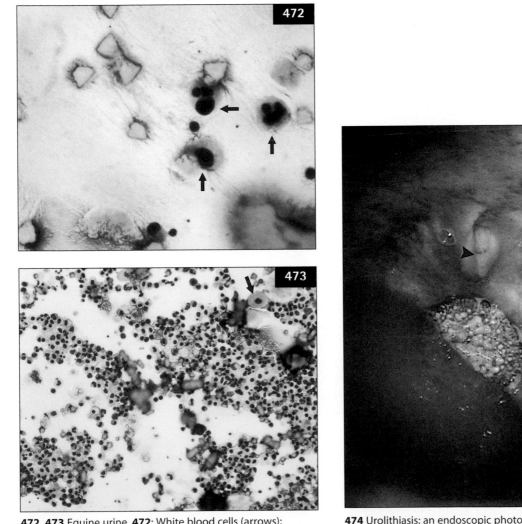

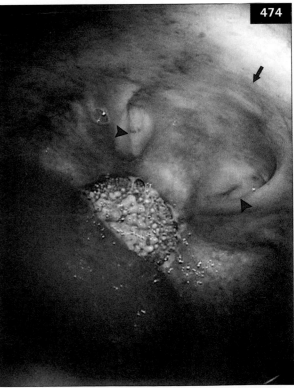

472, 473 Equine urine. **472**: White blood cells (arrows); **473**: a renal tubule cell (arrow) is seen following Giemsa staining. (**464–473** Courtesy of Dr E. Teske.)

474 Urolithiasis; an endoscopic photograph of a rough urolith within the urinary bladder. Note the trigone of bladder (arrow) and the ureteric orifices (arrowheads).

Coprological examination (475–481)

Parasite eggs are separated from the faecal mass by a flotation technique using solutions of high specific gravity. The results are calculated as eggs per gram (epg) of faeces. Oxyuris (pinworm) eggs may be identified on the anal sphincter by pressing a strip of transparent adhesive tape onto the mucosal folds of the external sphincter (Taylor & Hillyer 1997). Care should be taken to avoid the intercostal vessels and nerve which run along the caudal part of the rib by entering the pleural cavity just cranial to the rib margin.

The mere presence of a parasite in or on an animal cannot be considered adequate evidence that it is the aetiological agent of a disease that may exist. Diagnostic aids such as coprological examination are used to supplement, not supplant, clinical observations (Coles 1986).

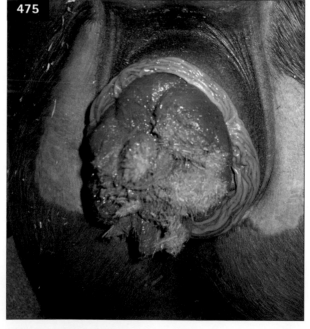

475 Examination of faeces.

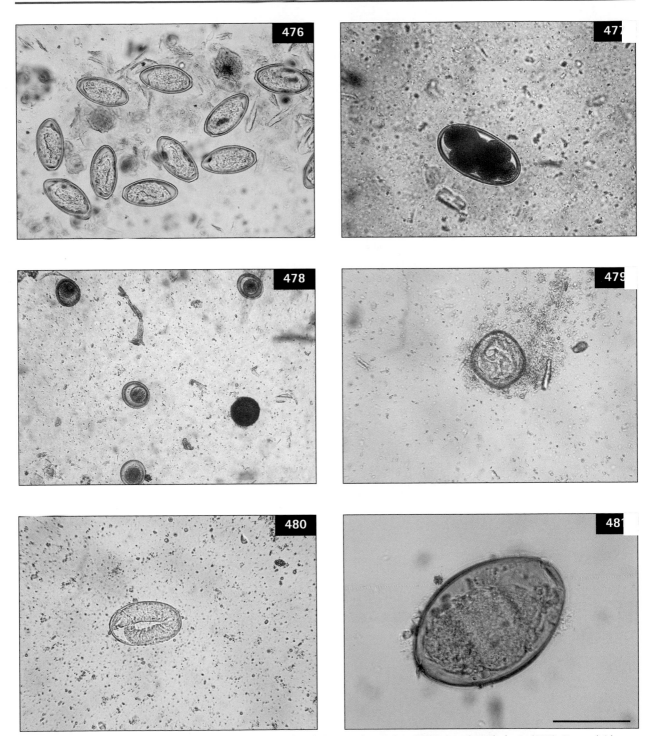

476–481 Parasite eggs: *Oxyuris equi* (**476**), *Strongylus* sp. (**477**), *Parascaris equorum* (**478**), *Anoplocephala* sp. (**479**), *Strongyloides westeri* (**480**) and, *Fasciola hepatica* (**481**).

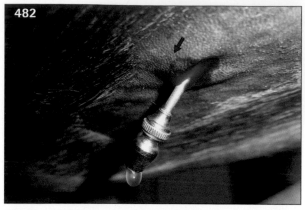

482 Abdominocentesis ideally is performed at the lowermost point of the belly, since this forms a natural basin in which peritoneal fluid accumulates. In all cases the point of insertion should be approximately a handsbreadth behind the xiphisternum to avoid damage to its cartilage (Taylor & Hillyer 1997).

Abdomino/thoracocentesis (482–484)

Abdominocentesis ideally is performed at the lowermost point of the belly, since this forms a natural basin in which peritoneal fluid accumulates. In all cases the point of insertion should be approximately a handsbreadth behind the xiphisternum to avoid damage to its cartilage (Taylor & Hillyer 1997).

Abdominocentesis performed within 10 days before foaling and again 12 hours, 3 days, and 7 days after foaling indicated that there were not any significant differences over time in specific gravity (1.011±0.0003 (SD) prior to foaling), total protein concentration (16.0±1.2 g/l), fibrinogen concentration (not quantified), total nucleated cell count (0.926±0.137 g/l), or number of small mononuclear cells (0.126±0.034 G/L). However, in samples collected before and after foaling there were significantly higher mean numbers of neutrophils (from 0.547±0.099 prior to foaling to 2.22±0.425 G/l 3 days after foaling) and large mononuclear cells (from 0.254±0.056 to 1.032±0.271 G/l 3 days after foaling) (van Hoogmoed *et al.* 1996).

The usual site of thoracocentesis is the 6th–7th intercostal spaces on the right, or the 8th–9th intercostals spaces on the left (Taylor & Hillyer 1997). Care should be taken to avoid the intercostal vessels and nerve which run along the caudal part of the rib by entering the pleural cavity just cranial to the rib margin.

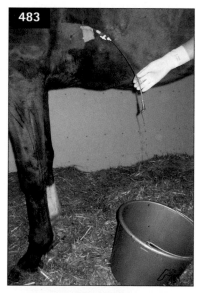

483 Thoracocentesis is generally performed in the ventral third of the chest, taking care to avoid damage to the heart. The usual site is the 6th–7th intercostal spaces on the right, or the 8th–9th intercostal spaces on the left (Taylor & Hillyer 1997).

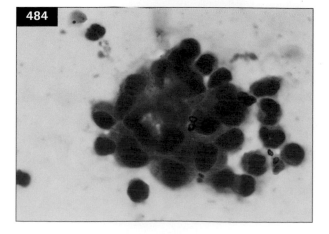

484 Abdominocentesis smear from a 12-year-old Thoroughbred horse that contains a cluster of large neoplastic lymphoblasts consistent with a large cell malignant lymphoma. (May–Grünwald–Giemsa stain.)

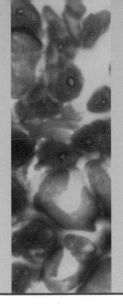

References

INTRODUCTION

Coles EH 1986. *Veterinary Clinical Pathology*, 4th edn. WB Saunders, London.

Fauquet CM, Mayo MA, Maniloff J, Desselberger U, Ball LA (eds) 2005. *Virus Taxonomy*. 8th Report of the International Committee on Taxonomy of Viruses. Academic Press, Elsevier, Amsterdam.

Garrity GM, Bell JA, Lilburn TG 2004. Taxonomic outline of the prokaryotes. In: *Bergey's Manual of Systematic Bacteriology*, 2nd edn. Springer, New York.

Kassai T 1999. *Veterinary Helminthology*. Butterworth-Heinemann, Oxford.

CHAPTER 1 BACTERIAL DISEASES

Anaplasma spp.

Bjoersdorff A, Bergström S, Massung RF, Haemig PD, Olsen B 2001. *Ehrlichia*-infected ticks on migrating birds. *Emerging Infectious Diseases* 7:877–879.

Butler CM, Nijhof AM, Jongejan F, van der Kolk JH 2008. *Anaplasma phagocytophilum* infection in horses in the Netherlands. *Veterinary Record* 162:216–218.

Chang YF, McDonough SP, Chang CF, Shin KS, Yen W, Divers T 2000. Human granulocytic ehrlichiosis agent infection in a pony vaccinated with a *Borrelia burgdorferi* recombinant OspA vaccine and challenged by exposure to naturally infected ticks. *Clinical and Diagnostic Laboratory Immunology* 7:68–71.

Dumler JS, Madigan JE, Pusterla N, Bakken JS 2007. Ehrlichioses in humans: epidemiology, clinical presentation, diagnosis, and treatment. *Clinical Infectious Diseases* 45 Suppl 1:S45–S51.

Foley JE, Nieto NC, Massung R, Barbet A, Madigan J, Brown RN 2009. Distinct ecologically relevant strains of *Anaplasma phagocytophilum*. *Emerging Infectious Diseases* 15:842–843.

Franzén P, Aspan A, Egenvall A, Gunnarsson A, Åberg L, Pringle J 2005. Acute clinical, hematologic, serologic, and polymerase chain reaction findings in horses experimentally infected with a European Strain of *Anaplasma phagocytophilum*. *Journal of Veterinary Internal Medicine* 19:232–239.

Franzén P, Aspan A, Egenvall A, Gunnarsson A, Karlstam E, Pringle J 2009. Molecular evidence for persistence of *Anaplasma phagocytophilum* in the absence of clinical abnormalities in horses after recovery from acute experimental infection. *Journal of Veterinary Internal Medicine* 23:636–642.

Gerhards H, Offeney F, Friedhoff KT 1987. *Ehrlichia*-Infektion beim Pferd. *Pferdeheilkunde* 6:283–291.

Gribble DH 1969. Equine ehrlichiosis. *Journal of the American Veterinary Medical Association* 155:462–469.

Hilton H, Madigan JE, Aleman M 2008. Rhabdomyolysis associated with *Anaplasma phagocytophilum* infection in a horse. *Journal of Veterinary Internal Medicine* 22:1061–1064.

Jubb KVF, Kennedy PC, Palmer N 2007. *Pathology of Domestic Animals*, 5th edn. WB Saunders Elsevier, Edinburgh 3:249, 309–310.

Lillini E, Macri G, Proietti G, Scarpulla M 2006. New findings on anaplasmosis caused by infection with *Anaplasma phagocytophilum*. *Annals of the New York Academy of Sciences* 1081:360–370.

Madigan JE 1993. Equine ehrlichiosis. *Veterinary Clinics of North America: Equine Practice* 9:423–428.

Madigan JE, Gribble DH 1987. Equine ehrlichiosis in northern California: 49 cases (1968–1981). *Journal of the American Veterinary Medical Association* 190:445–448.

Madigan JE, Hietala S, Chalmers S, DeRock E 1990. Seroepidemiologic survey of antibodies to *Ehrlichia equi* in horses of northern California. *Journal of the American Veterinary Medical Association* 196:1962–1964.

Madigan JE, Richter PJ, Kimsey RB, Barlough JE, Bakken JS, Dumler JS 1995. Transmission and passage in horses of the agent of human granulocytic ehrlichiosis. *Journal of Infectious Diseases* 172:1141–1144.

Magnarelli LA, Ijdo JW, Andel AE van, Wu C, Padula SJ, Fikrig E 2000. Serologic confirmation of *Ehrlichia equi* and *Borrelia burgdorferi* infections in horses from the northeastern United States. *Journal of the American Veterinary Medical Association* 217:1045–1050.

Nyindo MBA, Ristic M, Lewis GE, Huxsoll DL, Stephenson EH 1978. Immune response of ponies to experimental infection with *Ehrlichia equi*. *American Journal of Veterinary Research* **39**:15–18.

Skarphedinsson S, Jensen PM, Kristiansen K 2005. Survey of tickborne infections in Denmark. *Emerging Infectious Diseases* **11**:1055–1061.

Stannard A, Gribble D, Smith R 1969. Equine ehrlichiosis: a disease with similarities to tick-borne fever and bovine petechial fever. *Veterinary Record* **84**:149–150.

Vorou RM, Papavassiliou VG, Tsiodras S 2007. Emerging zoonoses and vector-borne infections affecting humans in Europe. Review article. *Epidemiology and Infection* **135**:1231–1247.

Zeman P, Jahn P 2009. An entropy-optimized multilocus approach for characterizing the strains of *Anaplasma phagocytophilum* infecting horses in the Czech Republic. *Journal of Medical Microbiology* **58**:423–429.

Neorickettsia risticii

Biswas B, Mukherjee D, Mattingly-Napier BL, Dutta SK 1991. Diagnostic application of polymerase chain reaction for detection of *Ehrlichia risticii* in equine monocytic ehrlichiosis (Potomac horse fever). *Journal of Clinical Microbiology* **29**:2228–2233.

Dawson JE, Ristic M, Holland CJ, Whitlock RH, Sessions J 1987. Isolation of *Ehrlichia risticii*, the causative agent of Potomac horse fever, from the fetus of an experimentally infected mare. *Veterinary Record* **121**:232.

Dutta SK, Penney BE, Myrup AC, Robl MG, Rice RM 1988. Disease features in horses with induced equine monocytic ehrlichiosis (Potomac horse fever). *American Journal of Veterinary Research* **49**:1747–1751.

Dutta SK, Vemulapalli R, Biswas B 1998. Association of deficiency in antibody response to vaccine and heterogeneity of *Ehrlichia risticii* strains with Potomac horse fever vaccine failure in horses. *Journal of Clinical Microbiology* **36**:506–512.

Gibson KE, Rikihisa Y, Zhang C, Martin C 2005. *Neorickettsia risticii* is vertically transmitted in the trematode *Acanthatrium oregonense* and horizontally transmitted to bats. *Environmental Microbiology* **7**:203–212.

Holland CJ, Ristic M, Cole AI, Johnson P, Baker G, Goetz T 1985. Isolation, experimental transmission, and characterization of causative agent of Potomac horse fever. *Science* **227**:522–524.

Jubb KVF, Kennedy PC, Palmer N 2007. *Pathology of Domestic Animals*, 5th edn. WB Saunders Elsevier, Edinburgh **2**:228.

Lin M, Zhang C, Gibson K, Rikihisa Y 2009. Analysis of complete genome sequence of *Neorickettsia risticii*: causative agent of Potomac horse fever. *Nucleic Acids Research* **37**:6076–6091.

Long MT, Goetz TE, Kakoma I, *et al*. 1992. Isolation of *Ehrlichia risticii* from the aborted fetus of an infected mare. *Veterinary Record* **131**:370.

Madigan JE, Pusterla N, Johnson E, *et al*. 2000. Transmission of *Ehrlichia risticii*, the agent of Potomac horse fever using naturally infected aquatic insects and helminth vectors: preliminary report. *Equine Veterinary Journal* **32**:275–279.

Mott J, Rikihisa Y, Zhang Y, Reed SM, Yu CY 1997. Comparison of PCR and culture to the indirect fluorescent antibody test for diagnosis of Potomac horse fever. *Journal of Clinical Microbiology* **35**:2215–2219.

Mott J, Muramatsu Y, Seaton E, Martin C, Reed SM, Rikihisa Y 2002. Molecular analysis of *Neorickettsia risticii* in adult aquatic insects in Pennsylvania, in horses infected by ingestion of insects, and isolated in cell culture. *Journal of Clinical Microbiology* **40**:690–693.

Palmer JE, Whitlock RH, Benson CE 1986. Equine ehrlichial colitis (Potomac horse fever): recognition of the disease in Pennsylvania, New Jersey, New York, Ohio, Idaho, and Connecticut. *Journal of the American Veterinary Medical Association* **189**:197–199.

Palmer JE, Whitlock RH, Benson CE 1988. Equine ehrlichial colitis: effect of oxytetracycline treatment during the incubation period of *Ehrlichia risticii* infection in ponies. *Journal of the American Veterinary Medical Association* **192**:343–345.

Palmer JE, Benson CE, Whitlock RH 1990. Resistance to development of equine ehrlichial colitis in experimentally inoculated horses and ponies. *American Journal of Veterinary Research* **51**:763–765.

Palmer JE, Benson CE, Whitlock RH 1992. Effect of treatment with oxytetracycline during the acute stages of experimentally induced equine ehrlichial colitis in ponies. *American Journal of Veterinary Research* **53**:2300–2304.

Rikihisa Y, Perry BD, Cordes DO 1985. Ultrastructural study of rickettsial organisms in the large colon of ponies experimentally infected with Potomac horse fever. *Infection and Immunology* **49**:505–512.

Rikihisa Y, Zhang C, Kanter M, Cheng Z, Ohashi N, Fukuda T 2004. Analysis of p51, groESL, and the major antigen P51 in various species of *Neorickettsia*, an obligatory intracellular bacterium that infects trematodes and mammals. *Journal of Clinical Microbiology* **42**:3823–3826.

Ristic M, Holland CJ, Dawson JE, Sessions JE, Palmer J 1986. Diagnosis of equine monocytic ehrlichiosis (Potomac horse fever) by indirect immunofluorescence. *Journal of the American Veterinary Medical Association* **189**:39–46.

Whitlock RH, Palmer JE 1986. Potomac horse fever: clinical signs, diagnosis and treatment. *Proceedings of the Annual Meeting of the American Association of Equine Practitioners* **32**:405–413.

Bartonella henselae

Chomel BB, Kasten RW, Williams C, *et al*. 2009. *Bartonella* endocarditis: a pathology shared by animal reservoirs and patients. *Annals of the New York Academy of Sciences* **1166**:120–126.

Johnson R, Ramos-Vara J, Vemulapalli R 2009. Identification of *Bartonella henselae* in an aborted equine fetus. *Veterinary Pathology* **46**:277–281.

Jones SL, Maggi R, Shuler J, Alward A, Breitschwerdt EB 2008. Detection of *Bartonella henselae* in the blood of 2 adult horses. *Journal of Veterinary Internal Medicine* **22**:495–498.

Maguiña C, Guerra H, Ventosilla P 2009. Bartonellosis. *Clinical Dermatology* 27:271–280.

Maurin M, Gasquet S, Ducco C, Raoult D 1995. MICs of 28 antibiotic compounds for 14 *Bartonella* (formerly *Rochalimaea*) isolates. *Antimicrobial Agents* and *Chemotherapeutics* 39:2387–2391.

Vorou RM, Papavassiliou VG, Tsiodras S 2007. Emerging zoonoses and vector-borne infections affecting humans in Europe. Review article. *Epidemiology and Infection* 135:1231–1247.

Brucella spp.

Abo-Shehada MN 2009. Seroprevalence of *Brucella* species in equids in Jordan. *Veterinary Record* 165:267–268.

Acosta-González RI, González-Reyes I, Flores-Gutiérrez GH 2006. Prevalence of *Brucella abortus* antibodies in equines of a tropical region of Mexico. *Canadian Journal of Veterinary Research* 70:302–304.

Al Dahouk S, Tomaso H, Nöckler K, Neubauer H 2004. The detection of *Brucella* spp. using PCR-ELISA and real-time PCR assays. Review. *Clinical Laboratory* 50:387–394.

Carrigan MJ, Cockram FA, Nash GV 1987. *Brucella abortus* biotype 1 arthritis in a horse. *Australian Veterinary Journal* 64:190.

Cohen ND, Carter GK, McMullan WC 1992. Fistulous withers in horses: 24 cases (1984–1990). *Journal of the American Veterinary Medical Association* 201:121–124.

Collins JD, Kelly WR, Twomey T, Farrelly BT, Whitty BT 1971. *Brucella*-associated vertebral osteomyelitis in a thoroughbred mare. *Veterinary Record* 88:321–326.

Cook DR, Kingston GC 1988. Isolation of *Brucella suis* biotype 1 from a horse. *Australian Veterinary Journal* 65:162–163.

Ekers BM 1978. *Brucella* cultures typed by the WHO Brucellosis Centre at the Commonwealth Serum Laboratories, Melbourne. *Australian Veterinary Journal* 54:440–443.

Lucero NE, Ayala SM, Escobar GI, Jacob NR 2008. *Brucella* isolated in humans and animals in Latin America from 1968 to 2006. *Epidemiology and Infection* 136:496–503.

MacMillan AP, Baskerville A, Hambleton P, Corbel MJ 1982. Experimental *Brucella abortus* infection in the horse: observations during the three months following inoculation. *Research in Veterinary Science* 33:351–359.

MacMillan AP, Cockrem DS 1986. Observations on the long term effects of *Brucella abortus* infection in the horse, including effects during pregnancy and lactation. *Equine Veterinary Journal* 18:388–390.

Mazokopakis E, Christias E, Kofteridis D 2003. Acute brucellosis presenting with erythema nodosum. *European Journal of Epidemiology* 18:913–915.

McCaughey WJ, Kerr WR 1967. Abortion due to brucellosis in a thoroughbred mare. *Veterinary Record* 80:186–187.

Mohandas N, Balasubramanian R, Prasad SB 2009. Can *Brucella* endocarditis be treated successfully with medical therapy alone? *Tropical Doctor* 39:123–124.

Pappas G, Papadimitriou P, Akritidis N, Christou L, Tsianos EV 2006. The new global map of human brucellosis. Review. *Lancet Infectious Diseases* 6:91–99.

Ranjbar M, Rezaiee AA, Hashemi SH, Mehdipour S 2009. Neurobrucellosis: report of a rare disease in 20 Iranian patients referred to a tertiary hospital. *East Mediterranean Health Journal* 15:143–148.

Refai M 2002. Incidence and control of brucellosis in the Near East region. Review. *Veterinary Microbiology* 90:81–110.

Rolando I, Vilchez G, Olarte L, *et al.* 2009. Brucellar uveitis: intraocular fluids and biopsy studies. *International Journal of Infectious Diseases* 13:e206–211.

Roop RM 2nd, Gaines JM, Anderson ES, Caswell CC, Martin DW 2009. Survival of the fittest: how *Brucella* strains adapt to their intracellular niche in the host. *Medical Microbiology and Immunology* 198:221–238.

Sakran W, Chazan B, Koren A 2006. Brucellosis: clinical presentation, diagnosis, complications and therapeutic options. Review. *Harefuah* 145:836–840, 860.

Seleem MN, Boyle SM, Sriranganathan N 2010. Brucellosis: A re-emerging zoonosis. *Veterinary Microbiology* 140:392–398.

Shortridge EH 1967. Two cases of suspected *Brucella abortus* abortion in mares. *New Zealand Veterinary Journal* 15:33–34.

Burkholderia mallei

Arun S, Neubauer H, Gürel A, *et al.* 1999. Equine glanders in Turkey. *Veterinary Record* 144:255–258.

Harvey SP, Minter JM 2005. Ribotyping of *Burkholderia mallei* isolates. *FEMS Immunology and Medical Microbiology* 44:91–97.

Jubb KVF, Kennedy PC, Palmer N 2007. *Pathology of Domestic Animals*, 5th edn. WB Saunders Elsevier, Edinburgh 2:633–634.

Katz J, Dewald R, Nicholson J 2000. Procedurally similar competitive immunoassay systems for the serodiagnosis of *Babesia equi*, *Babesia caballi*, *Trypanosoma equiperdum*, and *Burkholderia mallei* infection in horses. *Journal of Veterinary Diagnostic Investigation* 12:46–50.

Lehavi O, Aizenstien O, Katz LH, Hourvitz A 2002. Glanders – a potential disease for biological warfare in humans and animals. *Harefuah* 141:88–91, 119.

Lopez J, Copps J, Wilhelmsen C, *et al.* 2003. Characterization of experimental equine glanders. *Microbes and Infection* 5:1125–1131.

Mandell GL, Bennett JE, Dolin R 1995. *Pseudomonas Species (Including Melioidosis and Glanders)*. Churchill Livingstone, New York.

Ribot WJ, Ulrich RL 2006. The animal pathogen-like type III secretion system is required for the intracellular survival of *Burkholderia mallei* within J774.2 macrophages. *Infection and Immunity* 74:4349–4353.

Schell MA, Ulrich RL, Ribot WJ, *et al.* 2007. Type IV secretion is a major virulence determinant in *Burkholderia mallei*. *Molecular Microbiology* 64:1466–1485.

Sprague LD, Zachariah R, Neubauer H, *et al.* 2009. Prevalence-dependent use of serological tests for diagnosing glanders in horses. *BMC Veterinary Research* 5:32.

Thibault FM, Valade E, Vidal DR 2004. Identification and discrimination of *Burkholderia pseudomallei*, *B. mallei*, and *B. thailandensis* by real-time PCR targeting type III secretion system genes. *Journal of Clinical Microbiology* 42:5871–5874.

Verma RD, Venkateswaran KS, Sharma JK, Agarwal GS 1994. Potency of partially purified malleo-proteins for mallein test in the diagnosis of glanders in equines. *Veterinary Microbiology* 41:391–397.

Whitlock GC, Estes DM, Torres AG 2007. Glanders: off to the races with *Burkholderia mallei*. *FEMS Microbiology Letters* 277:115–122.

Burkholderia pseudomallei

Adler NR, Govan B, Cullinane M, Harper M, Adler B, Boyce JD 2009. The molecular and cellular basis of pathogenesis in melioidosis: how does *Burkholderia pseudomallei* cause disease? *FEMS Microbiology Reviews* 33:1079–1099.

Balder R, Lipski S, Lazarus JJ, et al. 2010. Identification of *Burkholderia mallei* and *Burkholderia pseudomallei* adhesins for human respiratory epithelial cells. *BMC Microbiology* 10:250.

Choy JL, Mayo M, Janmaat A, Currie BJ 2000. Animal melioidosis in Australia. Review. *Acta Tropica* 74:153–158.

Currie BJ, Fisher DA, Howard DM, et al. 2000a. Endemic melioidosis in tropical northern Australia: a 10-year prospective study and review of the literature. Review. *Clinical Infectious Diseases* 31:981–986.

Currie BJ, Fisher DA, Anstey NM, Jacups SP 2000b. Melioidosis: acute and chronic disease, relapse and re-activation. *Transactions of the Royal Society of Tropical Medicine and Hygiene* 94:301–304.

De Keulenaer BL, Van Hooland SR, Damodaran PR, Currie BJ, Powell BP, Jenkins IR 2008. *Burkholderia pseudomallei* sepsis presenting with pericardial effusion and tamponade. *Critical Care and Resuscitation* 10:137–139.

Gibney KB, Cheng AC, Currie BJ 2008. Cutaneous melioidosis in the tropical top end of Australia: a prospective study and review of the literature. Review. *Clinical Infectious Diseases* 47:603–609.

Ladds PW, Thomas AD, Pott B 1981. Melioidosis with acute meningoencephalomyelitis in a horse. *Australian Veterinary Journal* 57:36–38.

Li L, Lu Z, Han O 1994. Epidemiology of melioidosis in China. *Zhonghua Liu Xing Bing Xue Za Zhi* 15:292–295.

Neubauer H, Meyer H, Finke EJ 1997. Human glanders. *International Review of the Armed Forces Medical Services* 70:258–265.

Sarkar-Tyson M, Smither SJ, Harding SV, Atkins TP, Titball RW 2009. Protective efficacy of heat-inactivated *B. thailandensis*, *B. mallei* or *B. pseudomallei* against experimental melioidosis and glanders. *Vaccine* 27:4447–4451.

Thibault FM, Valade E, Vidal DR 2004. Identification and discrimination of *Burkholderia pseudomallei*, *B. mallei*, and *B. thailandensis* by real-time PCR targeting type III secretion system genes. *Journal of Clinical Microbiology* 42:5871–5874.

Trunck LA, Propst KL, Wuthiekanun V, et al. 2009. Molecular basis of rare aminoglycoside susceptibility and pathogenesis of *Burkholderia pseudomallei* clinical isolates from Thailand. *PLoS Neglected Tropical Diseases* 3:e519.

White NJ 2003. Melioidosis. *Lancet* 361:1715–1722.

Wiersinga WJ, van der Poll T 2009. Immunity to *Burkholderia pseudomallei*. Review. *Current Opinion in Infectious Diseases* 22:102–108.

Bordetella bronchiseptica

Christley RM, Hodgson DR, Rose RJ, et al. 2001. A case-control study of respiratory disease in Thoroughbred racehorses in Sydney, Australia. *Equine Veterinary Journal* 33:256–264.

Dousse F, Thomann A, Brodard I, et al. 2008. Routine phenotypic identification of bacterial species of the family *Pasteurellaceae* isolated from animals. *Journal of Veterinary Diagnostic Investigation* 20:716–724.

Hoffman AM, Viel L, Prescott JF, Rosendal S, Thorsen J 1993. Association of microbiologic flora with clinical, endoscopic, and pulmonary cytologic findings in foals with distal respiratory tract infection. *American Journal of Veterinary Research* 54:1615–1622.

Koehne GW, Herren CE, Gibson RB, Northington WA 1981. An outbreak of *Bordetella bronchiseptica* respiratory disease in foals. *Veterinary Medicine & Small Animal Clinician* 76:507–508.

Le Blay K, Gueirard P, Guiso N, Chaby R 1997. Antigenic polymorphism of the lipopolysaccharides from human and animal isolates of *Bordetella bronchiseptica*. *Microbiology* 143:1433–1441.

Mather EC, Addison B, Owens D, Bierschwal CJ, Martin CE 1973. *Bordetella bronchiseptica* associated with infertility in a mare. *Journal of the American Veterinary Medical Association* 163:76–77.

Mathewson JJ, Simpson RB 1982. Glucose-nonfermenting Gram-negative bacilli associated with clinical veterinary specimens. *Journal of Clinical Microbiology* 15:1016–1018.

Mohan K, Obwolo MJ 1991. *Bordetella bronchiseptica* from aborted equine foetus. *Tropical Animal Health and Production* 23:155–156.

Porter JF, Wardlaw AC 1994. Tracheobronchial washings from seven vertebrate species as growth media for the four species of *Bordetella*. *FEMS Immunology and Medical Microbiology* 8:259–269.

Register KB, Boisvert A, Ackermann MR 1997. Use of ribotyping to distinguish *Bordetella bronchiseptica* isolates. *International Journal of Systemic Bacteriology* 47:678–683.

Saxegaard F, Teige J Jr, Fjellheim P 1971. Equine bronchopneumonia caused by *Bordetella bronchiseptica*. A case report. *Acta Veterinaria Scandinavica* 12:114–115.

Taylorella equigenitalis

Båverud V, Nyström C, Johansson KE 2006. Isolation and identification of *Taylorella asinigenitalis* from the genital tract of a stallion, first case of a natural infection. *Veterinary Microbiology* 116:294–300.

Bleumink-Pluym NM, van Dijk L, van Vliet AH, van der Giessen JW, van der Zeijst BA 1993. Phylogenetic position of *Taylorella equigenitalis* determined by analysis of amplified 16S ribosomal DNA sequences. *International Journal of Systematic Bacteriology* 43:618–621.

Bleumink-Pluym NM, ter Laak EA, Houwers DJ, van der Zeijst BA 1996. Differences between *Taylorella equigenitalis* strains in their invasion of and replication in cultured cells. *Clinical and Diagnostic Laboratory Immunology* 3:47–50.

Brooks BW, Lutze-Wallace CL, Maclean LL, Vinogradov E, Perry MB 2010. Identification and differentiation of *Taylorella equigenitalis* and *Taylorella asinigenitalis* by lipopolysaccharide O-antigen serology using monoclonal antibodies. *Canadian Journal of Veterinary Research* 74:18–24.

Duquesne F, Pronost S, Laugier C, Petry S 2007. Identification of *Taylorella equigenitalis* responsible for contagious equine metritis in equine genital swabs by direct polymerase chain reaction. *Research in Veterinary Science* 82:47–49.

Fontijne P, Ter Laak EA, Hartman EG 1989. *Taylorella equigenitalis* isolated from an aborted foal. *Veterinary Record* 125:485.

Jubb KVF, Kennedy PC, Palmer N 2007. *Pathology of Domestic Animals*, 5th edn. WB Saunders Elsevier, Edinburgh 3:467–468.

Kagawa S, Klein F, Corboz L, Moore JE, Murayama O, Matsuda M 2001. Demonstration of heterogeneous genotypes of *Taylorella equigenitalis* isolated from horses in six European countries by pulsed-field gel electrophoresis. *Veterinary Research Communications* 25:565–575.

Katz JB, Evans LE, Hutto DL, *et al.* 2000. Clinical, bacteriologic, serologic, and pathologic features of infections with atypical *Taylorella equigenitalis* in mares. *Journal of the American Veterinary Medical Association* 216:1945–1948.

Katz J, Geer P 2001. An enzyme-linked immunosorbent assay for the convenient serodiagnosis of contagious equine metritis in mares. *Journal of Veterinary Diagnostic Investigation* 13:87–88.

Kristula MA, Smith BI 2004. Diagnosis and treatment of four stallions, carriers of the contagious metritis organism—case report. *Theriogenology* 61:595–601.

Matsuda M, Tazumi A, Kagawa S, *et al.* 2006. Homogeneity of the 16S rDNA sequence among geographically disparate isolates of *Taylorella equigenitalis*. *BMC Veterinary Research* 2:1.

Parlevliet JM, Bleumink-Pluym NM, Houwers DJ, Remmen JL, Sluijter FJ, Colenbrander B 1997. Epidemiologic aspects of *Taylorella equigenitalis*. *Theriogenology* 47:1169–1177.

Timoney PJ 1996. Contagious equine metritis. *Comparative Immunology, Microbiology and Infectious Diseases* 19:199–204.

Timoney PJ 2011. Contagious equine metritis: An insidious threat to the U.S. horse breeding industry. *Journal of Animal Science* 89:1552–1560.

Wakeley PR, Errington J, Hannon S, *et al.* 2006. Development of a real time PCR for the detection of *Taylorella equigenitalis* directly from genital swabs and discrimination from *Taylorella asinigenitalis*. *Veterinary Microbiology* 118:247–254.

Wood JL, Kelly L, Cardwell JM, Park AW 2005. Quantitative assessment of the risks of reducing the routine swabbing requirements for the detection of *Taylorella equigenitalis*. Review. *Veterinary Record* 157:41–46.

Zdovc I, Ocepek M, Gruntar I, Pate M, Klobucar I, Krt B 2005. Prevalence of *Taylorella equigenitalis* infection in stallions in Slovenia: bacteriology compared with PCR examination. *Equine Veterinary Journal* 37:217–221.

Francisella tularensis

Green JH, Bolin RC, Carver RK, Gross H, Pigott N, Harrell WK 1970. Preparation of agglutinating antisera and fluorescent-antibody conjugates against *Pasteurella tularensis* in equines. *Applied Microbiology* 19:894–897.

Greub G, Raoult D 2004. Microorganisms resistant to free-living amoebae. *Clinical Microbiology Reviews* 17:413–433.

Petersen JM, Mead PS, Schriefer ME 2009. *Francisella tularensis*: an arthropod-borne pathogen. *Veterinary Research* 40:7.

Vorou RM, Papavassiliou VG, Tsiodras S 2007. Emerging zoonoses and vector-borne infections affecting humans in Europe. Review article. *Epidemiology and Infection* 135:1231–1247.

Legionella pneumophila

Cho S-N, Collins MT, Reif JS, McChesney AE 1983. Experimental infections of horses with *Legionella pneumophila*. *American Journal of Veterinary Research* 44:662–668.

Cho S-N, Collins MT, Reif JS 1984. Serologic evidence of *Legionella* infection in horses. *American Journal of Veterinary Research* 45:2600–2602.

Collins MT, Cho S-N, Reif JS 1982. Prevalence of antibodies to *Legionella pneumophila* in animal populations. *Journal of Clinical Microbiology* 15:130–136.

Wilkins CA, Bergh N 1988. A review of *Legionella pneumophila* in horses and some South African serological results. *Journal of the South African Veterinary Association* 59:23–26.

Coxiella burnetii

Somma-Moreira RE, Caffarena RM, Somma S, Pérez G, Monteiro M 1987. Analysis of Q fever in Uruguay. *Reviews of Infectious Diseases* 9:386–387.

Moraxella spp.

Andrew SE, Nguyen A, Jones GL, Brooks DE 2003. Seasonal effects on the aerobic bacterial and fungal conjunctival flora of normal thoroughbred brood mares in Florida. *Veterinary Ophthalmology* 6:45–50.

Gemensky-Metzler AJ, Wilkie DA, Kowalski JJ, Schmall LM, Willis AM, Yamagata M 2005. Changes in bacterial and fungal ocular flora of clinically normal horses following experimental application of topical antimicrobial or antimicrobial-corticosteroid ophthalmic preparations. *American Journal of Veterinary Research* 66:800–811.

Hoquet F, Higgins R, Lessard P, Vrins A, Marcoux M 1985. Comparison of the bacterial and fungal flora in the pharynx of normal horses and horses affected with pharyngitis. *Canadian Veterinary Journal* 26:342–346.

Hughes DE, Pugh GW Jr 1970. Isolation and description of a *Moraxella* from horses with conjunctivitis. *American Journal of Veterinary Research* 31:457–462.

Huntington PJ, Coloe PJ, Bryden JD, Macdonald F 1987. Isolation of a *Moraxella* sp from horses with conjunctivitis. *Australian Veterinary Journal* 64:118–119.

Murphy TF, Parameswaran GI 2009. *Moraxella catarrhalis*, a human respiratory tract pathogen. Review. *Clinical Infectious Diseases* 49:124–131.

Escherichia coli

Ahmed MO, Clegg PD, Williams NJ, Baptiste KE, Bennett M 2010. Antimicrobial resistance in equine faecal *Escherichia coli* isolates from North West England. *Annals of Clinical Microbiology and Antimicrobials* 9:12.

Corley KTT, Pearce G, Magdesian KG, Wilson WD 2007. Bacteraemia in neonatal foals: clinicopathological differences between Gram-positive and Gram-negative infections, and single organism and mixed infections. *Equine Veterinary Journal* 39:84–89.

DebRoy C, Roberts E, Jayarao BM, Brooks JW 2008. Bronchopneumonia associated with extraintestinal pathogenic *Escherichia coli* in a horse. *Journal of Veterinary Diagnostic Investigation* 20:661–664.

Dunowska M, Morley PS, Traub-Dargatz JL, Hyatt DR, Dargatz DA 2006. Impact of hospitalization and antimicrobial drug administration on antimicrobial susceptibility patterns of commensal *Escherichia coli* isolated from the faeces of horses. *Journal of the American Veterinary Medical Association* 228:1909–1917.

LeBlanc MM 2010. Advances in the diagnosis and treatment of chronic infectious and post-mating-induced endometritis in the mare. *Reproduction in Domestic Animimals* 45 Suppl 2:21–27.

Lorenzo-Figueras M, Pusterla N, Byrne BA, Samitz EM 2006. *In vitro* evaluation of three bacterial culture systems for the recovery of *Escherichia coli* from equine blood. *American Journal of Veterinary Research* 67:2025–2029.

Meyer S, Giguère S, Rodriguez R, Zielinski RJ, Grover GS, Brown SA 2009. Pharmacokinetics of intravenous ceftiofur sodium and concentration in body fluids of foals. *Journal of Veterinary Pharmacology and Therapeutics* 32:309–316.

Netherwood T, Wood JL, Townsend HG, Mumford JA, Chanter N 1996. Foal diarrhoea between 1991 and 1994 in the United Kingdom associated with *Clostridium perfringens, rotavirus, Strongyloides westeri,* and *Cryptosporidium* spp. *Epidemiology and Infection* 117:375–383.

Pusterla N, Mapes S, Byrne BA, Magdesian KG 2009. Detection of bloodstream infection in neonatal foals with suspected sepsis using real-time PCR. *Veterinary Record* 165:114–117.

Rodriguez F, Kramer J, Fales W, Wilson D, Keegan K 2009. Evaluation of intraoperative culture results as a predictor for short-term incisional complications in 49 horses undergoing abdominal surgery. *Veterinary Therapeutics* 10:E1–E13.

Rouquet G, Porcheron G, Barra C, *et al.* 2009. A metabolic operon in extraintestinal pathogenic *Escherichia coli* promotes fitness under stressful conditions and invasion of eukaryotic cells. *Journal of Bacteriology* 191:4427–4440.

Russell CM, Axon JE, Blishen A, Begg AP 2008. Blood culture isolates and antimicrobial sensitivities from 427 critically ill neonatal foals. *Australian Veterinary Journal* 86:266–271.

Sanchez LC, Giguère S, Lester GD 2008. Factors associated with survival of neonatal foals with bacteremia and racing performance of surviving Thoroughbreds: 423 cases (1982–2007). *Journal of the American Veterinary Medical Association* 233:1446–1452.

Weaver RW, Entry JA, Graves A 2005. Numbers of faecal streptococci and *Escherichia coli* in fresh and dry cattle, horse, and sheep manure. *Canadian Journal of Microbiology* 51:847–851.

Wilson WD, Madigan JE 1989. Comparison of bacteriologic culture of blood and necropsy specimens for determining the cause of foal septicaemia: 47 cases (1978–1987). *Journal of the American Veterinary Medical Association* 195:1759–1763.

Salmonella spp.

Bruhn O, Cauchard J, Schlusselhuber M, *et al.* 2009. Antimicrobial properties of the equine alpha-defensin DEFA1 against bacterial horse pathogens. *Veterinary Immunology and Immunopathology* 130:102–106.

Dallap Schaer BL, Aceto H, Rankin SC 2010. Outbreak of salmonellosis caused by *Salmonella enterica* serovar *Newport* MDR-AmpC in a large animal veterinary teaching hospital. *Journal of Veterinary Internal Medicine* 24:1138–1146.

Dolente BA, Beech J, Lindborg S, Smith G 2005. Evaluation of risk factors for development of catheter-associated jugular thrombophlebitis in horses: 50 cases (1993–1998). *Journal of the American Veterinary Medical Association* 227:1134–1141.

Duijkeren E van, Houwers DJ 2000. A critical assessment of antimicrobial treatment in uncomplicated *Salmonella enteritis*. *Veterinary Microbiology* 73:61–73.

Ekiri AB, MacKay RJ, Gaskin JM, *et al.* 2009. Epidemiologic analysis of nosocomial *Salmonella* infections in hospitalized horses. *Journal of the American Veterinary Medical Association* 234:108–119.

Frederick J, Giguère S, Sanchez LC 2009. Infectious agents detected in the faeces of diarrheic foals: a retrospective study of 233 cases (2003–2008). *Journal of Veterinary Internal Medicine* 23:1254–1260.

Frye JG, Fedorka-Cray PJ 2007. Prevalence, distribution and characterisation of ceftiofur resistance in *Salmonella enterica* isolated from animals in the USA from 1999 to 2003. *International Journal of Antimicrobial Agents* 30:134–142.

Hird DW, Casebold DB, Carter JD, Pappaioanou M, Hjerpe CA 1986. Risk factors for salmonellosis in hospitalized horses. *Journal of the American Veterinary Medical Association* 188:173–177.

House JK, Smith BP, Wildman TR, Carrigan MJ, Kamiya DY 1999. Isolation of *Salmonella* organisms from the mesenteric lymph nodes of horses at necropsy. *Journal of the American Veterinary Medical Association* 215:507–510.

Humphrey TJ, Threlfall EJ, Cruickshank JG 1998. Salmonellosis. In: Palmer SR, Soulsby Lord Simpson DIH (eds). *Zoonoses*. Oxford Medical Publications, Oxford University Press, Oxford: 191–206.

Neil KM, Charman RE, Vasey JR 2010. Rib osteomyelitis in three foals. *Australian Veterinary Journal* 88:96–100.

Niwa H, Anzai T, Izumiya H, *et al*. 2009. Antimicrobial resistance and genetic characteristics of *Salmonella typhimurium* isolated from horses in Hokkaido, Japan. *Journal of Veterinary Medical Science* 71:1115–1119.

Plummer PJ 2006. Malabsorptive maldigestive disorder with concurrent *Salmonella* in a 3-year-old quarter horse. *Veterinary Clinics of North America: Equine Practice* 22:85–94.

Pusterla N, Byrne BA, Hodzic E, Mapes S, Jang SS, Magdesian KG 2009. Use of quantitative real-time PCR for the detection of *Salmonella* spp. in fecal samples from horses at a veterinary teaching hospital. *Veterinary Journal* 186:252–255.

Singh BR, Chandra M, Agrawal RK, Nagrajan B 2006. Antigenic competition among different 'O' antigens of *Salmonella enterica* subspecies enterica serovars during hyperimmunization in pony mares. *Indian Journal of Experimental Biology* 44:1022–1025.

Vo AT, van Duijkeren E, Fluit AC, Gaastra W 2007. A novel *Salmonella* genomic island 1 and rare integron types in *Salmonella typhimurium* isolates from horses in the Netherlands. *Journal of Antimicrobials and Chemotherapeutics* 59:594–599.

Zhao S, McDermott PF, White DG, *et al*. 2007. Characterization of multidrug resistant *Salmonella* recovered from diseased animals. *Veterinary Microbiology* 123:122–132.

Pasteurella spp.

Bailey GD, Love DN 1991. Oral associated bacterial infection in horses: studies on the normal anaerobic flora from the pharyngeal tonsillar surface and its association with lower respiratory tract and paraoral infections. *Veterinary Microbiology* 26:367–379.

Bourgault A, Bada R, Messier S 1994. Isolation of *Pasteurella canis* from a foal with polyarthritis. *Canadian Veterinary Journal* 35:244–245.

Burrows GE, Morton RJ, Fales WH 1993. Microdilution antimicrobial susceptibilities of selected gram-negative veterinary bacterial isolates. *Journal of Veterinary Diagnostic Investigation* 5:541–547.

Carrillo NA, Giguère S, Gronwall RR, Brown MP, Merritt KA, O'Kelley JJ 2005. Disposition of orally administered cefpodoxime proxetil in foals and adult horses and minimum inhibitory concentration of the drug against common bacterial pathogens of horses. *American Journal of Veterinary Research* 66:30–35.

Chapman PS, Green C, Main JP, *et al*. 2000. Retrospective study of the relationships between age, inflammation and the isolation of bacteria from the lower respiratory tract of thoroughbred horses. *Veterinary Record* 146:91–95.

Church S, Harrigan KE, Irving AE, Peel MM 1998. Endocarditis caused by *Pasteurella caballi* in a horse. *Australian Veterinary Journal* 76:528–530.

Crane SA, Ziemer EL, Sweeney CR 1989. Cytologic and bacteriologic evaluation of tracheobronchial aspirates from clinically normal foals. *American Journal of Veterinary Research* 50:2042–2048.

Hayakawa Y, Komae H, Ide H, *et al*.1993. An occurrence of equine transport pneumonia caused by mixed infection with *Pasteurella caballi*, *Streptococcus suis*, and *Streptococcus zooepidemicus*. *Journal of Veterinary Medical Science* 55:455–456.

Hunt ML, Adler B, Townsend KM 2000. The molecular biology of *Pasteurella multocida*. *Veterinary Microbiology* 72:23–25.

Kawashima S, Matsukawa N, Ueki Y, Hattori M, Ojika K 2010. *Pasteurella multocida* meningitis caused by kissing animals: a case report and review of the literature. *Journal of Neurology* 257:653–654.

Maxson AD, Reef VB 1997. Bacterial endocarditis in horses: ten cases (1984–1995). *Equine Veterinary Journal* 29:394–399.

Miller RM, Dresher LK 1981. Equine ulcerative lymphangitis caused by *Pasteurella hemolytica* (2 case reports). *Veterinary Medicine, Small Animal Clinician* 76:1335–1338.

Mizuno N, Itoh H 2009. Functions and regulatory mechanisms of Gq-signaling pathways. *Neurosignals* 17:42–54.

Newton JR, Wood JL 2002. Evidence of an association between inflammatory airway disease and EIPH in young Thoroughbreds during training. *Equine Veterinary Journal*. Supplement 34:417–424.

Newton JR, Wood JL, Chanter N 2003. A case control study of factors and infections associated with clinically apparent respiratory disease in UK Thoroughbred racehorses. *Preventive Veterinary Medicine* 60:107–132.

Raidal SL, Bailey GD, Love DN 1997a. Effect of transportation on lower respiratory tract contamination and peripheral blood neutrophil function. *Australian Veterinary Journal* 75:433–438.

Raidal SL, Taplin RH, Bailey GD, Love DN 1997b. Antibiotic prophylaxis of lower respiratory tract contamination in horses confined with head elevation for 24 or 48 hours. *Australian Veterinary Journal* 75:126–131.

Satomura A, Yanai M, Fujita T, *et al*. 2010. Peritonitis associated with *Pasteurella multocida*: molecular evidence of zoonotic etiology. *Therapeutic Apheresis and Dialysis* 14:373–376.

Saxegaard F, Svenkrud R 1974. *Pasteurella haemolytica* associated with pneumonia in a foal. A case report. *Acta Veterinaria Scandinavica* 15:439–441.

Sweeney CR, Holcombe SJ, Barningham SC, Beech J 1991. Aerobic and anaerobic bacterial isolates from horses with pneumonia or pleuropneumonia and antimicrobial susceptibility patterns of the aerobes. *Journal of the American Veterinary Medical Association* 198:839–842.

Ward CL, Wood JL, Houghton SB, Mumford JA, Chanter N 1998. *Actinobacillus* and *Pasteurella* species isolated from horses with lower airway disease. *Veterinary Record* 143:277–279.

Wilson BA, Ho M 2010. Recent insights into *Pasteurella multocida* toxin and other G-protein-modulating bacterial toxins. *Future Microbiology* 5:1185–1201.

Yersinia enterocolitica

Browning GF, Chalmers RM, Snodgrass DR, *et al.* 1991. The prevalence of enteric pathogens in diarrhoeic thoroughbred foals in Britain and Ireland. *Equine Veterinary Journal* 23:405–409.

Bucher M, Meyer C, Grötzbach B, Wacheck S, Stolle A, Fredriksson-Ahomaa M 2008. Epidemiological data on pathogenic *Yersinia enterocolitica* in Southern Germany during 2000–2006. *Foodborne Pathogens and Disease* 5:273–280.

Czernomysy-Furowicz D 1997. An outbreak of foal yersiniosis in Poland: pathological and bacteriological examination. *Zentralblatt für Bakteriologie* 286:542–546.

Derlet RW, Carlson JR 2002. An analysis of human pathogens found in horse/mule manure along the John Muir Trail in Kings Canyon and Sequoia and Yosemite National Parks. *Wilderness and Environmental Medicine* 13:113–118.

Katayama Y, Kuwano A, Yoshihara T 2001. Histoplasmosis in the lung of a race horse with yersiniosis. *Journal of Veterinary Medical Science* 63:1229–1231.

Kim DH, Lee BK, Kim YD, Rhee SK, Kim YC 2010. Detection of representative enteropathogenic bacteria, *Vibrio* spp., pathogenic *Escherichia coli*, *Salmonella* spp., *Shigella* spp., and *Yersinia enterocolitica*, using a virulence factor gene-based oligonucleotide microarray. *Journal of Microbiology* 48:682–688.

Leclerc H, Schwartzbrod L, Dei-Cas E 2002. Microbial agents associated with waterborne diseases. *Critical Reviews in Microbiology* 28:371–409.

Netherwood T, Wood JL, Townsend HG, Mumford JA, Chanter N 1996. Foal diarrhoea between 1991 and 1994 in the United Kingdom associated with *Clostridium perfringens*, rotavirus, *Strongyloides westeri* and *Cryptosporidium* spp. *Epidemiology and Infection* 117:375–383.

Räisänen S, Alavaikko A 1989. *Yersinia* infection from a horse bite. *Duodecim* 105:1496–1497.

Trülzsch K, Sporleder T, Igwe EI, Rüssmann H, Heesemann J 2004. Contribution of the major secreted yops of *Yersinia enterocolitica* O:8 to pathogenicity in the mouse infection model. *Infection and Immunity* 72:5227–5234.

Wooley RE, Shotts EB Jr, McConnell JW 1980. Isolation of *Yersinia enterocolitica* from selected animal species. *American Journal of Veterinary Research* 41:1667–1668.

Actinobacillus lignieresii

Baum KH, Shin SJ, Rebhun WC, Patten VH 1984. Isolation of *Actinobacillus lignieresii* from enlarged tongue of a horse. *Journal of the American Veterinary Medical Association* 185:792–793.

Benaoudia F, Escande F, Simonet M 1994. Infection due to *Actinobacillus lignieresii* after a horse bite. *European Journal of Clinical Microbiology and Infectious Diseases* 13:439–440.

Carmalt JL, Baptiste KE, Chirino-Trejo JM 1999. *Actinobacillus lignieresii* infection in two horses. *Journal of the American Veterinary Medical Association* 215:826–828.

Christensen H, Bisgaard M, Angen O, Olsen JE 2002. Final classification of Bisgaard taxon 9 as *Actinobacillus arthritidis* sp. nov. and recognition of a novel genomospecies for equine strains of *Actinobacillus lignieresii*. *International Journal of Systematic and Evolutionary Microbiology* 52:1239–1246.

Dibb WL, Digranes A, Tønjum S 1981. *Actinobacillus lignieresii* infection after a horse bite. *British Medical Journal (Clinical Research Edition)* 283:583–584.

Peel MM, Hornidge KA, Luppino M, Stacpoole AM, Weaver RE 1991. *Actinobacillus* spp. and related bacteria in infected wounds of humans bitten by horses and sheep. *Journal of Clinical Microbiology* 29:2535–2538.

Samitz EM, Biberstein EL 1991. *Actinobacillus suis*-like organisms and evidence of hemolytic strains of *Actinobacillus lignieresii* in horses. *American Journal of Veterinary Research* 52:1245–1251.

Ward CL, Wood JL, Houghton SB, Mumford JA, Chanter N 1998. *Actinobacillus* and *Pasteurella* species isolated from horses with lower airway disease. *Veterinary Record* 143:277–279.

Actinobacillus equuli

Aalbaek B, Ostergaard S, Buhl R, Jensen HE, Christensen H, Bisgaard M 2007. *Actinobacillus equuli* subsp. *equuli* associated with equine valvular endocarditis. *Acta Pathologica, Microbiologica et Immunologica Scandinavica* 115:1437–1442.

Al-Mashat RR, Taylor DJ 1986. Bacteria in enteric lesions of horses. *Veterinary Record* 118:453–458.

Ashhurst-Smith C, Norton R, Thoreau W, Peel MM 1998. *Actinobacillus equuli* septicemia: an unusual zoonotic infection. *Journal of Clinical Microbiology* 36:2789–2790.

Baker JR 1972. An outbreak of neonatal deaths in foals due to *Actinobacillus equuli*. *Veterinary Record* 90:630–632.

Belknap J, Arden W, Yamini B 1988. Septic periorchitis in a horse. *Journal of the American Veterinary Medical Association* 192:363–364.

Bolin DC, Donahue JM, Vickers ML, *et al.* 2005. Microbiologic and pathologic findings in an epidemic of equine pericarditis. *Journal of Veterinary Diagnostic Investigation* 17:38–44.

Castagnetti C, Rossi M, Parmeggiani F, Zanoni RG, Pirrone A, Mariella J 2008. Facial cellulitis due to *Actinobacillus equuli* infection in a neonatal foal. *Veterinary Record* 162:347–349.

Corley KTT, Pearce G, Magdesian KG, Wilson WD 2007. Bacteraemia in neonatal foals: clinicopathological differences between Gram-positive and Gram-negative infections, and single organism and mixed infections. *Equine Veterinary Journal* 39:84–89.

Dill SG, Simoncini DC, Bolton GR, *et al.* 1982. Fibrinous pericarditis in the horse. *Journal of the American Veterinary Medical Association* 180:266–271.

Gay CC, Lording PM 1980. Peritonitis in horses associated with *Actinobacillus equuli*. *Australian Veterinary Journal* 56:296–300.

Golland LC, Hodgson DR, Hodgson JL, *et al.* 1994. Peritonitis associated with *Actinobacillus equuli* in horses: 15 cases (1982–1992). *Journal of the American Veterinary Medical Association* 205:340–343.

Kuhnert P, Berthoud H, Christensen H, Bisgaard M, Frey J 2003. Phylogenetic relationship of equine *Actinobacillus* species and distribution of RTX toxin genes among clusters. *Veterinary Research* 34:353–359.

Matthews S, Dart AJ, Dowling BA, Hodgson JL, Hodgson DR 2001. Peritonitis associated with *Actinobacillus equuli* in horses: 51 cases. *Australian Veterinary Journal* 79:536–539.

Meyer W, Kacza J, Schnapper A, Verspohl J, Hornickel I, Seeger J 2010. A first report on the microbial colonisation of the equine oesophagus. *Annals of Anatomy* 192:42–51.

Peel MM, Hornidge KA, Luppino M, Stacpoole AM, Weaver RE 1991. *Actinobacillus* spp. and related bacteria in infected wounds of humans bitten by horses and sheep. *Journal of Clinical Microbiology* 29:2535–2538.

Pusterla N, Jones ME, Mohr FC, *et al.* 2008. Fatal pulmonary hemorrhage associated with RTX toxin producing *Actinobacillus equuli* subspecies *haemolyticus* infection in an adult horse. *Journal of Veterinary Diagnostic Investigation* 20:118–121.

Raisis AL, Hodgson JL, Hodgson DR 1996. Equine neonatal septicaemia: 24 cases. *Australian Veterinary Journal* 73:137–140.

Thomas E, Thomas V, Wilhelm C 2006. Antibacterial activity of cefquinome against equine bacterial pathogens. *Veterinary Microbiology* 115:140–147.

Ward CL, Wood JL, Houghton SB, Mumford JA, Chanter N 1998. *Actinobacillus* and *Pasteurella* species isolated from horses with lower airway disease. *Veterinary Record* 143:277–279.

Webb RF, Cockram FA, Pryde L 1976. The isolation of *Actinobacillus equuli* from equine abortion. *Australian Veterinary Journal* 52:100–101.

Zakopal J, Nesvadba J 1968. Actinobacillary septicaemia as an enzootic in a breeding stud of mares. *Zentralblatt für Veterinärmedizin Reihe A* 15:41–59.

Lawsonia intracellularis

Collins A, Love RJ, Pozo J, Smith SH, McOrist S 2000. Studies on the *ex-vivo* survival of *Lawsonia intracellularis*. *Journal of Swine Health and Production* 8:211–215.

Cooper DM, Gebhart CJ 1998. Comparative aspects of proliferative enteritis. *Journal of the American Veterinary Medical Association* 212:1446–1451.

Deprez P, Chiers K, Gebhart CJ, *et al.* 2005. *Lawsonia intracellularis* infection in a 12-month-old colt in Belgium. *Veterinary Record* 157:774–776.

Frazer ML 2008. *Lawsonia intracellularis* infection in horses: 2005–2007. *Journal of Veterinary Internal Medicine* 22:1243–1248.

Lavoie JP, Drolet R, Parsons D, *et al.* 2000. Equine proliferative enteropathy: a cause of weight loss, colic, diarrhoea and hypoproteinaemia in foals on three breeding farms in Canada. *Equine Veterinary Journal* 32:418–425.

McOrist S, Gebhart CJ, Boid R, Barns SM 1995. Characterization of *Lawsonia intracellularis* gen. nov., sp. nov., the obligately intracellular bacterium of porcine proliferative enteropathy. *International Journal of Systemic Bacteriology* 45:820–825.

McOrist S, Gebhart CJ 1999. Proliferative enteropathies. In: Straw BE, D'Allaire S, Mengeling WL, Taylor DJ, editors: *Diseases of Swine*, Ames, Iowa State University Press.

Pusterla N, Mapes S, Rejmanek D, Gebhart C 2008. Detection of *Lawsonia intracellularis* by real-time PCR in the feces of free-living animals from equine farms with documented occurrence of equine proliferative enteropathy. *Journal of Wildlife Diseases* 44:992–998.

Pusterla N, Hilton H, Wattanaphansak S, *et al.* 2009a. Evaluation of the humoral immune response and fecal shedding in weanling foals following oral and intra-rectal administration of an avirulent live vaccine of *Lawsonia intracellularis*. *Veterinary Journal* 182:458–462.

Pusterla N, Jackson R, Wilson R, Collier J, Mapes S, Gebhart C 2009b. Temporal detection of *Lawsonia intracellularis* using serology and real-time PCR in Thoroughbred horses residing on a farm endemic for equine proliferative enteropathy. *Veterinary Microbiology* 136:173–176.

Pusterla N, Collier J, Mapes SM, Wattanaphasak S, Gebhart C 2009c. Effects of administration of an avirulent live vaccine of *Lawsonia intracellularis* on mares and foals. *Veterinary Record* 164:783–785.

Pusterla N, Wattanaphansak S, Mapes S, *et al.* 2010a. Oral infection of weanling foals with an equine isolate of *Lawsonia intracellularis*, agent of equine proliferative enteropathy. *Journal of Veterinary Internal Medicine* 24:622–627.

Pusterla N, Mapes S, Johnson C, Slovis N, Page A, Gebhart C 2010b. Comparison of feces versus rectal swabs for the molecular detection of *Lawsonia intracellularis* in foals with equine proliferative enteropathy. *Journal of Veterinary Diagnostic Investigation* 22:741–744.

Reef VB 1998. Pediatric abdominal ultrasonography. In: *Equine Diagnostic Ultrasound*, 1st edn. WB Saunders, Philadelphia, 364–403.

Sampieri F, Hinchcliff KW, Toribio RE 2006. Tetracycline therapy of *Lawsonia intracellularis* enteropathy in foals. *Equine Veterinary Journal* 38:89–92.

Wong DM, Alcott CJ, Sponseller BA, Young JL, Sponseller BT 2009. Impaired intestinal absorption of glucose in 4 foals with *Lawsonia intracellularis* infection. *Journal of Veterinary Internal Medicine* 23:940–944.

Wuersch K, Huessy D, Koch C, Oevermann A 2006. *Lawsonia intracellularis* proliferative enteropathy in a filly. *Journal of Veterinary Medicine. Physiology, Pathology, Clinical Medicine* 53:17–21.

Campylobacter spp.

Al-Mashat RR, Taylor DJ 1986. Bacteria in enteric lesions of horses. *Veterinary Record* 118:453–458.

Browning GF, Chalmers RM, Snodgrass DR, *et al.* 1991. The prevalence of enteric pathogens in diarrhoeic thoroughbred foals in Britain and Ireland. *Equine Veterinary Journal* 23:405–409.

Haddad N, Burns CM, Bolla JM, et al. 2009. Long-term survival of *Campylobacter jejuni* at low temperature is dependent on polynucleotide phosphorylase activity. *Applied and Environmental Microbiology* 75:7310–7318.

Hong CB, Donahue JM 1989. Campylobacteriosis in an aborted equine fetus. *Journal of the American Veterinary Medical Association* 194:263–264.

Hurcombe SD, Fox JG, Kohn CW 2009. Isolation of *Campylobacter fetus* subspecies *fetus* in a two-year-old Quarterhorse with chronic diarrhea of an undetermined etiology. *Journal of Veterinary Diagnostic Investigation* 21:266–269.

Johnson PJ, Goetz TE 1993. Granulomatous enteritis and *Campylobacter* bacteremia in a horse. *Journal of the American Veterinary Medical Association* 203:1039–1042.

Kakoyiannis CK, Winter PJ, Marshall RB 1988. The relationship between intestinal *Campylobacter* species isolated from animals and humans as determined by BRENDA. *Epidemiology and Infection* 100:379–387.

Netherwood T, Wood JL, Townsend HG, Mumford JA, Chanter N 1996. Foal diarrhoea between 1991 and 1994 in the United Kingdom associated with *Clostridium perfringens, rotavirus, Strongyloides westeri* and *Cryptosporidium* spp. *Epidemiology and Infection* 117:375–383.

Putten JP van, van Alphen LB, Wösten MM, de Zoete MR 2009. Molecular mechanisms of campylobacter infection. *Current Topics in Microbiology and Immunology* 337:197–229.

Wysok B, Uradzinski J 2009. *Campylobacter* spp. – a significant microbiological hazard in food. I. Characteristics of *Campylobacter* species, infection source, epidemiology. Review. *Polish Journal of Veterinary Science* 12:141–148.

Helicobacter equorum

Euzéby JP 2007. List of prokaryotic names with standing in nomenclature – genus Helicobacter. URL: http://www.bacterio.cict.fr/h/helicobacter.html

Moyaert H, Decostere A, Vandamme P, et al. 2007a. *Helicobacter equorum* sp. *Nov.*, a urease-negative *Helicobacter* species isolated from horse faeces. *International Journal of Systematic and Evolutionary Microbiology* 57:213–218.

Moyaert H, Haesebrouck F, Baele M, et al. 2007b. Prevalence of *H. equorum* in faecal samples of horses and humans. *Veterinary Microbiology* 121:378–383.

Moyaert H, Decostere A, Pasmans F, et al. 2007c. Acute *in vivo* interactions of *Helicobacter equorum* with its equine host. *Equine Veterinary Journal* 39:370–372.

Moyaert H, Pasmans F, Decostere A, Ducatelle R, Haesebrouck F 2009. *Helicobacter equorum*: prevalence and significance for horses and humans. *FEMS Immunology and Medical Microbiology* 57:14–16.

Clostridium botulinum

Adam-Castrillo D, White NA 2nd, Donaldson LL, Furr MO 2004. Effects of injection of botulinum toxin type B into the external anal sphincter on anal pressure of horses. *American Journal of Veterinary Research* 65:26–30.

Atassi MZ, Dolimbek BZ, Hayakari M, Middlebrook JL, Whitney B, Oshima M 1996. Mapping of the antibody-binding regions on botulinum neurotoxin H-chain domain 855–1296 with antitoxin antibodies from three host species. *Journal of Protein Chemistry* 15:691–700.

Atassi MZ, Dolimbek BZ, Steward LE, Aoki KR 2007. Molecular bases of protective immune responses against botulinum neurotoxin A—how antitoxin antibodies block its action. *Critical Reviews in Immunology* 27:319–341.

Bernard W, Divers TJ, Whitlock RH, Messick J, Tulleners E 1987. Botulism as a sequel to open castration in a horse. *Journal of the American Veterinary Medical Association* 191:73–74.

Böhnel H, Wagner C, Gessler F 2008. Tonsils – place of botulinum toxin production: results of routine laboratory diagnosis in farm animals. *Veterinary Microbiology* 130:403–409.

Critchley EM 1991. A comparison of human and animal botulism: a review. *Journal of the Royal Society of Medicine* 84:295–298.

Dembek ZF, Smith LA, Rusnak JM 2007. Botulism: cause, effects, diagnosis, clinical and laboratory identification, and treatment modalities. *Disaster Medicine and Public Health Preparedness* 1:122–134.

Frey J, Eberle S, Stahl C, et al. 2007. Alternative vaccination against equine botulism (BoNT/C). *Equine Veterinary Journal* 39:516–520.

Furr MO, Tyler RD 1990. Cerebrospinal fluid creatine kinase activity in horses with central nervous system disease: 69 cases (1984–1989). *Journal of the American Veterinary Medical Association* 197:245–248.

Galey FD 2001. Botulism in the horse. *Veterinary Clinics of North America: Equine Practice* 17:579–588.

Gerber V, Straub R, Frey J 2006. Equine botulism and acute pasture myodystrophy: new soil-borne emerging diseases in Switzerland? *Schweizer Archiv für Tierheilkunde* 148:553–559.

Hahn CN, Mayhew IG 2000. Phenylephrine eyedrops as a diagnostic test in equine grass sickness. *Veterinary Record* 147:603–606.

Hunter LC, Miller JK, Poxton IR 1999. The association of *Clostridium botulinum* type C with equine grass sickness: a toxicoinfection? *Equine Veterinary Journal* 31:492–499.

Johnson AL, McAdams SC, Whitlock RH 2010. Type A botulism in horses in the United States: a review of the past ten years (1998–2008). *Journal of Veterinary Diagnostic Investigation* 22:165–173.

Kinde H, Bettey RL, Ardans A, et al. 1991. *Clostridium botulinum* type-C intoxication associated with consumption of processed alfalfa hay cubes in horses. *Journal of the American Veterinary Medical Association* 199:742–746.

Montal M 2010. Botulinum neurotoxin: a marvel of protein design. *Annual Review of Biochemistry* 79:591–617.

Nunn FG, Pirie RS, McGorum B, Wernery U, Poxton IR 2007. Preliminary study of mucosal IgA in the equine small intestine: specific IgA in cases of acute grass sickness and controls. *Equine Veterinary Journal* 39:457–460.

Padua L, Aprile I, Monaco ML, *et al.* 1999. Neurophysiological assessment in the diagnosis of botulism: usefulness of single-fiber EMG. *Muscle and Nerve* 22:1388–1392.

Peck MW 2009. Biology and genomic analysis of *Clostridium botulinum*. *Advances in Microbial Physiology* 55:183–265, 320.

Schoenbaum MA, Hall SM, Glock RD, *et al.* 2000. An outbreak of type C botulism in 12 horses and a mule. *Journal of the American Veterinary Medical Association* 217:365–368, 340.

Sobel J 2009. Diagnosis and treatment of botulism: a century later, clinical suspicion remains the cornerstone. *Clinical Infectious Diseases* 48:1674–1675.

Souayah N, Karim H, Kamin SS, McArdle J, Marcus S 2006. Severe botulism after focal injection of botulinum toxin. *Neurology* 67:1855–1856.

Stahl C, Unger L, Mazuet C, Popoff M, Straub R, Frey J 2009. Immune response of horses to vaccination with the recombinant Hc domain of botulinum neurotoxin types C and D. *Vaccine* 27:5661–5666.

Steinman A, Kachtan I, Levi O, Shpigel NY 2007. Seroprevalence of antibotulinum neurotoxin type C antibodies in horses in Israel. *Equine Veterinary Journal* 39:232–235.

Swerczek TW 1980*a*. Toxicoinfectious botulism in foals and adult horses. *Journal of the American Veterinary Medical Association* 176:217–220.

Swerczek TW 1980*b*. Experimentally induced toxicoinfectious botulism in horses and foals. *American Journal of Veterinary Research* 41:348–350.

Szabo EA, Pemberton JM, Gibson AM, Thomas RJ, Pascoe RR, Desmarchelier PM 1994. Application of PCR to a clinical and environmental investigation of a case of equine botulism. *Journal of Clinical Microbiology* 32:1986–1991.

Thomas RJ 1991. Detection of *Clostridium botulinum* types C and D toxin by ELISA. *Australian Veterinary Journal* 68:111–113.

Waggett BE, McGorum BC, Shaw DJ, *et al.* 2010. Evaluation of synaptophysin as an immunohistochemical marker for equine grass sickness. *Journal of Comparative Pathology* 42:284–290.

Wheeler C, Inami G, Mohle-Boetani J, Vugia D 2009. Sensitivity of mouse bioassay in clinical wound botulism. *Clinical Infectious Diseases* 48:1669–1673.

Whitlock RH, Buckley C 1997. Botulism. *Veterinary Clinics of North America: Equine Practice* 13:107–128.

Wijnberg ID, Franssen H, Jansen GH, van den Ingh TS, van der Harst MR, van der Kolk JH 2006. The role of quantitative electromyography (EMG) in horses suspected of acute and chronic grass sickness. *Equine Veterinary Journal* 38:230–237.

Wijnberg ID, Schrama SE, Elgersma AE, Maree JT, de Cocq P, Back W 2009. Quantification of surface EMG signals to monitor the effect of a Botox treatment in six healthy ponies and two horses with stringhalt: preliminary study. *Equine Veterinary Journal* 41:313–318.

Wijnberg ID, Sleutjens J, van der Kolk JH, Back W 2010. Effect of head and neck position on outcome of quantitative neuromuscular diagnostic techniques in Warmblood riding horses directly following moderate exercise. *Equine Veterinary Journal*. Supplement 42:261–267.

Wilkins PA, Palmer JE 2003*a*. Botulism in foals less than 6 months of age: 30 cases (1989–2002). *Journal of Veterinary Internal Medicine* 17:702–707.

Wilkins PA, Palmer JE 2003*b*. Mechanical ventilation in foals with botulism: 9 cases (1989–2002). *Journal of Veterinary Internal Medicine* 17:708–712.

Witoonpanich R, Vichayanrat E, Tantisiriwit K, Rattanasiri S, Ingsathit A 2009. Electrodiagnosis of botulism and clinico-electrophysiological correlation. *Clinical Neurophysiology* 120:1135–1138.

Clostridium difficile

Arroyo LG, Weese JS, Staempfli HR 2004. Experimental *Clostridium difficile* enterocolitis in foals. *Journal of Veterinary Internal Medicine* 18:734–738.

Arroyo LG, Staempfli H, Weese JS 2006. Potential role of *Clostridium difficile* as a cause of duodenitis-proximal jejunitis in horses. *Journal of Medical Microbiology* 55:605–608.

Arroyo LG, Staempfli H, Weese JS 2007. Molecular analysis of *Clostridium difficile* isolates recovered from horses with diarrhea. *Veterinary Microbiology* 120:179–183.

Båverud V, Gustafsson A, Franklin A, Lindholm A, Gunnarsson A 1997. *Clostridium difficile* associated with acute colitis in mature horses treated with antibiotics. *Equine Veterinary Journal* 29:279–284.

Jones RL, Adney WS, Alexander AF, Shideler RK, Traub-Dargatz JL 1988. Hemorrhagic necrotizing enterocolitis associated with *Clostridium difficile* infection in four foals. *Journal of the American Veterinary Medical Association* 193:76–79.

Keel MK, Songer JG 2006. The comparative pathology of *Clostridium difficile*-associated disease. Review. *Veterinary Pathology* 43:225–240.

Kuipers EJ, Surawicz CM 2008. *Clostridium difficile* infection. *Lancet* 371:1486–1488.

Magdesian KG, Dujowich M, Madigan JE, Hansen LM, Hirsh DC, Jang SS 2006. Molecular characterization of *Clostridium difficile* isolates from horses in an intensive care unit and association of disease severity with strain type. *Journal of the American Veterinary Medical Association* 228:751–755.

Magdesian KG, Leutenegger CM 2011. Real-time PCR and typing of *Clostridium difficile* isolates colonizing mare-foal pairs. *Veterinary Journal* 190:119–123.

McGavin MD, Zachary JF 2007. *Pathological Basis of Veterinary Disease*, 4th edn. Mosby, Elsevier, St Louis, 367.

Medina-Torres CE, Weese JS, Staempfli HR 2010. Validation of a commercial enzyme immunoassay for detection of *Clostridium difficile* toxins in feces of horses with acute diarrhea. *Journal of Veterinary Internal Medicine* 24:628–632.

Norén T 2005. Outbreak from a high-toxin intruder: *Clostridium difficile*. *Lancet* 366:1053–1054.

Ruby R, Magdesian KG, Kass PH 2009. Comparison of clinical, microbiologic, and clinicopathologic findings in horses positive and negative for *Clostridium difficile* infection. *Journal of the American Veterinary Medical Association* 234:777–784.

Songer JG, Trinh HT, Dial SM, Brazier JS, Glock RD 2009. Equine colitis X associated with infection by *Clostridium difficile* NAP1/027. *Journal of Veterinary Diagnostic Investigation* 21:377–380.

Taha S, Johansson O, Rivera Jonsson S, Heimer D, Krovacek K 2007. Toxin production by and adhesive properties of *Clostridium difficile* isolated from humans and horses with antibiotic-associated diarrhea. *Comparative Immunology, Microbiology and Infectious Diseases* 30:163–174.

Weese JS, Parsons DA, Staempfli HR 1999. Association of *Clostridium difficile* with enterocolitis and lactose intolerance in a foal. *Journal of the American Veterinary Medical Association* 214:229–232.

Weese JS, Staempfli HR, Prescott JF 2000a. Isolation of environmental *Clostridium difficile* from a veterinary teaching hospital. *Journal of Veterinary Diagnostic Investigation* 12:449–452.

Weese JS, Staempfli HR, Prescott JF 2000b. Survival of *Clostridium difficile* and its toxins in equine faeces: implications for diagnostic test selection and interpretation. *Journal of Veterinary Diagnostic Investigation* 12:332–336.

Weese JS, Anderson ME, Lowe A, et al. 2004. Screening of the equine intestinal microflora for potential probiotic organisms. *Equine Veterinary Journal* 36:351–355.

Clostridium perfringens

Bacciarini LN, Boerlin P, Straub R, Frey J, Gröne A 2003. Immunohistochemical localization of *Clostridium perfringens* beta2-toxin in the gastrointestinal tract of horses. *Veterinary Pathology* 40:376–381.

Bueschel D, Walker R, Woods L, Kokai-Kun J, McClane B, Songer JG 1998. Enterotoxigenic *Clostridium perfringens* type A necrotic enteritis in a foal. *Journal of the American Veterinary Medical Association* 213:1305–1307, 1280.

Choi YK, Kang MS, Yoo HS, Lee DY, Lee HC, Kim DY 2003. *Clostridium perfringens* type A myonecrosis in a horse in Korea. *Journal of Veterinary Medical Science* 65:1245–1247.

Donaldson MT, Palmer JE 1999. Prevalence of *Clostridium perfringens* enterotoxin and *Clostridium difficile* toxin A in faeces of horses with diarrhea and colic. *Journal of the American Veterinary Medical Association* 215:358–361.

East LM, Savage CJ, Traub-Dargatz JL, Dickinson CE, Ellis RP 1998. Enterocolitis associated with *Clostridium perfringens* infection in neonatal foals: 54 cases (1988–1997). *Journal of the American Veterinary Medical Association* 212:1751–1756.

East LM, Dargatz DA, Traub-Dargatz JL, Savage CJ 2000. Foaling-management practices associated with the occurrence of enterocolitis attributed to *Clostridium perfringens* infection in the equine neonate. *Preventive Veterinary Medicine* 46:61–74.

Frederick J, Giguère S, Sanchez LC 2009. Infectious agents detected in the feces of diarrheic foals: a retrospective study of 233 cases (2003–2008). *Journal of Veterinary Internal Medicine* 23:1254–1260.

Herholz C, Miserez R, Nicolet J, et al. 1999. Prevalence of beta2-toxigenic *Clostridium perfringens* in horses with intestinal disorders. *Journal of Clinical Microbiology* 37:358–361.

Hyman SS, Wilkins PA, Palmer JE, Schaer TP, Del Piero F 2002. *Clostridium perfringens* urachitis and uroperitoneum in 2 neonatal foals. *Journal of Veterinary Internal Medicine* 16:489–493.

Johansson A, Aspan A, Bagge E, Båverud V, Engström BE, Johansson KE 2006. Genetic diversity of *Clostridium perfringens* type A isolates from animals, food poisoning outbreaks and sludge. *BMC Microbiology* 6:47.

Jones RL 2000. Clostridial enterocolitis. Review. *Veterinary Clinics of North America: Equine Practice* 16:471–485.

Lawler JB, Hassel DM, Magnuson RJ, Hill AE, McCue PM, Traub-Dargatz JL 2008. Adsorptive effects of di-tri-octahedral smectite on *Clostridium perfringens* alpha, beta, and beta-2 exotoxins and equine colostral antibodies. *American Journal of Veterinary Research* 69:233–239.

May KA, Cheramie HS, Howard RD, et al. 2002. Purulent pericarditis as a sequela to clostridial myositis in a horse. *Equine Veterinary Journal* 34:636–640.

McGorum BC, Dixon PM, Smith DG 1998. Use of metronidazole in equine acute idiopathic toxaemic colitis. *Veterinary Record* 142:635–638.

Ochi S, Oda M, Nagahama M, Sakurai J 2003. *Clostridium perfringens* alpha-toxin-induced hemolysis of horse erythrocytes is dependent on Ca^{2+} uptake. *Biochimica et Biophysica Acta* 1613:79–86.

Peek SF, Semrad SD, Perkins GA 2003. Clostridial myonecrosis in horses (37 cases 1985–2000). *Equine Veterinary Journal* 35:86–92.

Popoff MR, Bouvet P 2009. Clostridial toxins. *Future Microbiology* 4:1021–1064.

Rebhun WC, Cho JO, Gaarder JE, Peek SF, Patten VH 1999. Presumed clostridial and aerobic bacterial infections of the cornea in two horses. *Journal of the American Veterinary Medical Association* 214:1519–1522, 1496.

Reef VB 1983. *Clostridium perfringens* cellulitis and immune-mediated hemolytic anemia in a horse. *Journal of the American Veterinary Medical Association* 182:251–254.

Songer JG 2010. Clostridia as agents of zoonotic disease. *Veterinary Microbiology* 140:399–404.

Stickle JE, McKnight CA, Williams KJ, Carr EA 2006. Diarrhea and hyperammonaemia in a horse with progressive neurologic signs. *Veterinary Clinical Pathology* 35:250–253.

Sting R 2009. Detection of beta2 and major toxin genes by PCR in *Clostridium perfringens* field isolates of domestic animals suffering from enteritis or enterotoxaemia. *Berliner und Münchener Tierärztliche Wochenschrift* 122:341–347.

Tillotson K, Traub-Dargatz JL, Dickinson CE, et al. 2002. Population-based study of fecal shedding of *Clostridium perfringens* in broodmares and foals. *Journal of the American Veterinary Medical Association* 220:342–348.

Timoney JF, Hartmann M, Fallon L, Fallon E, Walker J 2005. Antibody responses of mares to prepartum vaccination with *Clostridium perfringens* bacterin and beta2 toxin. *Veterinary Record* 157:810–812.

Vilei EM, Schlatter Y, Perreten V, et al. 2005. Antibiotic-induced expression of a cryptic cpb2 gene in equine beta2-toxigenic *Clostridium perfringens*. *Molecular Microbiology* 57:1570–1581.

Waggett BE, McGorum BC, Wernery U, Shaw DJ, Pirie RS 2010. Prevalence of *Clostridium perfringens* in faeces and ileal contents from grass sickness affected horses: comparisons with 3 control populations. *Equine Veterinary Journal* 42:494–499.

Waters M, Raju D, Garmory HS, Popoff MR, Sarker MR 2005. Regulated expression of the beta2-toxin gene (cpb2) in *Clostridium perfringens* type a isolates from horses with gastrointestinal diseases. *Journal of Clinical Microbiology* 43:4002–4009.

Weese JS, Staempfli HR, Prescott JF 2001. A prospective study of the roles of *Clostridium difficile* and enterotoxigenic *Clostridium perfringens* in equine diarrhoea. *Equine Veterinary Journal* 33:403–409.

Weese JS, Anderson ME, Lowe A, et al. 2004. Screening of the equine intestinal microflora for potential probiotic organisms. *Equine Veterinary Journal* 36:351–355.

Weiss DJ, Moritz A 2003. Equine immune-mediated hemolytic anemia associated with *Clostridium perfringens* infection. Review. *Veterinary Clinical Pathology* 32:22–26.

White G, Prior SD 1982. Comparative effects of oral administration of trimethoprim/sulphadiazine or oxytetracycline on the faecal flora of horses. *Veterinary Record* 111:316–318.

Clostridium piliforme

Borchers A, Magdesian KG, Halland S, Pusterla N, Wilson WD 2006. Successful treatment and polymerase chain reaction (PCR) confirmation of Tyzzer's disease in a foal and clinical and pathologic characteristics of 6 additional foals (1986–2005). *Journal of Veterinary Internal Medicine* 20:1212–1218.

Fosgate GT, Hird DW, Read DH, Walker RL 2002. Risk factors for *Clostridium piliforme* infection in foals. *Journal of the American Veterinary Medical Association* 220:785–790.

Hook RR, Riley LK, Franklin CL, Besch-Williford CL 1995. Seroanalysis of Tyzzer's disease in horses: implications that multiple strains can infect Equidae. *Equine Veterinary Journal* 27:8–12.

Sasseville VG, Simon MA, Chalifoux LV, Lin KC, Mansfield KG 2007. Naturally occurring Tyzzer's disease in cotton-top tamarins (*Saguinus oedipus*). *Comparative Medicine* 57:125–127.

Swerczek TW 1976. Multifocal hepatic necrosis and hepatitis in foals caused by *Bacillus piliformis* (Tyzzer's disease). *Veterinary Annual* 30:36–37.

Clostridium tetani

Altura BM, Altura BT 1981. Magnesium ions and contraction of vascular smooth muscles: relationship to some vascular diseases. *Federation Proceedings* 40:2672–2679.

Ansari MM, Matros LE 1982. Tetanus. *Compendium on Continuing Education for the Practicing Veterinarian* 11:S473–S477.

Brauner JS, Vieira SR, Bleck TP 2002. Changes in severe accidental tetanus mortality in the ICU during two decades in Brazil. *Intensive Care Medicine* 28:930–935.

Galen G van, Delguste C, Sandersen C, Verwilghen D, Grulke S, Amory H 2008. Tetanus in the equine species: a retrospective study of 31 cases. *Tijdschrift voor Diergeneeskunde* 133:512–517.

Green SL, Little CB, Baird JB, Tremblay RR, Smith-Maxie LL 1994. Tetanus in the horse: a review of 20 cases (1970–1990). *Journal of Veterinary Internal Medicine* 8:128–132.

Heldens JG, Pouwels HG, Derks CG, Van de Zande SM, Hoeijmakers MJ 2010. Duration of immunity induced by an equine influenza and tetanus combination vaccine formulation adjuvanted with ISCOM-Matrix. *Vaccine* 28:6989–6996.

Holmes MA, Townsend HGG, Kohler AK, et al. 2006. Immune responses to commercial equine vaccines against equine herpesvirus-1, equine influenza virus, eastern equine encephalomyelitis, and tetanus. *Veterinary Immunology and Immunopathology* 111:67–80.

Humeau Y, Doussau F, Grant NJ, Poulain B 2000. How botulinum and tetanus neurotoxins block neurotransmitter release. *Biochimie* 82:427–446.

Kay G, Knottenbelt DC 2007. Tetanus in equids: a report of 56 cases. *Equine Veterinary Education* 19:107–112.

Muylle E, Oyaert W, Ooms L, Decraemere H 1975. Treatment of tetanus in the horse by injections of tetanus antitoxin into the subarachnoid space. *Journal of the American Veterinary Medical Association* 167:47–48.

Roper MH, Vandelaer JH, Gasse FL 2007. Maternal and neonatal tetanus. *Lancet* 370:1947–1959.

Thwaites CL, Yen LM, Loan HT, et al. 2006. Magnesium sulphate for treatment of severe tetanus: a randomised controlled trial. *Lancet* 368:1436–1443.

Wassilak SGF, Roper MH, Murphy TV, Orenstein WA 2004. Tetanus toxoid. In: Plotkin SA, Orenstein WA (eds). *Vaccines*, 4th edn. WB Saunders, Philadelphia, 745–781.

Wilkins CA, Richter MB, Hobbs WB, Whitcomb M, Bergh N, Carstens J 1988. Occurrence of *Clostridium tetani* in soil and horses. *South African Medical Journal* 73:718–720.

Mycoplasma spp.

Baczynska A, Fedder J, Schougaard H, Christiansen G 2007. Prevalence of mycoplasmas in the semen and vaginal swabs of Danish stallions and mares. *Veterinary Microbiology* 121:138–143.

Bermudez V, Miller RB, Johnson W, Rosendal S, Ruhnke L 1988. Effect of sample freezing on the isolation of *Mycoplasma* spp. from the clitoral fossa of the mare. *Canadian Journal of Veterinary Research* 52:147–148.

Christley RM, Hodgson DR, Rose RJ, et al. 2001. A case-control study of respiratory disease in Thoroughbred racehorses in Sydney, Australia. *Equine Veterinary Journal* 33:256–264.

Cunha BA 2006. The atypical pneumonias: clinical diagnosis and importance. Review. *Clinical Microbiology and Infection* 12 Supplement 3:12–24.

Dieckmann SM, Winkler M, Groebel K, et al. 2010. Haemotrophic *Mycoplasma* infection in horses. *Veterinary Microbiology* 145:351–353.

Dussurget O, Roulland-Dussoix D 1994. Rapid, sensitive PCR-based detection of mycoplasmas in simulated samples of animal sera. *Applied and Environmental Microbiology* 60:953–959.

Fadiel A, Eichenbaum KD, El Semary N, Epperson B 2007. *Mycoplasma* genomics: tailoring the genome for minimal life requirements through reductive evolution. Review. *Frontiers in Bioscience* 12:2020–2028.

Hoffman AM, Baird JD, Kloeze HJ, Rosendal S, Bell M 1992. *Mycoplasma felis* pleuritis in two show-jumper horses. *Cornell Veterinarian* 82:155–162.

Jubb KVF, Kennedy PC, Palmer N 2007. *Pathology of Domestic Animals*, 5th edn. WB Saunders Elsevier, Edinburgh 2:634.

Nagatomo H, Tokita Y, Shimizu T 1997. Survival of mycoplasmas inoculated in horse sera. *Journal of Veterinary Medical Science* 59:487–490.

Newton JR, Wood JL, Chanter N 2003. A case control study of factors and infections associated with clinically apparent respiratory disease in UK Thoroughbred racehorses. *Preventive Veterinary Medicine* 60:107–132.

Pitcher DG, Nicholas RA 2005. *Mycoplasma* host specificity: fact or fiction? Review. *Veterinary Journal* 170:300–306.

Rosendal S, Lumsden JH, Viel L, Physick-Sheard PW 1987. Phagocytic function of equine neutrophils exposed to *Mycoplasma felis in vitro* and *in vivo*. *American Journal of Veterinary Research* 48:758–762.

Shams Eldin HE, Kirchhoff H 1994. Detection of mycoplasmas in horses with respiratory diseases and their biochemical and serologic characterization. *Berliner und Münchener Tierärztliche Wochenschrift* 107:52–55.

Spergser J, Aurich C, Aurich JE, Rosengarten R 2002. High prevalence of mycoplasmas in the genital tract of asymptomatic stallions in Austria. *Veterinary Microbiology* 87:119–129.

Szeredi L, Tenk M, Schiller I, Révész T 2003. Study of the role of *Chlamydia*, *Mycoplasma*, *Ureaplasma* and other microaerophilic and aerobic bacteria in uterine infections of mares with reproductive disorders. *Acta Veterinaria Hungarica* 51:45–52.

Tortschanoff M, Aurich C, Rosengarten R, Spergser J 2005. Phase and size variable surface-exposed proteins in equine genital mycoplasmas. *Veterinary Microbiology* 110:301–306.

Waites KB, Balish MF, Atkinson TP 2008. New insights into the pathogenesis and detection of *Mycoplasma pneumoniae* infections. Review. *Future Microbiology* 3:635–648.

Wood JL, Chanter N, Newton JR, *et al.* 1997. An outbreak of respiratory disease in horses associated with *Mycoplasma felis* infection. *Veterinary Record* 140:388–391.

Wood JL, Newton JR, Chanter N, Mumford JA 2005. Association between respiratory disease and bacterial and viral infections in British racehorses. *Journal of Clinical Microbiology* 43:120–126.

Erysipelothrix rhusiopathiae

Azofra J, Torres R, Gómez Garcés JL, Górgolas M, Fernández Guerrero ML, Jiménez Casado M 1991. Endocarditis caused by *Erysipelothrix rhusiopathiae*. Study of 2 cases and review of the literature. *Enfermedades Infecciosas y Microbiologia Clinica* 9:102–105.

Groschup MH, Cussler K, Weiss R, Timoney JF 1991. Characterization of a protective protein antigen of *Erysipelothrix rhusiopathiae*. *Epidemiology and Infection* 107:637–649.

McCormick BS, Peet RL, Downes K 1985. *Erysipelothrix rhusiopathiae* vegetative endocarditis in a horse. *Australian Veterinary Journal* 62:392.

Seahorn TL, Brumbaugh GW, Carter GK, Wood RL 1989. *Erysipelothrix rhusiopathiae* bacteremia in a horse. *Cornell Veterinarian* 79:151–156.

Veraldi S, Girgenti V, Dassoni F, Gianotti R 2009. Erysipeloid: a review. *Clinical and Experimental Dermatology* 34:859–862.

Wang Q, Chang BJ, Riley TV 2010. *Erysipelothrix rhusiopathiae*. *Veterinary Microbiology* 140:405–417.

Bacillus anthracis

Aikembayev AM, Lukhnova L, Temiraliyeva G, *et al.* 2010. Historical distribution and molecular diversity of *Bacillus anthracis*, Kazakhstan. *Emerging Infectious Diseases* 16:789–796.

Constable PD, Gay CC, Hindcliff KW, Radostits OM 2007. *Veterinary Medicine: A Textbook of the Diseases of Cattle, Horses, Sheep, Pigs and Goats*, 10th edn. WB Saunders, Edinburgh, 816–819.

Devrim I, Kara A, Tezer H, Cengiz AB, Ceyhan M, Seçmeer G 2009. Animal carcass and eyelid anthrax: a case report. *Turkish Journal of Pediatrics* 51:67–68.

Duriez E, Goossens PL, Becher F, Ezan E 2009. Femtomolar detection of the anthrax edema factor in human and animal plasma. *Analytical Chemistry* 81:5935–5941.

Fasanella A, Garofolo G, Galante D, *et al.* 2010a. Severe anthrax outbreaks in Italy in 2004: considerations on factors involved in the spread of infection. *New Microbiologica* 33:83–86.

Fasanella A, Galante D, Garofolo G, Jones MH 2010b. Anthrax undervalued zoonosis. *Veterinary Microbiology* 140:318–331.

Friedlander AM, Welkos SL, Pitt ML, *et al.* 1993. Postexposure prophylaxis against experimental inhalation anthrax. *Journal of Infectious Diseases* 167:1239–1243.

Guidi-Rontani C 2002. The alveolar macrophage: the Trojan horse of *Bacillus anthracis*. *Trends in Microbiology* 10:405–409.

Himsworth CG, Argue CK 2009. Clinical impressions of anthrax from the 2006 outbreak in Saskatchewan. *Canadian Veterinary Journal* 50:291–294.

Narayan SK, Sreelakshmi M, Sujatha S, Dutta TK 2009. Anthrax meningoencephalitis – declining trends in an uncommon but catastrophic CNS infection in rural Tamil Nadu, South India. *Journal of Neurological Science* 281:41–45.

Parkinson R, Rajic A, Jenson C 2003. Investigation of an anthrax outbreak in Alberta in 1999 using a geographic information system. *Canadian Veterinary Journal* 44:315–318.

Listeria monocytogenes

Dussurget O 2008. New insights into determinants of *Listeria monocytogenes* virulence. *International Review of Cell and Molecular Biology* 270:1–38.

Edman DC, Pollock MB, Hall ER 1968. *Listeria monocytogenes* L forms. I. Induction maintenance, and biological characteristics. *Journal of Bacteriology* 96:352–357.

Evans K, Smith M, McDonough P, Wiedmann M 2004. Eye infections due to *Listeria monocytogenes* in three cows and one horse. *Journal of Veterinary Diagnostic Investigation* 16:464–469.

Greub G, Raoult D 2004. Microorganisms resistant to free-living amoebae. Review. *Clinical Microbiology Reviews* 17:413–433.

Gudmundsdottir KB, Svansson V, Aalbæk B, Gunnarsson E, Sigurdarson S 2004. *Listeria monocytogenes* in horses in Iceland. *Veterinary Record* 155:456–459.

Jose-Cunilleras E, Hinchcliff KW 2001. *Listeria monocytogenes* septicaemia in foals. *Equine Veterinary Journal* 33:519–522.

Jubb KVF, Kennedy PC, Palmer N 2007. *Pathology of Domestic Animals*, 5th edn. WB Saunders Elsevier, Edinburgh, 1:407–408.

Korthals M, Ege MJ, Tebbe CC, von Mutius E, Bauer J 2008. Application of PCR-SSCP for molecular epidemiological studies on the exposure of farm children to bacteria in environmental dust. *Journal of Microbiological Methods* 73:49–56.

Rütten M, Lehner A, Pospischil A, Sydler T 2006. Cerebral listeriosis in an adult Freiberger gelding. *Journal of Comparative Pathology* 134:249–253.

Sanchez S, Studer M, Currin P, Barlett P, Bounous D 2001. Listeria keratitis in a horse. *Veterinary Ophthalmology* 4:217–219.

Methicillin-resistant *Staphylococcus aureus*

Abbott Y, Leggett B, Rossney AS, Leonard FC, Markey BK 2010. Isolation rates of methicillin-resistant *Staphylococcus aureus* in dogs, cats and horses in Ireland. *Veterinary Record* 166:451–455.

Anderson MEC, Lefebvre SL, Weese JS 2008. Evaluation of prevalence and risk factors for methicillin-resistant *Staphylococcus aureus* colonization in veterinary personnel attending an international equine veterinary conference. *Veterinary Microbiology* 129:410–417.

Anderson ME, Lefebvre SL, Rankin SC, et al. 2009. Retrospective multicentre study of methicillin-resistant *Staphylococcus aureus* infections in 115 horses. *Equine Veterinary Journal* 41:401–405.

Baptiste KE, Williams K, Williams NJ, et al. 2005. Methicillin-resistant staphylococci in companion animals. *Emerging Infectious Diseases* 11:1942–1944.

Busscher JF, Duijkeren E van, Sloet van Oldruitenborgh-Oosterbaan MM 2005. The prevalence of methicillin-resistant staphylococci in healthy horses in the Netherlands. *Veterinary Microbiology* 113:131–136.

Casewell MW, Hill RL 1986. The carrier state: methicillin-resistant *Staphylococcus aureus*. *Journal of Antimicrobials and Chemotherapeutics* 18 Supplement A:1–12.

Catry B, Van Duijkeren E, Pomba MC, et al., Scientific Advisory Group on Antimicrobials (SAGAM) 2010. Reflection paper on MRSA in food-producing and companion animals: epidemiology and control options for human and animal health. *Epidemiology and Infection* 138:626–644.

Christianson S, Golding GR, Campbell J, Mulvey MR 2007. Canadian Nosocomial Infection Surveillance Program. Comparative genomics of Canadian epidemic lineages of methicillin-resistant *Staphylococcus aureus*. *Journal of Clinical Microbiology* 45:1904–1911.

De Martino L, Lucido M, Mallardo K, et al. 2010. Methicillin-resistant staphylococci isolated from healthy horses and horse personnel in Italy. *Journal of Veterinary Diagnostic Investigation* 22:77–82.

Duijkeren E van, Moleman M, Sloet van Oldruitenborgh-Oosterbaan MM, et al. 2010. Methicillin-resistant *Staphylococcus aureus* in horses and horse personnel: An investigation of several outbreaks. *Veterinary Microbiology* 141:96–102.

Eede A Van den, Martens A, Lipinska U, et al. 2009. High occurrence of methicillin-resistant *Staphylococcus aureus* ST398 in equine nasal samples. *Veterinary Microbiology* 133:138–144.

Grundmann H, Aires-de-Sousa M, Boyce J, Tiemersma E 2006. Emergence and resurgence of methicillin-resistant *Staphylococcus aureus* as a public-health threat. *Lancet* 368:874–885.

Haenni M, Targant H, Forest K, et al. 2010. Retrospective study of necropsy-associated coagulase-positive staphylococci in horses. *Journal of Veterinary Diagnostic Investigation* 22:953–956.

Loeffler A, Pfeiffer DU, Lindsay JA, Magalhães RJ, Lloyd DH 2011. Prevalence of and risk factors for MRSA carriage in companion animals: a survey of dogs, cats, and horses. *Epidemiology and Infection* 139:1019–1028.

Morgan M 2008. Methicillin-resistant *Staphylococcus aureus* and animals: zoonosis or humanosis? Review. *Journal of Antimicrobials and Chemotherapeutics* 62:1181–1187.

Tacconelli E, De Angelis G, de Waure C, Cataldo MA, La Torre G, Cauda R 2009. Rapid screening tests for methicillin-resistant *Staphylococcus aureus* at hospital admission: systematic review and meta-analysis. Review. *Lancet Infectious Diseases* 9:546–554.

Tokateloff N, Manning ST, Weese JS, et al. 2009. Prevalence of methicillin-resistant *Staphylococcus aureus* colonization in horses in Saskatchewan, Alberta, and British Columbia. *Canadian Veterinary Journal* 50:1177–1180.

Walther B, Monecke S, Ruscher C, et al. 2009. Comparative molecular analysis substantiates zoonotic potential of equine methicillin-resistant *Staphylococcus aureus*. *Journal of Clinical Microbiology* 47:704–710.

Weese JS, Rousseau J 2005. Attempted eradication of methicillin-resistant *Staphylococcus aureus* colonisation in horses on two farms. *Equine Veterinary Journal* 37:510–514.

Weese JS, Lefebvre SL 2007. Risk factors for methicillin-resistant *Staphylococcus aureus* colonization in horses admitted to a veterinary teaching hospital. *Canadian Veterinary Journal* 48:921–926.

Weese JS, Archambault M, Willey BM, et al. 2005a. Methicillin-resistant *Staphylococcus aureus* in horses and horse personnel, 2000–2002. *Emerging Infectious Diseases* 11:430–435.

Weese JS, Rousseau J, Traub-Dargatz JL, Willey BM, McGeer A, Low DE 2005b. Community-associated methicillin-resistant *Staphylococcus aureus* in horses and humans who work with horses. *Journal of the American Veterinary Medical Association* 226:580–583.

Weese JS, Caldwell F, Willey BM, et al. 2006a. An outbreak of methicillin-resistant *Staphylococcus aureus* skin infections resulting from horse to human transmission in a veterinary hospital. *Veterinary Microbiology* 114:160–164.

Weese SJ, Rousseau J, Willey BM, Archambault M, McGeer A, Low DE 2006b. Methicillin-resistant *Staphylococcus aureus* in horses at a veterinary teaching hospital: Frequency, characterization, and association with clinical disease. *Journal of Veterinary Internal Medicine* 20:182–186.

Streptococcus equi subsp. *equi*

Albini S, Korczak BM, Abril C, et al. 2008. Mandibular lymphadenopathy caused by *Actinomyces denticolens* mimicking strangles in three horses. *Veterinary Record* 162:158–159.

Breiman RF, Silverblatt FJ 1986. Systemic *Streptococcus equi* infection in a horse handler – a case of human strangles. *Western Journal of Medicine* 145:385–386.

Chanter N, Newton JR, Wood JL, Verheyen K, Hannant D 1998. Detection of strangles carriers. *Veterinary Record* 142:496.

Chiesa OA, Lopez C, Domingo M, Cuenca R, Timoney JF 2000. A percutaneous technique for guttural pouch lavage. *Equine Practice* 22:8–11.

De Clercq D, Loon G van, Nollet H, Delesalle C, Lefère L, Deprez P 2003. Percutaneous puncture technique for treating persistent retropharyngeal lymph node infections in seven horses. *Veterinary Record* 152:169–172.

Elsayed S, Hammerberg O, Massey V, Hussain Z 2003. *Streptococcus equi* subspecies *equi* (Lancefield group C) meningitis in a child. *Clinical Microbiology and Infection* 9:869–872.

Evers WD 1968. Effect of furaltadone on strangles in horses. *Journal of the American Veterinary Medical Association* 152:1394–1398.

Facklam R 2002. What happened to the streptococci: overview of taxonomic and nomenclature changes. Review. *Clinical Microbiology Reviews* 15:613–630.

Ford J, Lokai MD 1980. Complications of *Streptococcus equi* infection. *Equine Practice* 4:41–44.

Guss B, Flock M, Frykberg L, et al. 2009. Getting to grips with strangles: an effective multi-component recombinant vaccine for the protection of horses from *Streptococcus equi* infection. *PLoS Pathogens* 5:e1000584.

Hamlen HJ, Timoney JF, Bell RJ 1994. Epidemiologic and immunologic characteristics of *Streptococcus equi* infection in foals. *Journal of the American Veterinary Medical Association* 204:768–775.

Ivens PAS, Waller A, Robinson C, Slater JD 2009. Molecular epidemiology of strangles out-breaks in the UK: the use of M-protein typing of *Streptococcus equi* subspecies *equi*, to track isolates within and between field outbreaks. *Proceedings of the 3rd ECEIM Congress*, 28–30 Jan 2009. Barcelona, Spain:14.

Jubb KVF, Kennedy PC, Palmer N 2007. *Pathology of Domestic Animals*, 5th edn. WB Saunders Elsevier, Edinburgh, 2:633.

Knowles EJ, Mair TS, Butcher N, Waller AS, Wood JL 2010. Use of a novel serological test for exposure to *Streptococcus equi* subspecies *equi* in hospitalised horses. *Veterinary Record* 166:294–297.

Lanka S, Borst LB, Patterson SK, Maddox CW 2010. A multiphasic typing approach to subtype *Streptococcus equi* subspecies *equi*. *Journal of Veterinary Diagnostic Investigation* 22:928–936.

Lindsay AM, Zhang M, Mitchell Z, et al. 2009. The *Streptococcus equi* prophage-encoded protein SEQ2045 is a hyaluronan-specific hyaluronate lyase that is produced during equine infection. *Microbiology* 155(Pt 2):443–449.

Newton JR, Wood JLN, Dunn KA, Brauwere MN de, Chanter N 1997. Naturally occurring persistent and asymptomatic infection of the guttural pouches of horses with *Streptococcus equi*. *Veterinary Record* 140:84–90.

Newton JR, Verheyen K, Talbot NC, et al. 2000. Control of strangles outbreaks by isolation of guttural pouch carriers identified using PCR and culture of *Streptococcus equi*. *Equine Veterinary Journal* 32:515–526.

Popescu G-A, Fuerea R, Benea E 2006. Meningitis due to an unusual human pathogen: *Streptococcus equi* subspecies *equi*. *Southern Medical Journal* 99:190–191.

Spoormakers TJ, Ensink JM, Goehring LS, et al. 2003. Brain abscesses as a metastatic manifestation of strangles: symptomatology and the use of magnetic resonance imaging as a diagnostic aid. *Equine Veterinary Journal* 35:146–151.

Sweeney CR 1996. Strangles: *Streptococcus equi* infection in horses. *Equine Veterinary Education* 8:317–322.

Sweeney CR, Benson CE, Whitlock RH, Barningham SO 1987a. Strangles (*Streptococcus equi*) infection in horses. *Compendium on Continuing Education for the Practicing Veterinarian* 9:689–693.

Sweeney CR, Whitlock RH, Meirs DA, Whitehead SC, Barningham SO 1987b. Complications associated with *Streptococcus equi* infection on a horse farm. *Journal of the American Veterinary Medical Association* 191:1446–1448.

Sweeney CR, Timoney JF, Newton JR, Hines MT 2005. *Streptococcus equi* infections in horses: guidelines for treatment, control, and prevention of strangles. *Journal of Veterinary Internal Medicine* 19:123–134.

Timoney JF 2004. The pathogenic equine streptococci. *Veterinary Research* 35:397–409.

Timoney JF, Eggers D 1985. Serum bactericidal responses to *Streptococcus equi* of horses following infection or vaccination. *Equine Veterinary Journal* 17:306–310.

Timoney JF, Artiushin SC, Boschwitz JS 1997. Comparison of the sequences and functions of *Streptococcus equi* M-like proteins SeM and SzPSe. *Infection and Immunology* 65:3600–3605.

Timoney JF, Kumar P 2008. Early pathogenesis of equine *Streptococcus equi* infection (strangles). *Equine Veterinary Journal* 40:637–642.

Timoney JF, DeNegri R, Sheoran A, Forster N 2010. Affects of N-terminal variation in the SeM protein of *Streptococcus equi* on antibody and fibrinogen binding. *Vaccine* 28:1522–1527.

Todd TG 1910. Strangles. *Journal of Comparative Pathology and Therapeutics* 23:212–229.

Verheyen K, Newton JR, Talbot NC, Brauwere MN de, Chanter N 2000. Elimination of guttural pouch infection and inflammation in asymptomatic carriers of *Streptococcus equi*. *Equine Veterinary Journal* 32:527–532.

Streptococcus equi subsp. *zooepidemicus*

Barquero N, Chanter N, Laxton R, Wood JL, Newton JR 2009. Molecular epidemiology of *Streptococcus zooepidemicus* isolated from the respiratory tracts of Thoroughbred racehorses in training. *Veterinary Journal* 183:348–351.

Båverud V, Johansson SK, Aspan A 2007. Real-time PCR for detection and differentiation of *Streptococcus equi* subsp. *equi* and *Streptococcus equi* subsp. *zooepidemicus*. *Veterinary Microbiology* 124:219–229.

Bordes-Benítez A, Sánchez-Oñoro M, Suárez-Bordón P, et al. 2006. Outbreak of *Streptococcus equi* subsp. *zooepidemicus* infections on the island of Gran Canaria associated with the consumption of inadequately pasteurized cheese. *European Journal of Clinical Microbiology and Infectious Diseases* 25:242–246.

Caballero AR, Lottenberg R, Johnston KH 1999. Cloning, expression, sequence analysis, and characterization of streptokinases secreted by porcine and equine isolates of *Streptococcus equisimilis*. *Infection and Immunology* 67:6478–6486.

Causey RC, Weber JA, Emmans EE, et al. 2006. The equine immune response to *Streptococcus equi* subspecies *zooepidemicus* during uterine infection. *Veterinary Journal* 172:248–257.

Downar J, Willey BM, Sutherland JW, Mathew K, Low DE 2001. Streptococcal meningitis resulting from contact with an infected horse. *Journal of Clinical Microbiology* 39:2358–2359.

Ensink JM, Bosch G, van Duijkeren E 2005. Clinical efficacy of prophylactic administration of trimethoprim/sulfadiazine in a *Streptococcus equi* subsp. *zooepidemicus* infection model in ponies. *Journal of Veterinary Pharmacology and Therapeutics* 28:45–49.

Eyre DW, Kenkre JS, Bowler IC, McBride SJ 2010. *Streptococcus equi* subspecies *zooepidemicus* meningitis—a case report and review of the literature. *European Journal of Clinical Microbiology and Infectious Diseases* 29:1459–1463.

Facklam R 2002. What happened to the streptococci: overview of taxonomic and nomenclature changes. Review. *Clinical Microbiology Reviews* 15:613–630.

Feary DJ, Hyatt D, Traub-Dargatz J, et al. 2005. Investigation of falsely reported resistance of *Streptococcus equi* subsp. *zooepidemicus* isolates from horses to trimethoprim–sulfamethoxazole. *Journal of Veterinary Diagnostic Investigation* 17:483–486.

Friederichs J, Hungerer S, Werle R, Militz M, Bühren V 2010. Human bacterial arthritis caused by *Streptococcus zooepidemicus*: report of a case. *International Journal of Infectious Diseases* Supplement 14(Suppl3):e233–235.

Gaede W, Reckling KF, Schliephake A, Missal D, Hotzel H, Sachse K 2010. Detection of *Chlamydophila caviae* and *Streptococcus equi* subsp. *zooepidemicus* in horses with signs of rhinitis and conjunctivitis. *Veterinary Microbiology* 142:440–444.

Hong K 2006. Characterization of the arginine deiminase of *Streptococcus equi* subsp. *zooepidemicus*. *Canadian Journal of Microbiology* 52:868–876.

Jovanovic M, Stevanovic G, Tosic T, Stosovic B, Zervos MJ 2008. *Streptococcus equi* subsp. *zooepidemicus* meningitis. *Journal of Medical Microbiology* 57(Pt 3):373–375.

Jubb KVF, Kennedy PC, Palmer N 2007. *Pathology of Domestic Animals*, 5th edn. WB Saunders Elsevier, Edinburgh, 3:28.

Keller RL, Hendrix DV 2005. Bacterial isolates and antimicrobial susceptibilities in equine bacterial ulcerative keratitis (1993–2004). *Equine Veterinary Journal* 37:207–211.

Kuusi M, Lahti E, Virolainen A, et al. 2006. An outbreak of *Streptococcus equi* subspecies *zooepidemicus* associated with consumption of fresh goat cheese. *BMC Infectious Diseases* 6:36.

Laus F, Preziuso S, Spaterna A, Beribè F, Tesei B, Cuteri V 2007. Clinical and epidemiological investigation of chronic upper respiratory diseases caused by beta-haemolytic *Streptococci* in horses. *Comparative Immunology, Microbiology and Infectious Diseases* 30:247–260.

Lee AS, Dyer JR 2004. Severe *Streptococcus zooepidemicus* infection in a gardener. *Medical Journal of Australia* 180:366.

Newton JR, Wood JL, Chanter N 2003. A case control study of factors and infections associated with clinically apparent respiratory disease in UK Thoroughbred racehorses. *Preventive Veterinary Medicine* 60:107–132.

Newton JR, Laxton R, Wood JL, Chanter N 2008. Molecular epidemiology of *Streptococcus zooepidemicus* infection in naturally occurring equine respiratory disease. *Veterinary Journal* 175:338–345.

Paillot R, Darby AC, Robinson C, et al. 2010. Identification of three novel superantigen-encoding genes in *Streptococcus equi* subsp. *zooepidemicus*, szeF, szeN, and szeP. *Infection and Immunology* 78:4817–4827.

Riddle WT, LeBlanc MM, Stromberg AJ 2007. Relationships between uterine culture, cytology and pregnancy rates in a Thoroughbred practice. *Theriogenology* 68:395–402.

Ryu SH, Koo HC, Park YK, et al. 2009. Etiologic and immunologic characteristics of thoroughbred horses with bacterial infectious upper respiratory disease at the Seoul race park. *Journal of Microbiology and Biotechnology* 19:1041–1050.

Samper JC, Tibary A 2006. Disease transmission in horses. *Theriogenology* 66:551–559.

Speck S, Höner OP, Wachter B, Fickel J 2008. Characterization of *Streptococcus equi* subsp. *ruminatorum* isolated from spotted hyenas (*Crocuta crocuta*) and plains zebras (*Equus burchelli*), and identification of a M-like protein (SrM) encoding gene. *Veterinary Microbiology* 128:148–159.

Thorley AM, Campbell D, Moghal NE, Hudson S 2007. Post streptococcal acute glomerulonephritis secondary to sporadic *Streptococcus equi* infection. *Pediatric Nephrology* 22:597–599.

Timoney JF 2004. The pathogenic equine *streptococci*. Review. *Veterinary Research* 35:397–409.

Tiwari R, Timoney JF 2009. *Streptococcus equi* bacteriophage SeP9 binds to group C carbohydrate but is not infective for the closely related *S. zooepidemicus*. *Veterinary Microbiology* **135**:304–307.

Ural O, Tuncer I, Dikici N, Aridogan B 2003. *Streptococcus zooepidemicus* meningitis and bacteraemia. *Scandinavian Journal of Infectious Diseases* **35**:206–207.

Webb K, Jolley KA, Mitchell Z, *et al.* 2008. Development of an unambiguous and discriminatory multilocus sequence typing scheme for the *Streptococcus zooepidemicus* group. *Microbiology* **154**(Pt 10):3016–3024.

Wood JL, Newton JR, Chanter N, Mumford JA 2005. Association between respiratory disease and bacterial and viral infections in British racehorses. *Journal of Clinical Microbiology* **43**:120–126.

Yoshikawa H, Yasu T, Ueki H, *et al.* 2003. Pneumonia in horses induced by intrapulmonary inoculation of *Streptococcus equi* subsp. *zooepidemicus*. *Journal of Veterinary Medical Science* **65**:787–792.

Actinomyces spp.

Albini S, Korczak BM, Abril C, *et al.* 2008. Mandibular lymphadenopathy caused by *Actinomyces denticolens* mimicking strangles in three horses. *Veterinary Record* **162**:158–159.

Bonenberger TE, Ihrke PJ, Naydan DK, Affolter VK 2001. Rapid identification of tissue micro-organisms in skin biopsy specimens from domestic animals using polyclonal BCG antibody. *Veterinary Dermatology* **12**:41–47.

Fielding CL, Magdesian KG, Morgan RA, Ruby RE, Sprayberry KA 2008. *Actinomyces* species as a cause of abscesses in nine horses. *Veterinary Record* **162**:18–20.

Ledbetter EC, Scarlett JM 2008. Isolation of obligate anaerobic bacteria from ulcerative keratitis in domestic animals. *Veterinary Ophthalmology* **11**:114–122.

Lynch M, O'Leary J, Murnaghan D, Cryan B 1998. *Actinomyces pyogenes* septic arthritis in a diabetic farmer. *Journal of Infection* **37**:71–73.

Robinson JA, Allen GK, Green EM, Fales WH, Loch WE, Wilkerson CG 1993. A prospective study of septicaemia in colostrum-deprived foals. *Equine Veterinary Journal* **25**:214–219.

Rumbaugh GE 1977. Disseminated septic meningitis in a mare. *Journal of the American Veterinary Medical Association* **171**:452–454.

Specht TE, Breuhaus BA, Manning TO, Miller RT, Cochrane RB 1991. Skin pustules and nodules caused by *Actinomyces viscosus* in a horse. *Journal of the American Veterinary Medical Association* **198**:457–459.

Sullivan DC, Chapman SW 2010. Bacteria that masquerade as fungi: actinomycosis/nocardia. *Proceedings of the American Thoracic Society* **7**:216–221.

Vos NJ 2007. Actinomycosis of the mandible, mimicking a malignancy in a horse. *Canadian Veterinary Journal* **48**:1261–1263.

Dermatophilus congolensis

Albrecht R, Horowitz S, Gilbert E, Hong R, Richard J, Connor DH 1974. *Dermatophilus congolensis* chronic nodular disease in man. *Pediatrics* **53**:907–912.

Ambrose NC, Mijinyawa MS, Hermoso de Mendoza J 1998. Preliminary characterisation of extracellular serine proteases of *Dermatophilus congolensis* isolates from cattle, sheep and horses. *Veterinary Microbiology* **62**:321–335.

Burd EM, Juzych LA, Rudrik JT, Habib F 2007. Pustular dermatitis caused by *Dermatophilus congolensis*. *Journal of Clinical Microbiology* **45**:1655–1658.

Byrne BA, Rand CL, McElliott VR, Samitz EM, Brault SA 2010. Atypical *Dermatophilus congolensis* infection in a three-year-old pony. *Journal of Veterinary Diagnostic Investigation* **22**:141–143.

DeVriese LA, Vlaminck K, Nuytten J, De Keersmaecker P 1983. *Staphylococcus hyicus* in skin lesions of horses. *Equine Veterinary Journal* **15**:263–265.

Hänel H, Kalisch J, Keil M, Marsch WC, Buslau M 1991. Quantification of keratinolytic activity from *Dermatophilus congolensis*. *Medical Microbiology and Immunology* **180**:45–51.

How SJ, Lloyd DH, Lida J 1988. Use of a monoclonal antibody in the diagnosis of infection by *Dermatophilus congolensis*. *Research in Veterinary Science* **45**:416–417.

Jubb KVF, Kennedy PC, Palmer N 2007. *Pathology of Domestic Animals*, 5th edn. WB Saunders Elsevier, Edinburgh, 1:683.

Krüger B, Siesenop U, Böhm KH 1998. Phenotypic characterization of equine *Dermatophilus congolensis* field isolates. *Berliner und Münchener Tierärztliche Wochenschrift* **111**:374–378.

Larrasa J, Garcia A, Ambrose NC, *et al.* 2002. A simple random amplified polymorphic DNA genotyping method for field isolates of *Dermatophilus congolensis*. *Journal of Veterinary Medicine, B. Infectious Diseases and Veterinary Public Health* **49**:135–141.

Makinde AA, Gyles CL 1999. A comparison of extracted proteins of isolates of *Dermatophilus congolensis* by sodium dodecyl sulphate-polyacrylamide gel electrophoresis and Western blotting. *Veterinary Microbiology* **67**:251–262.

Pal M 1995. Prevalence in India of *Dermatophilus congolensis* infection in clinical specimens from animals and humans. *Revue Scientifique et Technique* **14**:857–863.

Richard JL, Pier AC 1966. Transmission of *Dermatophilus congolensis* by *Stomoxys calcitrans* and *Musca domestica*. *American Journal of Veterinary Research* **27**:419–423.

Sebastian MM, Giles RC, Donahu JM, Sells SF, Fallon L, Vickers ML 2008. *Dermatophilus congolensis*-associated placentitis, funisitis and abortion in a horse. *Transboundary and Emerging Diseases* **55**:183–185.

Stannard AA 2000. Alopecia in the horse – an overview. *Veterinary Dermatology* **11**:191–203.

Corynebacterium pseudotuberculosis

Aleman M, Spier SJ, Wilson WD, Doherr M 1996. Retrospective study of *Corynebacterium pseudotuberculosis* infection in horses: 538 cases. *Journal of the American Veterinary Medical Association* **209**:804–809.

Costa LR, Spier SJ, Hirsh DC 1998. Comparative molecular characterization of *Corynebacterium pseudotuberculosis* of different origin. *Veterinary Microbiology* **62**:135–143.

Doherr MG, Carpenter TE, Wilson WD, Gardner IA 1999. Evaluation of temporal and spatial clustering of horses with *Corynebacterium pseudotuberculosis* infection. *American Journal of Veterinary Research* 60:284–291.

Gonzalez M, Tibary A, Sellon DC, Daniels J 2008. Unilateral orchitis and epididymitis caused by *Corynebacterium pseudotuberculosis* in a stallion. *Equine Veterinary Education* 20:30–36.

Henricson B, Segarra M, Garvin J, *et al.* 2000. Toxigenic *Corynebacterium diphtheriae* associated with an equine wound infection. *Journal of Veterinary Diagnostic Investigation* 12:253–257.

Jubb KVF, Kennedy PC, Palmer N 2007. *Pathology of Domestic Animals*, 5th edn. WB Saunders Elsevier, Edinburgh, 3:100–101, 292.

Knight HD 1978. A serologic method for the detection of *Corynebacterium pseudotuberculosis* infection in horses. *Cornell Veterinarian* 68:220–237.

Peel MM, Palmer GG, Stacpoole AM, Kerr TG 1997. Human lymphadenitis due to *Corynebacterium pseudotuberculosis*: report of ten cases from Australia and review. *Clinical Infectious Diseases* 24:185–191.

Pratt SM, Spier SJ, Vaughan B, Whitcomb MB, Wilson WD 2005. Clinical characteristics and diagnostic test results in horses with internal infection caused by *Corynebacterium pseudotuberculosis*: 30 cases (1995–2003). *Journal of the American Veterinary Medical Association* 227:441–448.

Pusterla N, Watson JL, Affolter VK, Magdesian KG, Wilson WD, Carlson GP 2003. Purpura haemorrhagica in 53 horses. *Veterinary Record* 153:118–121.

Spier SJ 2008. *Corynebacterium pseudotuberculosis* infection in horses: an emerging disease associated with climate change? *Equine Veterinary Education* 20:37–39.

Spier SJ, Leutenegger CM, Carroll SP, *et al.* 2004. Use of real-time polymerase chain reaction-based fluorogenic 5' nuclease assay to evaluate insect vectors of *Corynebacterium pseudotuberculosis* infections in horses. *American Journal of Veterinary Research* 65:829–834.

Vaughan B, Whitcomb MB, Pratt SM, Spier SJ 2004. Ultrasonographic appearance of abdominal organs in 14 horses with systemic *Corynebacterium pseudotuberculosis* infection. *Proceedings of the American Association of Equine Practitioners* 50:63–68.

Mycobacterium spp.

Binkhorst GJ, Gaag I van der, Aalfs RGH, Smidt AC 1972. Aviaire tuberculose bij pony's. *Tijdschrift voor Diergeneeskunde* 97:1268–1284.

Chang HJ, Huang MY, Yeh CS, *et al.* 2010. Rapid diagnosis of tuberculosis directly from clinical specimens by gene chip. *Clinical Microbiology and Infection* 16:1090–1096.

Cline JM, Schlafer DW, Callihan DR, Vanderwall D, Drazek FJ 1991. Abortion and granulomatous colitis due to *Mycobacterium avium* complex infection in a horse. *Veterinary Pathology* 28:89–91.

Collinson A, Harrill C, Kealy M, Robertson S, Sheldon C 2007. *Mycobacterium bovis*: guidance on BCG vaccination is needed. *Lancet* 369:2076–2077.

Flores JM, Sanchez J, Castano M 1991. Avian tuberculosis dermatitis in a young horse. *Veterinary Record* 128:407–408.

Francis J 1958. *Tuberculosis in Animals and Man*. A study in comparative pathology. Cassell and Company, London.

Gunnes G, Nord K, Vatn S, Saxegaard F 1995. A case of generalised avian tuberculosis in a horse. *Veterinary Record* 136:565–566.

Hélie P, Higgins R 1996. *Mycobacterium avium* complex abortion in a mare. *Journal of Veterinary Diagnostic Investigation* 8:257–258.

Helke KL, Mankowski JL, Manabe YC 2006. Animal models of cavitation in pulmonary tuberculosis. *Tuberculosis (Edinburgh)* 86:337–348.

Jubb KVF, Kennedy PC, Palmer N 2007. *Pathology of Domestic Animals*, 5th edn. WB Saunders Elsevier, Edinburgh, 2:610.

Keck N, Dutruel H, Smyej F, Nodet M, Boschiroli ML 2010. Tuberculosis due to *Mycobacterium bovis* in a Camargue horse. *Veterinary Record* 166:499–500.

Konyha LD, Kreier JP 1971. The significance of tuberculin tests in the horse. *American Review of Respiratory Disease* 103:91–99.

Kriz P, Jahn P, Bezdekova B, *et al.* 2010. *Mycobacterium avium* subsp. *hominissuis* infection in horses. *Emerging Infectious Diseases* 16:1328–1329.

Leifsson PS, Olsen SN, Larsen S 1997. Ocular tuberculosis in a horse. *Veterinary Record* 141:651–654.

Lofstedt J, Jakowski RM 1989. Diagnosis of avian tuberculosis in a horse by use of liver biopsy. *Journal of the American Veterinary Medical Association* 194:260–262.

Luke D 1958. Tuberculosis in the horse, pig, sheep, and goat. *Veterinary Record* 70:529–536.

Mair TS, Taylor FGR, Gibbs C, Lucke VM 1986. Generalized avian tuberculosis in a horse. *Equine Veterinary Journal* 18:226.

Malipeddi A, Rajendran R, Kallarackal G 2007. Disseminated tuberculosis after anti-TNFα treatment. *Lancet* 369:162.

Monreal L, Segura D, Segalés J, Garrido JM, Prades M 2001. Diagnosis of *Mycobacterium bovis* infection in a mare. *Veterinary Record* 149:712–714.

Sills RC, Mullaney TP, Stickle RL, Darien BJ, Brown CM 1990. Bilateral granulomatous guttural pouch infection due to *Mycobacterium avium complex* in a horse. *Veterinary Pathology* 27:133–135.

Tasler GRW, Hartley WJ 1981. Foal abortion associated with *Mycobacterium terrae* infection. *Veterinary Pathology* 18:122–125.

Thoen CO, LoBue PA 2007. *Mycobacterium bovis* tuberculosis: forgotten, but not gone. *Lancet* 369:1236–1237.

Nocardia spp.

Biberstein EL, Jang SS, Hirsh DC 1985. *Nocardia asteroides* infection in horses: a review. *Journal of the American Veterinary Medical Association* 186:273–277.

Kjelstrom JA, Beaman BL 1993. Development of a serologic panel for the recognition of nocardial infections in a murine model. *Diagnostic Microbiology and Infectious Diseases* 16:291–301.

Nakagawa Y, Fukushima Y, Sakata T 1996. Chronic pulmonary nocardiosis with eosinophilia in an immunocompetent host. *Nihon Kyobu Shikkan Gakkai Zasshi* 34:916–920.

Volkmann DH, Williams JH, Henton JH, Donahue JM, Williams NM 2001. The first reported case of equine nocardioform placentitis in South Africa. *Journal of the South African Veterinary Association* 72:235–238.

Rhodococcus equi

Bain AM 1963. *Corynebacterium equi* infections in the equine. *Australian Veterinary Journal* 39:116–121.

Barton MD, Embury DH 1987. Studies of the pathogenesis of *Rhodococcus equi* infection in foals. *Australian Veterinary Journal* 64:332–339.

Båverud V, Franklin A, Gunnarsson A, Gustafsson A, Hellander-Edman A 1998. *Clostridium difficile* associated with acute colitis in mares when their foals are treated with erythromycin and rifampicin (rifampin) for *Rhodococcus equi* pneumonia. *Equine Veterinary Journal* 30:482–488.

Bolton T, Kuskie K, Halbert N, *et al.* 2010. Detection of strain variation in isolates of *Rhodococcus equi* from an affected foal using repetitive sequence-based polymerase chain reaction. *Journal of Veterinary Diagnostic Investigation* 22:611–615.

Caston SS, McClure SR, Martens RJ, *et al.* 2006. Effect of hyperimmune plasma on the severity of pneumonia caused by *Rhodococcus equi* in experimentally infected foals. *Veterinary Therapeutics* 7:361–375.

Giguère S, Lee E, Williams E, *et al.* 2010. Determination of the prevalence of antimicrobial resistance to macrolide antimicrobials or rifampicin (rifampin) in *Rhodococcus equi* isolates and treatment outcome in foals infected with antimicrobial-resistant isolates of *R equi*. *Journal of the American Veterinary Medical Association* 237:74–81.

Giguère S, Jacks S, Roberts GD, Hernandez J, Long MT, Ellis C 2004. Retrospective comparison of azithromycin, clarithromycin, and erythromycin for the treatment of foals with *Rhodococcus equi* pneumonia. *Journal of Veterinary Internal Medicine* 18:568–573.

Giguère S, Gaskin JM, Miller C, Bowman JL 2002. Evaluation of a commercially available hyperimmune plasma product for prevention of naturally acquired pneumonia caused by *Rhodococcus equi* in foals. *Journal of the American Veterinary Medical Association* 220:59–63.

Giguère S, Prescott JF 1997. Clinical manifestations, diagnosis, treatment, and prevention of *Rhodococcus equi* infections in foals. Review. *Veterinary Microbiology* 56:313–334.

Goodfellow M, Alderson G 1977. The actinomycete-genus *Rhodococcus*: a home for the 'rhodochrous' complex. *Journal of General Microbiology* 100:99–122.

Hébert L, Cauchard J, Doligez P, Quitard L, Laugier C, Petry S 2009. Viability of *Rhodococcus equi* and *Parascaris equorum* eggs exposed to high temperatures. *Current Microbiology* 60:38–41.

Higuchi T, Hashikura S, Gojo C, *et al.* 1997. Clinical evaluation of the serodiagnostic value of enzyme-linked immunosorbent assay for *Rhodococcus equi* infection in foals. *Equine Veterinary Journal* 29:274–278.

Hillidge CJ 1987. Use of erythromycin-rifampicin (rifampin)combination in treatment of *Rhodococcus equi* pneumonia. *Veterinary Microbiology* 14:337–342.

Johnson JA, Prescott JF, Markham RJF 1983a. The pathology of experimental *Corynebacterium equi* infection in foals following intrabronchial challenge. *Veterinary Pathology* 20:440–449.

Johnson JA, Prescott JF, Markham RJF 1983b. The pathology of experimental *Corynebacterium equi* infection in foals following intragastric challenge. *Veterinary Pathology* 20:450–459.

Kolk JH van der, Kraus H, Vink-Nooteboom M 1999. *Rhodococcus equi* pneumonia in a foal. *Equine Practice* 21:6–9.

Magnusson H 1938. Pyaemia in foals caused by *Corynebacterium equi*. *Veterinary Record* 50:1459–1468.

Makrai L, Dénes B, Hajtós I, Fodor L, Varga J 2008. Serotypes of *Rhodococcus equi* isolated from horses, immunocompromised human patients and soil in Hungary. *Acta Veterinaria Hungarica* 56:271–279.

Martens RJ, Fiske RA, Renshaw HW 1982. Experimental subacute foal pneumonia induced by aerosol administration of *Corynebacterium equi*. *Equine Veterinary Journal* 14:111–116.

Meijer WG, Prescott JF 2004. *Rhodococcus equi*. *Veterinary Research* 35:383–396.

Morresey PR, Waldridge BM 2010. Successful treatment of *Rhodococcus equi* pneumonia in an adult horse. *Journal of Veterinary Internal Medicine* 24:436–438.

Prescott JF, Nicholson VM, Patterson MC, *et al.* 1997. Use of *Rhodococcus equi* virulence-associated protein for immunization of foals against *R. equi* pneumonia. *American Journal of Veterinary Research* 58:356–359.

Prescott JF, Travers M, Yager YA 1984. Epidemiological survey of *Corynebacterium equi* infections on five Ontario horse farms. *Canadian Journal of Comparative Medicine* 48:10–13.

Reuss SM, Chaffin MK, Cohen ND 2009. Extrapulmonary disorders associated with *Rhodococcus equi* infection in foals: 150 cases (1987–2007). *Journal of the American Veterinary Medical Association* 235:855–863.

Smith BP, Robinson RC 1981. Studies of an outbreak of *Corynebacterium equi* pneumonia in foals. *Equine Veterinary Journal* 13:223–228.

Sweeney CR, Sweeney RW, Divers TJ 1987. *Rhodococcus equi* pneumonia in 48 foals: responses to antimicrobial therapy. *Veterinary Microbiology* 14:329–336.

Venner M 2009. *Rhodococcus equi* pneumonia: treatment strategies. *4th World Equine Airways Symposium (WEAS)* August 5–7, 2009. Berne, Switzerland. Abstract:132–134.

Chlamydophila spp.

Abdelrahman YM, Belland RJ 2005. The chlamydial developmental cycle. *FEMS Microbiology Reviews* 29:949–959.

Baghian A, Schnorr KL 1992. Detection and antigenicity of chlamydial proteins that bind eukaryotic cell membrane proteins. *American Journal of Veterinary Research* 53:980–986.

Blunden AS, Mackintosh ME 1991. The microflora of the lower respiratory tract of the horse: an autopsy study. *British Veterinary Journal* 147:238–250.

Bocklisch H, Ludwig C, Lange S 1991. *Chlamydia* as the cause of abortions in horses. *Berliner und Münchener Tierarztliche Wochenschrift* **104**:119–124.

Bodetti TJ, Jacobson E, Wan C, *et al.* 2002. Molecular evidence to support the expansion of the hostrange of *Chlamydophila pneumoniae* to include reptiles as well as humans, horses, koalas, and amphibians. *Systematic and Applied Microbiology* **25**:146–152.

Forster JL, Wittenbrink MM, Häni HJ, Corboz L, Pospischil A 1997. Absence of *Chlamydia* as an aetiological factor in aborting mares. *Veterinary Record* **141**:424.

Gaede W, Reckling KF, Schliephake A, Missal D, Hotzel H, Sachse K 2010. Detection of *Chlamydophila caviae* and *Streptococcus equi* subsp. *zooepidemicus* in horses with signs of rhinitis and conjunctivitis. *Veterinary Microbiology* **142**:440–444.

Henning K, Sachse K, Sting R 2000. Demonstration of *Chlamydia* from an equine abortion. *Deutsche Tierärztliche Wochenschrift* **107**:49–52.

Jubb KVF, Kennedy PC, Palmer N 2007. *Pathology of Domestic Animals*, 5th edn. WB Saunders Elsevier, Edinburgh **3**:502–503.

Khorvash F, Keshteli AH, Salehi H, Szeredi L, Morré SA 2008. Unusual transmission route of lymphogranuloma venereum; following sexual contact with a female donkey. *International Journal of STD and AIDS* **19**:563–564.

Mair TS, Wills JM 1992. *Chlamydia psittaci* infection in horses: results of a prevalence survey and experimental challenge. *Veterinary Record* **130**:417–419.

McChesney AE, Becerra V, England JJ 1974. Chlamydial polyarthritis in a foal. *Journal of the American Veterinary Medical Association* **165**:259–261.

McChesney SL, England JJ, McChesney AE 1982. *Chlamydia psittaci* induced pneumonia in a horse. *Cornell Veterinarian* **72**:92–97.

McGavin MD, Zachary JF 2007. *Pathologic Basis of Veterinary Disease*, 4th edn. Mosby Elsevier, St. Louis, 520.

Miyamoto C, Takashima I, Karaiwa H, Sugiura T, Kamada M, Hashimoto N 1993. Seroepidemiological survey of chlamydial infections in Light horses in Japan. *Journal of Veterinary Medical Science* **55**:333–335.

Moorthy AR, Spradbrow PB 1978. *Chlamydia psittaci* infection of horses with respiratory disease. *Equine Veterinary Journal* **10**:38–42.

Pantchev A, Sting R, Bauerfeind R, Tyczka J, Sachse K 2010. Detection of all *Chlamydophila* and *Chlamydia* spp. of veterinary interest using species-specific real-time PCR assays. *Comparative Immunology, Microbiology and Infectious Diseases* **33**:473–484.

Sachse K, Grossmann E 2002. Chlamydial diseases of domestic animals - zoonotic potential of the agents and diagnostic issues. Review. *Deutsche Tierrztliche Wochenschrift* **109**:142–148.

Shewen PE 1980. Chlamydial infection in animals: a review. *Canadian Veterinary Journal* **21**:2–11.

Szeredi L, Tenk M, Schiller I, Révész T 2003. Study of the role of *Chlamydia, Mycoplasma, Ureaplasma* and other microaerophilic and aerobic bacteria in uterine infections of mares with reproductive disorders. *Acta Veterinaria Hungarica* **51**:45–52.

Theegarten D, Sachse K, Mentrup B, Fey K, Hotzel H, Anhenn O 2008. *Chlamydophila* spp. infection in horses with recurrent airway obstruction: similarities to human chronic obstructive disease. *Respiratory Research* **9**:14.

Vězník Z, Svecová D, Pospísil L, Diblíková I 1996. Detection of chlamydiae in animal and human semen using direct immunofluorescence. *Veterinary Medicin (Praha)* **41**:201–206.

Wills JM, Watson G, Lusher M, Mair TS, Wood D, Richmond SJ 1990. Characterisation of *Chlamydia psittaci* isolated from a horse. *Veterinary Microbiology* **24**:11–19.

Borrelia burgdorferi

Alekseev AN, Arumova EA, Vasilieva IS 1995. *Borrelia burgdorferi* sensu lato in female cement plug of *Ixodes persulcatus* ticks (*Acari, Ixodidae*). *Experimental and Applied Acarology* **19**:519–522.

Bhide M, Yilmaz Z, Golcu E, Torun S, Mikula I 2008. Seroprevalence of anti-*Borrelia burgdorferi* antibodies in dogs and horses in Turkey. *Annals of Agricultural and Environmental Medicine* **15**:85–90.

Browning A, Carter SD, Barnes A, May C, Bennett D 1993. Lameness associated with *Borrelia burgdorferi* infection in the horse. *Veterinary Record* **132**:610–611.

Burgess EC, Gillette D, Pickett JP 1986. Arthritis and panuveitis as manifestations of *Borrelia burgdorferi* infection in a Wisconsin pony. *Journal of the American Veterinary Medical Association* **189**:1340–1342.

Burgess EC, Gendron-Fitzpatrick A, Mattison M 1987a. Foal mortality associated with natural infection of pregnant mares with *Borrelia burgdorferi* (Abstract). *5th International Conference of Equine Infectious Diseases*:217.

Burgess EC, Mattison M 1987b. Encephalitis associated with *Borrelia burgdorferi* infection in a horse. *Journal of the American Veterinary Medical Association* **191**:1457–1458.

Butler CM, Houwers DJ, Jongejan F, Kolk JH van der 2005. *Borrelia burgdorferi* infections with special reference to horses. A review. *Veterinary Quarterly* **27**:146–156.

Chang YF, Novosol V, McDonough SP, *et al.* 2000. Experimental infection of ponies with *Borrelia burgdorferi* by exposure to Ixodid ticks. *Veterinary Pathology* **37**:68–76.

Divers TJ, Chang YF, Jacobson RH, McDonough SP 2001. Lyme disease in horses. *Compendium on Continuing Education for the Practicing Veterinarian* **23**:375–380.

Divers TJ, Chang YF, McDonough PL 2003. Equine Lyme disease: a review of experimental disease production, treatment efficacy, and vaccine protection. *49th Annual Convention of the American Association of Equine Practitioners*, November 2003, New Orleans, Louisiana, USA.

Gern L, Estrada-Pena A, Frandsen F, *et al.* 1998. European reservoir hosts of *Borrelia burgdorferi* sensu lato. *Zentralblatt für Bakteriologie* **287**:196–204.

Hahn CN, Mayhew IG, Whitwell KE, *et al.* 1996. A possible case of Lyme borreliosis in a horse in the UK. *Equine Veterinary Journal* **28**:84–88.

Hansen MG, Christoffersen M, Thuesen LR, Petersen MR, Bojesen AM 2010. Seroprevalence of *Borrelia burgdorferi* sensu lato and *Anaplasma phagocytophilum* in Danish horses. *Acta Veterinaria Scandinavica* 52:49.

Hasle G, Bjune G, Edvardsen E, *et al.* 2009. Transport of ticks by migratory passerine birds to Norway. *Journal of Parasitology* 95:1342–1351.

Humair PF, Rais O, Gern L 1999. Transmission of *Borrelia afzelii* from *Apodemus* mice and *Clethrionomys* voles to *Ixodes ricinus* ticks: differential transmission pattern and overwintering maintenance. *Parasitology* 118:33–42.

Humair PF 2002. Birds and *Borrelia*. *International Journal of Medical Microbiology* 291:70–74.

James FM, Engiles JB, Beech J 2010. Meningitis, cranial neuritis, and radiculoneuritis associated with *Borrelia burgdorferi* infection in a horse. *Journal of the American Veterinary Medical Assciation* 237:1180–1185.

Johnson AL, Divers TJ, Chang YF 2008. Validation of an in-clinic enzyme-linked immunosorbent assay kit for diagnosis of *Borrelia burgdorferi* infection in horses. *Journal of Veterinary Diagnostic Investigation* 20:321–324.

Magnarelli LA, Anderson JF, Shaw E, Post JE, Palka FC 1988. Borreliosis in equids in northeastern United States. *American Journal of Veterinary Research* 49:359–362.

Magnarelli LA, Flavell RA, Padula SJ, Anderson JF, Fikrig E 1997. Serologic diagnosis of canine and equine borreliosis: use of recombinant antigens in enzyme-linked immunosorbent assays. *Journal of Clinical Microbiology* 35:169–173.

Magnarelli LA, Ijdo JW, Andel AE van, Wu C, Padula SJ, Fikrig E 2000. Serologic confirmation of *Ehrlichia equi* and *Borrelia burgdorferi* infections in horses from the northeastern United States. *Journal of the American Veterinary Medical Association* 217:1045–1050.

Manion TB, Khan MI, Dinger J, Bushmich SL 1998. Viable *Borrelia burgdorferi* in the urine of two clinically normal horses. *Journal of Veterinary Diagnostic Investigation* 10:196–199.

Marie-Angèle P, Lommano E, Humair PF, *et al.* 2006. Prevalence of *Borrelia burgdorferi* sensu lato in ticks collected from migratory birds in Switzerland. *Applied and Environmental Microbiology* 72:976–979.

Maurizi L, Marié JL, Aoun O, *et al.* 2010. Seroprevalence survey of equine Lyme borreliosis in France and in sub-Saharan Africa. *Vector Borne and Zoonotic Diseases* 10:535–537.

Muller I, Khanakah G, Kundi M, Stanek G 2002. Horses and *Borrelia*: immunoblot patterns with five *Borrelia burgdorferi* sensu lato strains and sera from horses of various stud farms in Austria and from the Spanish Riding School in Vienna. *International Journal of Medical Microbiology* 291 Supplement 33:80–87.

Ogden NH, Lindsay LR, Hanincová K, *et al.* 2008. Role of migratory birds in introduction and range expansion of *Ixodes scapularis* ticks and of *Borrelia burgdorferi* and *Anaplasma phagocytophilum* in Canada. *Applied and Environmental Microbiology* 74:1780–1790.

Pal U, Li X, Wang T, *et al.* 2004. TROSPA, an *Ixodes scapularis* receptor for *Borrelia burgdorferi*. *Cell* 119:457–468.

Persing DH 1997. The cold zone: a curious convergence of tick-transmitted diseases. *Clinical Infectious Diseases* 25 Supplement 1:S35–S42.

Piesman J, Mather TN, Sinsky RJ, Spielman A 1987. Duration of tick attachment and *Borrelia burgdorferi* transmission. *Journal of Clinical Microbiology* 25:557–558.

Qiu WG, Schutzer SE, Bruno JF, *et al.* 2004. Genetic exchange and plasmid transfers in *Borrelia burgdorferi* sensu stricto revealed by three-way genome comparisons and multilocus sequence typing. *Proceedings of the National Academy of Sciences of the United States of America* 101:14150–14155.

Sorensen K, Neely DP, Grappell PM, Read W 1990. Lyme disease antibodies in Thoroughbred mares, correlation to early pregnancy failure. *Equine Veterinary Journal* 10:166–168.

Stanek G, Gray J, Strle F, Wormser G 2004. Lyme borreliosis. *Lancet Infectious Diseases* 4:197–199.

Steere AC 2006. Lyme borreliosis in 2005, 30 years after initial observations in Lyme Connecticut. *Wiener Klinische Wochenschrift* 118:625–633.

Stefancikova A, Adaszek Ł, Pet'ko B, Winiarczyk S, Dudinák V 2008. Serological evidence of *Borrelia burgdorferi* sensu lato in horses and cattle from Poland and diagnostic problems of Lyme borreliosis. *Annals of Agricultural and Environmental Medicine* 15:37–43.

Stricker RB, Lautin A, Burrascano JJ 2005. Lyme disease: point/counterpoint. *Expert Review of Anti-Infective Therapy* 3:155–165.

Thanassi WT, Schoen RT 2000. The Lyme disease vaccine: conception, development, and implementation. *Annals of Internal Medicine* 132:661–667.

Trevejo RT, Krause PJ, Sikand VK, *et al.* 1999. Evaluation of two-test serodiagnostic method for early Lyme disease in clinical practice. *Journal of Infectious Diseases* 179:931–938.

Wang G, Dam AP van, Schwartz I, Dankert J 1999. Molecular typing of *Borrelia burgdorferi* sensu lato: taxonomic, epidemiological, and clinical implications. *Clinical Microbiology Reviews* 12:633–653.

Wodecka B 2003. Detection of *Borrelia burgdorferi* sensu lato DNA in *Ixodes ricinus* ticks in North-Western Poland. *Annals of Agricultural and Environmental Medicine* 10:171–178.

Leptospira interrogans

Ahmad SN, Shah S, Ahmad FM 2005. Laboratory diagnosis of leptospirosis. *Journal of Postgraduate Medicine* 51:195–200.

Båverud V, Gunnarsson A, Engvall EO, Franzén P, Egenvall A 2009. Leptospira seroprevalence and associations between seropositivity, clinical disease and host factors in horses. *Acta Veterinaria Scandinavica* 51:15–25.

Bernard WV, Williams D, Tuttle PA, Pierce S 1993. Hematuria and leptospiruria in a foal. *Journal of the American Veterinary Medical Association* 203:276–278.

Blackmore DK, Bahaman AR, Marshall RB 1982. The epidemiological interpretation of serological responses to leptospiral serovars in sheep. *New Zealand Veterinary Journal* 30:38–42.

Charon NW, Goldstein SF 2002. Genetics of motility and chemotaxis of a fascinating group of bacteria: the spirochetes. *Annual Review of Genetics* **36**:47–73.

Divers TJ, Irby NL, Mohammed HO, Schwark WS 2008. Ocular penetration of intravenously administered enrofloxacin in the horse. *Equine Veterinary Journal* **40**:167–170.

Donahue JM, Williams NM 2000. Emergent causes of placentitis and abortion. *Veterinary Clinics of North America: Equine Practice* **16**:443–456.

Ellis WA, Bryson DG, O'Brien JJ, Neil SD 1983. Leptospiral infection in aborted equine foetuses. *Equine Veterinary Journal* **15**:321–324.

Frazer ML 1999. Acute renal failure from leptospirosis in a foal. *Australian Veterinary Journal* **77**:499–500.

Ingh TSGAM van den, Hartman FG, Bercovich Z 1989. Clinical *Leptospira interrogans* serogroup *australis* serovar *lora* infection in a stud farm in The Netherlands. *Veterinary Quarterly* **11**:175–182.

Jung BY, Lee KW, Ha TY 2010. Seroprevalence of *Leptospira* spp. in clinically healthy racing horses in Korea. *Journal of Veterinary Medical Science* **72**:197–201.

Leon A, Pronost S, Tapprest J, *et al.* 2006. Identification of pathogenic *Leptospira* strains in tissues of a premature foal by use of polymerase chain reaction analysis. *Journal of Veterinary Diagnostic Investigation* **18**:218–221.

Nagamine CM, Castro F, Buchanan B, Schumacher J, Craig LE 2005. Proliferative pododermatitis (canker) with intralesional spirochetes in three horses. *Journal of Veterinary Diagnostic Investigation* **17**:269–271.

Poonacha KB, Donahue JM, Giles RC, *et al.* 1993. Leptospirosis in equine fetuses, stillborn foals, and placentas. *Veterinary Pathology* **30**:362–369.

Rimpau W 1947. Leptospirose beim Pferde. *Tierarztliche Umschau* **2**:177.

Rocha T, Ellis WA, Montgomery J, Gilmore C, Regalla J, Brem S 2004. Microbiological and serological study of leptospirosis in horses at slaughter: first isolations. *Research in Veterinary Science* **76**:199–202.

Rohrbach BW, Ward DA, Hendrix DVH, Cawrse-Foss M, Moyers TD 2005. Effect of vaccination against leptospirosis on the frequency, days to recurrence and progression of disease in horses with equine recurrent uveitis. *Veterinary Ophthalmology* **8**:171–179.

Sebastian M, Giles R, Roberts J, *et al.* 2005. Funisitis associated with leptospiral abortion in an equine placenta. *Veterinary Pathology* **42**:659–662.

Szeredi L, Haake DA 2006. Immunohistochemical identification and pathologic findings in natural cases of equine abortion caused by leptospiral infection. *Veterinary Pathology* **43**:755–761.

Torfs S, Goossens E, Bauwens C, Durie I, Loon G van 2009. Leptospirosis as a cause of acute respiratory distress and renal failure in two foals. *Proc 3rd ECEIM Congress*, Barcelona, Spain. 28–30 January 2009:13–14.

Verma A, Rathinam SR, Priya CG, Muthukkaruppan VR, Stevenson B, Timoney JF 2008. LruA and LruB antibodies in sera of humans with leptospiral uveitis. *Clinical and Vaccine Immunology* **15**:1019–1023.

Whitwell KE, Blunden AS, Miller J, Errington J 2009. Two cases of equine pregnancy loss associated with *Leptospira* infection in England. *Veterinary Record* **165**:377–378.

Williams RD, Morter RL, Freeman MJ, Lavignette AM 1971. Experimental chronic uveitis. Ophthalmic signs following equine leptospirosis. *Investigative Ophthalmology* **10**:948–954.

Wollanke B, Rohrbach BW, Gerhards H 2001. Serum and vitreous humor antibody titers in and isolation of *Leptospira interrogans* from horses with recurrent uveitis. *Journal of the American Veterinary Medical Association* **219**:795–800.

Yan W, Faisal SM, Divers T, McDonough SP, Akey B, Chang YF 2010. Experimental *Leptospira interrogans* serovar *kennewicki* infection of horses. *Journal of Veterinary Internal Medicine* **24**:912–917.

Bacteroidaceae and Fusobacteriaceae

Bailey GD, Love DN 1991. Oral associated bacterial infection in horses: studies on the normal anaerobic flora from the pharyngeal tonsillar surface and its association with lower respiratory tract and paraoral infections. *Veterinary Microbiology* **26**:367–379.

Bienert A, Bartmann CP, Verspohl J, Deegen E 2003. Bacteriological findings for endodontical and apical molar dental diseases in the horse. *Deutsche Tierärztliche Wochenschrift* **110**:358–361.

Bramanti TE, Holt SC 1991. Roles of porphyrins and host iron transport proteins in regulation of growth of *Porphyromonas gingivalis* W50. *Journal of Bacteriology* **173**:7330–7339.

Carlson GP, O'Brien MA 1990. Anaerobic bacterial pneumonia with septicemia in two racehorses. *Journal of the American Veterinary Medical Association* **196**:941–943.

Dorsch M, Lovet DN, Bailey GD 2001. *Fusobacterium equinum* sp. *nov.*, from the oral cavity of horses. *International Journal of Systemic Evolutionary Microbiology* **51**:1959–1963.

Ledbetter EC, Scarlett JM 2008. Isolation of obligate anaerobic bacteria from ulcerative keratitis in domestic animals. *Veterinary Ophthalmology* **11**:114–122.

Mair TS 1996. Bacterial pneumonia associated with corticosteroid therapy in three horses. *Veterinary Record* **138**:205–207.

Milinovich GJ, Trott DJ, Burrell PC, *et al.* 2007. Fluorescence *in situ* hybridization analysis of hindgut bacteria associated with the development of equine laminitis. *Environmental Microbiology* **9**:2090–2100.

Myers LL, Shoop DS, Byars TD 1987. Diarrhea associated with enterotoxigenic *Bacteroides fragilis* in foals. *American Journal of Veterinary Research* **48**:1565–1567.

Peek SF, Divers TJ 2000. Medical treatment of cholangiohepatitis and cholelithiasis in mature horses: 9 cases (1991–1998). *Equine Veterinary Journal* **32**:301–306.

Racklyeft DJ, Love DN 2000. Bacterial infection of the lower respiratory tract in 34 horses. *Australian Veterinary Journal* **78**:549–559.

Botryomycosis

Bersoff-Matcha SJ, Roper CC, Liapis H, Little JR 1998. Primary pulmonary botryomycosis: case report and review. *Clinical Infectious Diseases* **26**:620–624.

Bollinger O 1870. Mycosis der Lunge beim Pferde. *Virchows Archive A: Pathological Anatomy and Histology* **49**:583–586.

CHAPTER 2 VIRAL DISEASES

Equine adenovirus

Corrier DE, Montgomery D, Scutchfield WL 1982. *Adenovirus* in the intestinal epithelium of a foal with prolonged diarrhea. *Veterinary Pathology* **19**:564–567.

Davison AJ, Benko M, Harrach B 2003. Genetic content and evolution of *adenoviruses*. Review. *Journal of General Virology* **84**(Pt 11):2895–2908.

Giles C, Cavanagh HM, Noble G, Vanniasinkam T 2010. Prevalence of equine adenovirus antibodies in horses in New South Wales, Australia. *Veterinary Microbiology* **143**:401–404.

Mair TS, Taylor FG, Harbour DA, Pearson GR 1990. Concurrent *cryptosporidium* and *coronavirus* infections in an Arabian foal with combined immunodeficiency syndrome. *Veterinary Record* **126**:127–130.

McChesney AE, England JJ, Whiteman CE, Adcock JL, Rich LJ, Chow TL 1974. Experimental transmission of equine adenovirus in Arabian and non-Arabian foals. *American Journal of Veterinary Research* **35**:1015–1023.

Moro MR, Bonville CA, Suryadevara M, *et al.* 2009. Clinical features, adenovirus types, and local production of inflammatory mediators in *adenovirus* infections. *Pediatric Infectious Disease Journal* **28**:376–380.

Newton JR, Wood JLN, Chanter N 2003. A case control study of factors and infections associated with clinically apparent respiratory disease in UK Thoroughbred racehorses. *Preventive Veterinary Medicine* **60**:107–132.

Phan TG, Shimizu H, Nishimura S, Okitsu S, Maneekarn N, Ushijima H 2006. Human adenovirus type 1 related to feline adenovirus: evidence of interspecies transmission. *Clinical Laboratory* **52**:515–518.

Sentsui H, Wu D, Murakami K, Kondo T, Matsumura T 2010. Antiviral effect of recombinant equine interferon-gamma on several equine viruses. *Veterinary Immunology and Immunopathology* **135**:93–99.

Studdert MJ, Blackney MH 1982. Isolation of an adenovirus antigenically distinct from equine adenovirus type 1 from diarrheic foal faeces. *American Journal of Veterinary Research* **43**:543–544.

Thompson DB, Studdert MJ, Beilharz RG, Littlejohns IR 1975. Inheritance of a lethal immunodeficiency disease of Arabian foals. *Australian Veterinary Journal* **51**:109–113.

Webb RF, Knight PR, Walker KH 1981. Involvement of adenovirus in pneumonia in a thoroughbred foal. *Australian Veterinary Journal* **57**:142–143.

Equine herpesvirus

Allen GP, Breathnach CC 2006. Quantification by real-time PCR of the magnitude and duration of leucocyte-associated viraemia in horses infected with neuropathogenic *vs.* non-neuropathogenic strains of EHV-1. *Equine Veterinary Journal* **38**:252–257.

Allen GP, Kydd JH, Slater JD, Smith KC 1998. Advances in understanding of the pathogenesis, epidemiology and immunological control of equine herpesvirus abortion. *Proceedings of the 8th International Conference on Equine Infectious Diseases*. Dubai:129–146.

Borchers K, Wolfinger U, Ludwig H, *et al.* 1998. Virological and molecular biological investigations into equine herpes virus type 2 (EHV-2) experimental infections. *Virus Research* **55**:101–106.

Borchers K, Wolfinger U, Ludwig H 1999. Latency-associated transcripts of equine herpesvirus type 4 in trigeminal ganglia of naturally infected horses. *Journal of General Virology* **80**:2165–2171.

Browning GF, Bulach DM, Ficorilli N, Roy EA, Thorp BH, Studdert MJ 1988. Latency of equine herpesvirus 4 (equine rhinopneumonitis virus). *Veterinary Record* **123**:518–519.

Carvalho R, Oliveira AM, Souza AM, Passos LM, Martins AS 2000. Prevalence of equine herpesvirus type 1 latency detected by polymerase chain reaction. *Archives of Virology* **145**:1773–1787.

Crabb BS, Studdert MJ 1993. Epitopes of glycoprotein G of equine herpesviruses 4 and 1 located near the C termini elicit type-specific antibody responses in the natural host. *Journal of Virology* **67**:6332–6338.

Crabb BS, Studdert MJ 1995. Equine herpesviruses 4 (equine rhinopneumonitis virus) and 1 (equine abortion virus). *Advances in Virus Research* **45**:153–190.

Crabb BS, MacPherson CM, Reubel GH, Browning GF, Studdert MJ, Drummer HE 1995. A type-specific serological test to distinguish antibodies to equine herpesviruses 4 and 1. *Archives of Virology* **140**:245–258.

Croubels S 2009. A pharmacokinetic and pharmacodynamic approach for dosing valacyclovir against equine herpesvirus type 1 infections. *4th World Equine Airways Symposium (WEAS)* August 5–7, 2009. Berne, Switzerland. Abstract:138–140.

Dinter Z, Klingeborn B 1976. Serological study of an outbreak of paresis due to equid herpesvirus 1 (EHV-1). *Veterinary Record* **99**:10–12.

Edington N, Welch HM, Griffiths L 1994. The prevalence of latent equid herpesviruses in the tissues of 40 abattoir horses. *Equine Veterinary Journal* **26**:140–142.

Flore PH, Minke JM, Mumford JA, *et al.* 1998. Studies on efficacy of an inactivated, carbomer-adjuvated equine herpes-virus vaccine in pregnant mares in face of a challenge with an abortigenic strain of EHV-1. *Proceedings of the 8th International Conference on Equine Infectious Diseases*. Dubai:422–423.

Frampton AR Jr, Stolz DB, Uchida H, Goins WF, Cohen JB, Glorioso JC 2007. Equine herpesvirus 1 enters cells by two different pathways, and infection requires the activation of the cellular kinase ROCK1. *Journal of Virology* **81**:10879–10889.

Gilkerson JR, Love DN, Whalley JM 1997. Serological evidence of equine herpesvirus 1 (EHV-1) infection in Thoroughbred foals 30–120 days of age. *Australian Equine Veterinarian* **15**:128–134.

Gilkerson JR, Whalley JM, Drummer HE, Studdert MJ, Love DN 1999. Epidemiological studies of equine herpesvirus-1 (EHV-1) in Thoroughbred foals: a review of studies conducted in the Hunter Valley of New South Wales between 1995 and 1997. *Veterinary Microbiology* **68**:15–25.

Goehring LS, van Winden SC, van Maanen C, Sloet van Oldruitenborgh-Oosterbaan MM 2006. Equine herpesvirus type 1-associated myeloencephalopathy in The Netherlands: a four-year retrospective study (1999–2003). *Journal of Veterinary Internal Medicine* 20:601–607.

Goehring LS, Landolt GA, Morley PS 2010a. Detection and management of an outbreak of equine herpesvirus type 1 infection and associated neurological disease in a veterinary teaching hospital. *Journal of Veterinary Internal Medicine* 24:1176–1183.

Goehring LS, Wagner B, Bigbie R, et al. 2010b. Control of EHV-1 viremia and nasal shedding by commercial vaccines. *Vaccine* 28:5203–5211.

Goehring LS, Hussey GS, Ashton LV, Schenkel AR, Lunn DP 2011. Infection of central nervous system endothelial cells by cell-associated EHV-1. *Veterinary Microbiology* 148:389–395.

Goodman LB, Loregian A, Perkins GA, et al. 2007. A point mutation in a herpesvirus polymerase determines neuropathogenicity. *PLoS Pathogens* 3:e160.

Heldens JG, Hannant D, Cullinane AA, et al. 2001. Clinical and virological evaluation of the efficacy of an inactivated EHV1 and EHV4 whole virus vaccine (Duvaxyn EHV1,4). Vaccination/challenge experiments in foals and pregnant mares. *Vaccine* 19:4307–4317.

Holmes MA, Townsend HGG, Kohler AK, et al. 2006. Immune responses to commercial equine vaccines against equine herpesvirus-1, equine influenza virus, eastern equine encephalomyelitis, and tetanus. *Veterinary Immunology and Immunopathology* 111:67–80.

Jackson TA, Osburn BI, Cordy DR, Kendrick JW 1977. Equine herpesvirus 1 infection of horses: studies on the experimentally induced neurologic disease. *American Journal of Veterinary Research* 38:709–719.

Jesset DM, Schrag D, Mumford JA 1998. Protection provided by an attenuated EHV-1 vaccine against challenge with the virulent AB4 isolate. *Proceedings of the 8th International Conference on Equine Infectious Diseases*. Dubai:414.

Jubb KVF, Kennedy PC, Palmer N 2007. *Pathology of Domestic Animals*, 5th edn. WB Saunders Elsevier, Edinburgh, 2:532–533.

Lunn DP, Davis-Poynter N, Flaminio MJ, et al. 2009. Equine herpesvirus-1 consensus statement. *Journal of Veterinary Internal Medicine* 23:450–461.

Maanen C van 2001. Equine herpesvirus 1 and 4 and equine influenza virus infections: diagnosis, epidemiology and vaccinology. PhD Thesis Utrecht University, Utrecht, the Netherlands.

Maanen C van 2002. Equine herpesvirus 1 and 4: an update. *Veterinary Quarterly* 24:57–78.

Maanen C van, Vreeswijk J, Moonen P, Brinkhof J, Boer-Luijtze E de, Terpstra C 2000. Differentiation and genomic and antigenic variation among fetal, respiratory, and neurological isolates from EHV1 and EHV4 infections in the Netherlands. *Veterinary Quarterly* 22:83–87.

Maanen C van, Sloet van Oldruitenborgh-Oosterbaan MM, Damen EA, Derksen AG 2001. Neurological disease associated with EHV-1-infection in a riding school: clinical and virological characteristics. *Equine Veterinary Journal* 33:191–196.

Mackie JT, Macleod GA, Reubel GH, Studdert MJ 1996. Diagnosis of equine herpesvirus 1 abortion using polymerase chain reaction. *Australian Veterinary Journal* 74:390–391.

Malik P, Pálfi V, Bálint A 2010. Development of a new primer-probe energy transfer method for the differentiation of neuropathogenic and non-neuropathogenic strains of equine herpesvirus-1. *Journal of Virological Methods* 169:425–427.

Murray MJ, Del Piero F, Jeffrey SC, et al. 1998. Neonatal equine herpesvirus type 1 infection on a Thoroughbred breeding farm. *Journal of Veterinary Internal Medicine* 12:36–41.

Nugent J, Birch-Machin I, Smith KC, et al. 2006. Analysis of equid herpesvirus 1 strain variation reveals a point mutation of the DNA polymerase strongly associated with neuropathogenic versus nonneuropathogenic disease outbreaks. *Journal of Virology* 80:4047–4060.

Patel JR, Heldens J 2005. Equine herpesviruses 1 (EHV-1) and 4 (EHV-4) – epidemiology, disease and immunoprophylaxis: a brief review. *Veterinary Journal* 170:14–23.

Perkins GA, Goodman LB, Dubovi EJ, Kim SG, Osterrieder N 2008. Detection of equine herpesvirus-1 in nasal swabs of horses by quantitative real-time PCR. *Journal of Veterinary Internal Medicine* 22:1234–1238.

Pusterla N, Mapes S, Wilson WD 2008. Diagnostic sensitivity of nasopharyngeal and nasal swabs for the molecular detection of EHV-1. *Veterinary Record* 162:520–521.

Pusterla N, Mapes S, Wilson WD 2010. Prevalence of equine herpesvirus type 1 in trigeminal ganglia and submandibular lymph nodes of equids examined postmortem. *Veterinary Record* 167:376–378.

Slater J 2007. Equine herpesviruses. In: Sellon DC, Long MT, eds. *Equine Infectious Diseases*. Saunders Elsevier, St. Louis:134–152.

Slater JD, Borchers K, Thackray AM, Field HJ 1994. The trigeminal ganglion is a location for equine herpesvirus 1 latency and reactivation in the horse. *Journal of General Virology* 75:2007–2016.

Thein P 1981. Infection of the central nervous system of horses with equine herpesvirus serotype 1. *Journal of the South African Veterinary Association* 52:239–241.

Thorsteinsdóttir L, Torfason EG, Torsteinsdóttir S, Svansson V 2010. Isolation and partial sequencing of equid herpesvirus 5 from a horse in Iceland. *Journal of Veterinary Diagnostic Investigation* 22:420–423.

Welch HM, Bridges CG, Lyon AM, Griffiths L, Edington N 1992. Latent equid herpesvirus 1 and 4 detection and distinction using the polymerase chain reaction and co-cultivation from lymphoid tissues. *Journal of General Virology* 73:261–268.

Williams KJ, Maes R, Del Piero F, et al. 2007. Equine multinodular pulmonary fibrosis: a newly recognized herpesvirus-associated fibrotic lung disease. *Veterinary Pathology* 44:849–862.

Wilson WD 1997. Equine herpesvirus 1 myeloencephalopathy. *Veterinary Clinics of North America: Equine Practice* 13:53–72.

Suid herpesvirus 1

Ingh TSGAM van den, Binkhorst GJ, Kimman TG, Vreeswijk J, Pol JMA, Oirschot JT van 1990. Aujeszky's disease in a horse. *Zentralblatt für Veterinaermedizin Reihe B* 37:532–538.

Kimman TG, Binkhorst GJ, Ingh TSGAM van den, Pol JM, Gielkens AL, Roelvink ME 1991. Aujeszky's disease in horses fulfils Koch's postulates. *Veterinary Record* 128:103–106.

Bovine and equine papillomavirus

Bogaert L, Van Poucke M, De Baere C, *et al.* 2007. Bovine papillomavirus load and mRNA expression, cell proliferation and p53 expression in four clinical types of equine sarcoid. *Journal of General Virology* 88:2155–2161.

Bogaert L, Martens A, Kast WM, Van Marck E, De Cock H 2010. Bovine papillomavirus DNA can be detected in keratinocytes of equine sarcoid tumors. *Veterinary Microbiology* 146:269–275.

Boom R van den, Veldhuis Kroeze EJ, Klein WR, Houwers DJ, van der Zanden AG, Sloet van Oldruitenborgh-Oosterbaan MM 2008. Granulomatous pneumonia, lymphadenopathy, and hepatopathy in an adult horse with repeated injection of BCG. *Journal of Veterinary Internal Medicine* 22:1056–1060.

Brandt S, Haralambus R, Schoster A, Kirnbauer R, Stanek C 2008. Peripheral blood mononuclear cells represent a reservoir of bovine papillomavirus DNA in sarcoid-affected equines. *Journal of General Virology* 89:1390–1395.

Carr EA, Theon AP, Madewell BR, Hitchcock ME, Schlegel R, Schiller JT 2001. Expression of a transforming gene (E5) of bovine papillomavirus in sarcoids obtained from horses. *American Journal of Veterinary Research* 62:1212–1217.

Dyk E van, Oosthuizen MC, Bosman AM, Nel PJ, Zimmerman D, Venter EH 2009. Detection of bovine papillomavirus DNA in sarcoid-affected and healthy free-roaming zebra (*Equus zebra*) populations in South Africa. *Journal of Virological Methods* 158:141–151.

Dzirlo L, Hubner M, Müller C, *et al.* 2007. A mimic of sarcoidosis. *Lancet* 369:1832.

Gobcil PA, Yuan Z, Gault EA, Morgan IM, Campo MS, Nasir L 2009. Small interfering RNA targeting bovine papillomavirus type 1 E2 induces apoptosis in equine sarcoid transformed fibroblasts. *Virus Research* 145:162–165.

Hallamaa RE 2008. Ultrastructural changes in regressing equine sarcoid tumours—mysterious role of mitochondria. *In Vivo* 22:519–523.

Haralambus R, Burgstaller J, Klukowska-Rötzler J, *et al.* 2010. Intralesional bovine papillomavirus DNA loads reflect severity of equine sarcoid disease. *Equine Veterinary Journal* 42:327–331.

Lancaster WD, Theilen GH, Olson C 1979. Hybridisation of bovine papillomavirus type 1 and type 2 DNA to DNA from virus-induced hamster tumours and naturally occurring equine tumours. *Intervirology* 11:227–233.

Lange CE, Tobler K, Ackermann M, Favrot C 2011. Identification of two novel equine papillomavirus sequences suggests three genera in one cluster. *Veterinary Microbiology* 149:85–90.

Marth T, Raoult D 2003. Whipple's disease. *Lancet* 361:239–246.

Nixon C, Chambers G, Ellsmore V, *et al.* 2005. Expression of cell cycle associated proteins cyclin A, CDK-2, p27kip1 and p53 in equine sarcoids. *Cancer Letters* 221:237–245.

Relman DA, Schmidt TM, MacDermott RP, Falkow S 1992. Identification of the uncultured bacillus of Whipple's disease. *New England Journal of Medicine* 327:293–301.

Vanderstraeten E, Bogaert L, Bravo IG, Martens A 2011. EcPV2 DNA in equine squamous cell carcinomas and normal genital and ocular mucosa. *Veterinary Microbiology* 147:292–299.

Villiers EM de, Fauquet C, Broker TR, Bernard HU, Hausen H zur 2004. Classification of papillomaviruses. *Virology* 324:17–27.

Yuan Z, Gallagher A, Gault EA, Campo MS, Nasir L 2007. Bovine papillomavirus infection in equine sarcoids and in bovine bladder cancers. *Veterinary Journal* 174:599–604.

Horsepox virus

Ellenberger C, Schüppel KF, Möhring M, *et al.* 2005. Cowpox virus infection associated with a streptococcal septicaemia in a foal. *Journal of Comparative Pathology* 132:101–105.

Jubb KVF, Kennedy PC, Palmer N 2007. *Pathology of Domestic Animals*, 5th edn. WB Saunders Elsevier, Edinburgh, 1:669–670.

Kaminjolo JS Jr, Johnson LW, Frank H, Gicho JN 1974. Vaccinia like Pox virus identified in a horse with a skin disease. *Zentralblatt Veterinärmedizin Reihe B* 21:202–206.

Lange L, Marett S, Maree C, Gerdes T 1991. Molluscum contagiosum in three horses. *Journal of the South African Veterinary Association* 62:68–71.

Rensburg IB van, Collett MG, Ronen N, Gerdes T 1991. Molluscum contagiosum in a horse. *Journal of the South African Veterinary Association* 62:72–74.

Scheinfeld N 2007. Treatment of molluscum contagiosum: a brief review and discussion of a case successfully treated with adapelene. *Dermatology Online Journal* 13:15.

Thompson CH, Yager JA, Rensburg IB van 1998. Close relationship between equine and human molluscum contagiosum virus demonstrated by *in situ* hybridisation. *Research in Veterinary Science* 64:157–161.

Tulman ER, Delhon G, Afonso CL, *et al.* 2006. Genome of horsepox virus. *Journal of Virology* 80:9244–9258.

Wouden JC van der, Menke J, Gajadin S, *et al.* 2006. Interventions for cutaneous molluscum contagiosum. Review. *Cochrane Database Systematic Reviews* 2:CD004767.

Zhang L, Villa NY, McFadden G 2009. Interplay between poxviruses and the cellular ubiquitin/ubiquitin-like pathways. Review. *FEBS Letters* 583:607–614.

Equine arteritis virus

Balasuriya UB, Hedges JF, Nadler SA, McCollum WH, Timoney PJ, MacLachlan NJ 1999. Genetic stability of equine arteritis virus during horizontal and vertical transmission in an outbreak of equine viral arteritis. *Journal of General Virology* 80:1949–1958.

Belak S, Stade T, Bjorklund H, *et al.* 1999. Genetic diversity among field isolates of equine arteritis virus. *Proceedings of the 8th International Conference on Equine Infectious Diseases* 8:177–183.

Cavanagh D, Brien DA, Brinton M, *et al.* 1994. Revision of the taxonomy of the coronavirus, togavirus and arterivirus genera. *Archives of Virology* 135:227–237.

Del Piero F 2000. Equine viral arteritis. *Veterinary Pathology* 37:287–296.

Doll ER, Bryans JT, McCollum WH, Crowe MEW 1957*a*. Isolation of a filterable agent causing arteritis of horses and abortion by mares. Its differentiation from equine abortion (influenza) virus. *Cornell Veterinarian* 47:3–41.

Doll ER, Knappenberger RE, Bryans JT 1957*b*. An outbreak of abortion caused by the equine arteritis virus. *Cornell Veterinarian* 47:69–75.

Duthie S, Mills H, Burr P 2008. The efficacy of a commercial ELISA as an alternative to virus neutralisation test for the detection of antibodies to EAV. *Equine Veterinary Journal* 40:182–183.

Fukunaga Y, Imagawa H, Tabuchi E 1981. Clinical and virological findings on experimental equine viral arteritis in horses. *Bulletin of the Equine Research Institute* 18:110–113.

Fukunaga Y, Wada R, Imagawa H, Kanemaru T 1997. Venereal infection of mares by equine arteritis virus and use of killed vaccine against the infection. *Journal of Comparative Pathology* 117:201–208.

Glaser AL, Chirnside ED, Horzinek MC, de Vries AA 1997. Equine arteritis virus. *Theriogenology* 47:1275–1295.

Jones TC, Doll ER, Bryans JT 1957. The lesions of equine viral arteritis. *Cornell Veterinarian* 47:52–68.

MacLachlan NJ, Balasuriya UB 2006. Equine viral arteritis. Review. *Advances in Experimental Medicine and Biology* 581:429–433.

McCollum WH, Little TV, Timoney PJ, Swerczek TW 1994. Resistance of castrated male horses to attempted establishment of the carrier state with equine arteritis virus. *Journal of Comparative Pathology* 111:383–388.

Moore BD, Balasuriya UB, Watson JL, Bosio CM, MacKay RJ, MacLachlan NJ 2003. Virulent and avirulent strains of equine arteritis virus induce different quantities of TNF-alpha and other proinflammatory cytokines in alveolar and blood-derived equine macrophages. *Virology* 314:662–670.

Neu SM, Timoney PJ, McCollum WH 1987. Persistent infection of the reproductive tract in stallions experimentally infected with equine arteritis virus. *Proceedings of the 5th International Conference on Equine Infectious Diseases* 5:14.

Newton JR, Wood JL, Castillo-Olivares FJ, Mumford JA 1999. Serological surveillance of equine viral arteritis in the United Kingdom since the outbreak in 1993. *Veterinary Record* 145:511–516.

Pronost S, Pitel PH, Miszczak F, *et al.* 2010. Description of the first recorded major occurrence of equine viral arteritis in France. *Equine Veterinary Journal* 42:713–720.

Sentsui H, Wu D, Murakami K, Kondo T, Matsumura T 2010. Antiviral effect of recombinant equine interferon-gamma on several equine viruses. *Veterinary Immunology and Immunopathology* 135:93–99.

Timoney PJ, McCollum WH 1993. Equine viral arteritis. *Veterinary Clinics of North America: Equine Practice* 9:295–309.

Timoney PJ, McCollum WH, Murphy TW 1987. The carrier state in equine arteritis virus infection in the stallion with specific emphasis on the venereal mode of virus transmission. *Journal of Reproduction and Fertility* 35 (Supplement 1):95.

Vaala WE, Hamir AN, Dubovi EJ, Timoney PJ, Ruiz B 1992. Fatal congenitally acquired infection with equine arteritis virus in a neonatal Thoroughbred. *Equine Veterinary Journal* 24:155–158.

Wilkins PA, Del Piero F, Lopez J, Cline M 1995. Recognition of bronchopulmonary dysplasia in a newborn foal. *Equine Veterinary Journal* 27:398.

Zhang J, Timoney PJ, Shuck KM, *et al.* 2010. Molecular epidemiology and genetic characterization of equine arteritis virus isolates associated with the 2006–2007 multi-state disease occurrence in the USA. *Journal of General Virology* 91:2286–2301.

West Nile virus/Kunjin virus

Barzon L, Squarzon L, Cattai M, *et al.* 2009. West Nile virus infection in Veneto region, Italy, 2008–2009. *Euro Surveillance* 14:19289.

Bowen RA, Nemeth NM 2007. Experimental infections with West Nile virus. *Current Opinion in Infectious Diseases* 20:293–297.

Bunning ML, Bowen RA, Cropp CB, *et al.* 2002. Experimental infection of horses with West Nile virus. *Emerging Infectious Diseases* 8:380–386.

Cantile C, Di Guardo G, Eleni C, Arispici M 2000. Clinical and neuropathological features of West Nile virus equine encephalomyelitis in Italy. *Equine Veterinary Journal* 32:31–35.

Davis BS, Chang GJ, Cropp B, *et al.* 2001. West Nile virus recombinant DNA vaccine protects mouse and horse from virus challenge and expresses *in vitro* a noninfectious recombinant antigen that can be used in enzyme-linked immunosorbent assays. *Journal of Virology* 75:4040–4047.

Davis EG, Zhang Y, Tuttle J, Hankins K, Wilkerson M 2008. Investigation of antigen specific lymphocyte responses in healthy horses vaccinated with an inactivated West Nile virus vaccine. *Veterinary Immunology and Immunopathology* 126:293–301.

Durand B, Chevalier V, Pouillot R, *et al.* 2002. West Nile virus outbreak in horses, southern France, 2000: results of a serosurvey. *Emerging Infectious Diseases* 8:777–782.

Epp T, Waldner C, Townsend HG 2007. A case-control study of factors associated with development of clinical disease due to West Nile virus, Saskatchewan 2003. *Equine Veterinary Journal* 39:498–503.

Hall RA, Scherret JH, Mackenzie JS 2001. Kunjin virus: an Australian variant of West Nile? Review. *Annals of the New York Academy of Sciences* 951:153–160.

Hobson-Peters J, Toye P, Sánchez MD, *et al.* 2008. A glycosylated peptide in the West Nile virus envelope protein is immunogenic during equine infection. *Journal of General Virology* 89:3063–3072.

Hubálek Z, Halouzka J 1999. West Nile fever – a reemerging mosquito-borne viral disease in Europe. *Emerging Infectious Diseases* 5:643–650.

Jubb KVF, Kennedy PC, Palmer N 2007. *Pathology of Domestic Animals*, 5th edn. WB Saunders Elsevier, Edinburgh, 1:421–422.

Kitai Y, Kondo T, Konishi E 2011. Non-structural protein 1 (NS1) antibody-based assays to differentiate West Nile (WN) virus from Japanese encephalitis virus infections in horses: Effects of WN virus NS1 antibodies induced by inactivated WN vaccine. *Journal of Virological Methods* 171:123–128.

Laperriere V, Brugger K, Rubel F 2011. Simulation of the seasonal cycles of bird, equine, and human West Nile virus cases. *Preventive Veterinary Medicine* 98:99–110.

Lim AK, Dunne G, Gurfield N 2009. Rapid bilateral intraocular cocktail sampling method for West Nile virus detection in dead corvids. *Journal of Veterinary Diagnostic Investigation* 21:516–519.

López G, Jiménez-Clavero MA, Tejedor CG, Soriguer R, Figuerola J 2008. Prevalence of West Nile virus neutralizing antibodies in Spain is related to the behavior of migratory birds. *Vector Borne Zoonotic Diseases* 8:615–621.

Minke JM, Siger L, Karaca K, et al. 2004. Recombinant canarypoxvirus vaccine carrying the prM/E genes of West Nile virus protects horses against a West Nile virus-mosquito challenge. *Archives of Virology Supplement* 18:221–230.

Monaco F, Lelli R, Teodori L, et al. 2010. Re-Emergence of West Nile Virus in Italy. *Zoonoses and Public Health* 57:476–486.

Murray KO, Mertens E, Despres P 2010. West Nile virus and its emergence in the United States of America. *Veterinary Research* 41:67.

Nielsen CF, Reisen WK, Armijos MV, Maclachlan NJ, Scott TW 2008. High subclinical West Nile virus incidence among nonvaccinated horses in northern California associated with low vector abundance and infection. *American Journal of Tropical Medicine and Hygiene* 78:45–52.

Ostlund EN, Crom RL, Pedersen DD, Johnson DJ, Williams WO, Schmitt BJ 2001. Equine West Nile encephalitis, United States. *Emerging Infectious Diseases* 7:665–669.

Porter MB, Long MT, Getman LM, et al. 2003. West Nile virus encephalomyelitis in horses: 46 cases (2001). *Journal of the American Veterinary Medical Association* 222:1241–1247.

Rios JJ, Fleming JG, Bryant UK, et al. 2010. OAS1 polymorphisms are associated with susceptibility to West Nile encephalitis in horses. *PLoS One* 5:e10537.

Schmidt JR, El Mansoury HK 1963. Natural and experimental infection of Egyptian equines with West Nile virus. *Annals of Tropical Medicine and Parasitology* 57:415–427.

Sejvar JJ 2007. The long-term outcomes of human West Nile virus infection. *Clinical Infectious Diseases* 44:1617–1624.

Shirafuji H, Kanehira K, Kamio T, et al. 2009. Antibody responses induced by experimental West Nile virus infection with or without previous immunization with inactivated Japanese encephalitis vaccine in horses. *Journal of Veterinary Medical Science* 71:969–974.

Snook CS, Hyman SS, del Piero F, et al. 2001. West Nile virus encephalomyelitis in eight horses. *Journal of the American Veterinary Medical Association* 218:1576–1579.

Trock SC, Meade BJ, Glaser AL, et al. 2001. West Nile virus outbreak among horses in New York State, 1999 and 2000. *Emerging Infectious Diseases* 7:745–747.

Venter M, Swanepoel R 2010. West Nile virus lineage 2 as a cause of zoonotic neurological disease in humans and horses in southern Africa. *Vector Borne Zoonotic Diseases* 10:659–664.

Verma S, Lo Y, Chapagain M, et al. 2009. West Nile virus infection modulates human brain microvascular endothelial cells tight junction proteins and cell adhesion molecules: Transmigration across the *in vitro* blood–brain barrier. *Virology* 385:425–433.

Vorou RM, Papavassiliou VG, Tsiodras S 2007. Emerging zoonoses and vector-borne infections affecting humans in Europe. Review article. *Epidemiology and Infection* 135:1231–1247.

Ward MP, Levy M, Thacker HL, et al. 2004. Investigation of an outbreak of encephalomyelitis caused by West Nile virus in 136 horses. *Journal of the American Veterinary Medical Association* 225:84–89.

Zeller HG, Schuffenecker I 2004. West Nile virus: an overview of its spread in Europe and the Mediterranean basin in contrast to its spread in the Americas. *European Journal of Clinical Microbiology and Infectious Diseases* 23:147–156.

Japanese encephalitis virus/Murray Valley encephalitis virus

Chang GJ, Davis BS, Hunt AR, Holmes DA, Kuno G 2001. *Flavivirus* DNA vaccines: current status and potential. Review. *Annals of the New York Academy of Sciences* 951:272–285.

Dung NM, Turtle L, Chong WK, et al. 2009. An evaluation of the usefulness of neuroimaging for the diagnosis of Japanese encephalitis. *Journal of Neurology* 256:2052–2060.

Hall RA, Scherret JH, Mackenzie JS 2001. Kunjin virus: an Australian variant of West Nile? Review. *Annals of the New York Academy of Sciences* 951:153–160.

Hayasaka D, Nagata N, Fujii Y, et al. 2009. Mortality following peripheral infection with tick-borne encephalitis virus results from a combination of central nervous system pathology, systemic inflammatory and stress responses. *Virology* 390:139–150.

Hirota J, Nishi H, Matsuda H, Tsunemitsu H, Shimiz S 2010. Cross-reactivity of Japanese encephalitis virus-vaccinated horse sera in serodiagnosis of West Nile virus. *Journal of Veterinary Medical Science* 72:369–372.

Jubb KVF, Kennedy PC, Palmer N 2007. *Pathology of Domestic Animals*, 5th edn. WB Saunders Elsevier, Edinburgh, 1:422–423.

Kay BH, Pollitt CC, Fanning ID, Hall RA 1987. The experimental infection of horses with Murray Valley encephalitis and Ross River viruses. *Australian Veterinary Journal* 64:52–55.

Kitai Y, Shoda M, Kondo T, Konishi E 2007. Epitope-blocking enzyme-linked immunosorbent assay to differentiate West Nile virus from Japanese encephalitis virus infections in equine sera. *Clinical and Vaccine Immunology* 14:1024–1031.

Konishi E, Shoda M, Kondo T 2006. Analysis of yearly changes in levels of antibodies to Japanese encephalitis virus nonstructural 1 protein in racehorses in central Japan shows high levels of natural virus activity still exist. *Vaccine* 24:516–524.

Konishi E, Shoda M, Ajiro N, Kondo T 2004. Development and evaluation of an enzyme-linked immunosorbent assay for quantifying antibodies to Japanese encephalitis virus nonstructural 1 protein to detect subclinical infections in vaccinated horses. *Journal of Clinical Microbiology* 42:5087–5093.

Lam KH, Ellis TM, Williams DT, *et al.* 2005. Japanese encephalitis in a racing thoroughbred gelding in Hong Kong. *Veterinary Record* 157:168–173.

Lelli R, Savini G, Teodori L, *et al.* 2008. Serological evidence of USUTU virus occurrence in north-eastern Italy. *Zoonoses and Public Health* 55:361–367.

Pant GR, Lunt RA, Rootes CL, Daniels PW 2006. Serological evidence for Japanese encephalitis and West Nile viruses in domestic animals of Nepal. *Comparative Immunology, Microbiology and Infectious Diseases* 29:166–175.

Satou K, Nishiura H 2007. Evidence of the partial effects of inactivated Japanese encephalitis vaccination: analysis of previous outbreaks in Japan from 1953 to 1960. *Annals of Epidemiology* 17:271–277.

Solomon T, Mallewa M 2001. Dengue and other emerging flaviviruses. Review. *Journal of Infection* 42:104–115.

Yamanaka T, Tsujimura K, Kondo T, *et al.* 2006. Isolation and genetic analysis of *Japanese encephalitis virus* from a diseased horse in Japan 2006. *Journal of Veterinary Medical Science* 68:293–295.

Yang DK, Kim BH, Kweon CH, *et al.* 2008. Serosurveillance for Japanese encephalitis, Akabane, and Aino viruses for Thoroughbred horses in Korea. *Journal of Veterinary Science* 9:381–385.

Equine influenza virus

Bryant NA, Paillot R, Rash AS, *et al.* 2009. Comparison of two modern vaccines and previous influenza infection against challenge with an equine influenza virus from the Australian 2007 outbreak. *Veterinary Research* 41:19.

Chambers TM, Holland RE jr, Lai ACK 1995. Equine influenza – current veterinary perspectives, part 2. *Equine Practice* 17:26–30.

Chen JM, Sun YX, Chen JW, *et al.* 2009. Panorama phylogenetic diversity and distribution of type A influenza viruses based on their six internal gene sequences. *Virology Journal* 6:137.

Daly JM, Lai ACK, Binns MM, Chambers TM, Barrandeguy M, Mumford JA 1996. Antigenic and genetic evolution of equine H3N8 influenza A viruses. *Journal of General Virology* 77:661–671.

Daly JM, Macrae S, Newton JR, Wattrang E, Elton DM 2010. Equine influenza: A review of an unpredictable virus. *Veterinary Journal* 189:7–14.

Gerber H, Lohrer J 1966. Influenza A/equi-2 in der Schweitz 1965. In: *Symptomatologie Reine Virusinfection. Zentralblatt für Veterinärmedizin Reihe B* 13:438.

Holmes MA, Townsend HGG, Kohler AK, Hussey S, Breathnach C, Barnett C, Holland R, Lunn DP 2006. Immune responses to commercial equine vaccines against equine herpesvirus-1, equine influenza virus, eastern equine encephalomyelitis, and tetanus. *Veterinary Immunology and Immunopathology* 111:67–80.

Ilobi CP, Nicolson C, Taylor J, Mumford JA, Wood JM, Robertson JS 1998. Direct sequencing of the HA gene of clinical equine H3N8 influenza virus and comparison with laboratory derived virus. *Archives of Virology* 143:891–901.

Jubb KVF, Kennedy PC, Palmer N 2007. *Pathology of Domestic Animals*, 5th edn. WB Saunders Elsevier, Edinburgh, 2:628–629.

Kittelberger R, McFadden AM, Hannah MJ, *et al.* 2011. Comparative evaluation of four competitive/blocking ELISAs for the detection of influenza A antibodies in horses. *Veterinary Microbiology* 148:377–383.

Maanen C van 2001. Equine herpesvirus 1 and 4 and equine influenza virus infections: diagnosis, epidemiology and vaccinology. PhD Thesis Utrecht University, Utrecht, the Netherlands.

Maanen C van, Cullinane A 2002. Equine influenza virus infections: an update. *Veterinary Quarterly* 24:79–94.

Maanen C van, Bruin G, De Boer-Luijtze E, Smolders G, De Boer GF 1992. Interference of maternal antibodies with the immune response of foals after vaccination against equine influenza. *Veterinary Quarterly* 14:13–17.

McGavin MD, Zachary JF 2007. *Pathologic Basis of Veterinary Disease*, 4th edn. Mosby Elsevier, St. Louis, 477, 518.

Muirhead TL, McClure JT, Wichtel JJ, *et al.* 2008. The effect of age on serum antibody titers after rabies and influenza vaccination in healthy horses. *Journal of Veterinary Internal Medicine* 22:654–661.

Mumford JA 1990. The diagnosis and control of equine influenza. *Proceedings of the American Association of Equine Practitioners* 36:377–385.

Mumford JA 1991. Progress in the control of equine influenza. *Proceedings of the 6th International Conference on Equine Infectious Diseases*, Newmarket, 207–219.

Mumford JA 1992. Respiratory viral disease. In: Robinson NE (ed). *Current Therapy in Equine Medicine 3*. WB Saunders, Philadelphia, 316–324.

Mumford JA, Rossdale PD 1980. Virus and its relationship to the 'poor performance' syndrome. *Equine Veterinary Journal* 12:3–9.

Mumford JA, Wood J, Chambers T 1995. Consultation of OIE and WHO experts on progress in surveillance of equine influenza and application to vaccine strain selection. Report of a meeting held at the Animal Health Trust, Newmarket, UK, 18–19 September 1995.

Mumford EL, Traub-Dargatz JL, Salman MD, Collins JK, Getzy DM, Carman J 1998. Monitoring and detection of acute viral respiratory tract disease in horses. *Journal of the American Veterinary Medical Association* 231:385–390.

Richt JA, García-Sastre A 2009. Attenuated influenza virus vaccines with modified NS1 proteins. Review. *Current Topics in Microbiology and Immunology* 333:177–195.

Rivailler P, Perry IA, Jang Y, *et al.* 2010. Evolution of canine and equine influenza (H3N8) viruses co-circulating between 2005 and 2008. *Virology* **408**:71–79.

Rooney JR 1966. The pathology of respiratory diseases of foals. *Proceedings of the first International Conference on Equine Infectious Diseases*, Stresa, 70–75.

Sergeant ES, Kirkland PD, Cowled BD 2009. Field evaluation of an equine influenza ELISA used in New South Wales during the 2007 Australian outbreak response. *Preventive Veterinary Medicine* **92**:382–385.

Spokes PJ, Marich AJ, Musto JA, Ward KA, Craig AT, McAnulty JM 2009. Investigation of equine influenza transmission in NSW: walk, wind or wing? *New South Wales Public Health Bulletin* **20**:152–156.

Sugiura T, Sugita S, Imagawa H, *et al.* 2001. Serological diagnosis of equine influenza using the hemagglutinin protein produced in a baculovirus expression system. *Journal of Virological Methods* **98**:1–8.

Walle GR van de, May MA, Peters ST, Metzger SM, Rosas CT, Osterrieder N 2010. A vectored equine herpesvirus type 1 (EHV-1) vaccine elicits protective immune responses against EHV-1 and H3N8 equine influenza virus. *Vaccine* **28**:1048–1055.

Webster R, Guo YJ 1991. New influenza virus in horses. *Nature* **351**:527.

Willoughby R, Ecker G, McKee S, *et al.* 1992. The effects of equine rhinovirus, influenza virus and herpesvirus infection on tracheal clearance rate in horses. *Canadian Journal of Veterinary Research* **56**:115–121.

Wilson WD 1993. Equine influenza. *Veterinary Clinics of North America: Equine Practice* **9**:257–281.

Wood JM, Gaines-Das RE, Taylor J, Chakraverty P 1994. Comparison of influenza serological techniques by international collaborative study. *Vaccine* **12**:167–174.

Borna disease virus

Dauphin G, Legay V, Pitel P-H, Zientara S 2002. Borna disease: current knowledge and virus detection in France. *Veterinary Research* **33**:127–138.

Dieckhöfer R 2008. Infections in horses: diagnosis and therapy. *Acta Pathologica, Microbiologica et Immunologica Supplement* **124**:40–43.

Dürrwald R, Ludwig H 1997. Borna disease virus (BDV), a (zoonotic?) worldwide pathogen. A review of the history of the disease and the virus infection with comprehensive bibliography. *Journal of Veterinary Medicine B* **44**:147–184.

Flower RL, Kamhieh S, McLean L, Bode L, Ludwig H, Ward CM 2008. Human Borna disease virus infection in Australia: serological markers of infection in multi-transfused patients. *Acta Pathologica, Microbiologica et Immunologica Supplement* **124**:89–93.

Gosztonyi G, Ludwig H 1995. Borna disease – neuropathology and pathogenesis. *Current Topics in Microbiology and Immunology* **190**:39–73.

Grabner A, Fischer A 1991. Symptomatology and diagnosis of Borna encephalitis of horses. A case analysis of the last 13 years. *Tierärztliche Praxis* **19**:68–73.

Hagiwara K, Kamitani W, Takamura S, *et al.* 2000. Detection of Borna disease virus in a pregnant mare and her fetus. *Veterinary Microbiology* **72**:207–216.

Herzog S, Frese K, Richt JA, Rott R 1994. Ein Beitrag zur Epizootiologie der Bornaschen Krankheit beim Pferd. *Wiener Tierärztliche Monatschrift* **81**:374–379.

Jordan I, Lipkin WI 2001. Borna disease virus. *Reviews in Medical Virology* **11**:37–57.

Jubb KVF, Kennedy PC, Palmer N 2007. *Pathology of Domestic Animals*, 5th edn. WB Saunders Elsevier, Edinburgh, **1**:425–426.

Puorger ME, Hilbe M, Müller JP, *et al.* 2010. Distribution of Borna disease virus antigen and RNA in tissues of naturally infected bicolored white-toothed shrews, *Crocidura leucodon*, supporting their role as reservoir host species. *Veterinary Pathology* **47**:236–244.

Richt JA, Grabner A, Herzog S 2000. Borna disease in horses. *Veterinary Clinics of North America: Equine Practice* **16**:579–595.

Richt JA, Rott R 2000. Borna disease virus: a mystery as an emerging zoonotic pathogen. *Veterinary Journal* **161**:24–40.

Staeheli P, Rinder M, Kaspers B 2010. Avian Bornavirus associated with fatal disease in psittacine birds. *Journal of Virology* **84**:6269–6275.

Hendra virus

Barker SC 2003. The Australian paralysis tick may be the missing link in the transmission of Hendra virus from bats to horses to humans. *Medical Hypotheses* **60**:481–483.

Black PF, Cronin JP, Morrissy CJ, Westbury HA 2001. Serological examination for evidence of infection with Hendra and Nipah viruses in Queensland piggeries. *Australian Veterinary Journal* **79**:424–426.

Field HE, Barratt PC, Hughes RJ, Shield J, Sullivan ND 2000. A fatal case of Hendra virus infection in a horse in North Queensland: clinical and epidemiological features. *Australian Veterinary Journal* **78**:279–280.

Field HE, Young P, Yob JM, Mills J, Hall L, Mackenzie J 2001. The natural history of Hendra and Nipah viruses. *Microbes and Infection* **3**:307–314.

Field H, Schaaf K, Kung N, *et al.* 2010. Hendra virus outbreak with novel clinical features, Australia. *Emerging Infectious Diseases* **16**:338–340.

Hanna JN, McBride WJ, Brookes DL, *et al.* 2006. Hendra virus infection in a veterinarian. *Medical Journal of Australia* **185**:562–564.

Jubb KVF, Kennedy PC, Palmer N 2007. *Pathology of Domestic Animals*, 5th edn. WB Saunders Elsevier, Edinburgh, **2**:630.

Li M, Embury-Hyatt C, Weingartl HM 2010. Experimental inoculation study indicates swine as a potential host for Hendra virus. *Veterinary Research* **41**:33.

McCormack JG, Allworth AM 2002. Emerging viral infections in Australia. Review. *Medical Journal of Australia* **177**:45–49.

McGavin MD, Zachary JF 2007. *Pathologic Basis of Veterinary Disease*, 4th edn. Mosby Elsevier, St. Louis, 519.

Playford EG, McCall B, Smith G, *et al.* 2010. Human Hendra virus encephalitis associated with equine outbreak, Australia, 2008. *Emerging Infectious Diseases* **16**:219–223.

Pringle CR 1998. Virus taxonomy. *Archives of Virology* **143**:1449–1459.

Prociv P 2007. Hendra virus infection in a veterinarian. *Medical Journal of Australia* **186**:325–326.

Selvey LA, Wells RM, McCormack JG, *et al.* 1995. Infection of humans and horses by a newly described morbillivirus. *Medical Journal of Australia* **162**:642–645.

Uppal PK 2000. Emergence of Nipah virus in Malaysia. *Annals of the New York Academy of Sciences* **916**:354–357.

Weingartl HM, Berhane Y, Czub M 2009. Animal models of henipavirus infection: a review. *Veterinary Journal* **181**:211–220.

Williamson MM, Hooper PT, Selleck PW, *et al.* 1998. Transmission studies of Hendra virus (equine morbillivirus) in fruit bats, horses and cats. *Australian Veterinary Journal* **76**:813–818.

Young PL, Halpin K, Selleck P, *et al.* 1996. Serological evidence for the presence in *Pteropus* bats of a paramyxovirus related to equine morbillivirus. *Emerging Infectious Diseases* **2**:239–240.

Equine rhinitis virus

Black WD, Wilcox RS, Stevenson RA, *et al.* 2007. Prevalence of serum neutralising antibody to equine rhinitis A virus (ERAV), equine rhinitis B virus 1 (ERBV1) and ERBV2. *Veterinary Microbiology* **119**:65–71.

Black WD, Studdert MJ 2006. Formerly unclassified, acid-stable equine picornaviruses are a third equine rhinitis B virus serotype in the genus Erbovirus. *Journal of General Virology* **87**:3023–3027.

Dynon K, Black WD, Ficorilli N, Hartley CA, Studdert MJ 2007. Detection of viruses in nasal swab samples from horses with acute, febrile, respiratory disease using virus isolation, polymerase chain reaction and serology. *Australian Veterinary Journal* **85**:46–50.

Huang J-A, Ficorilli N, Hartley CA, Wilcox RS, Weiss M, Studdert MJ 2001. Equine rhinitis B virus: a new serotype. *Journal of General Virology* **82**:2641–2645.

Kriegshäuser G, Deutz A, Kuechler E, Skern T, Lussy H, Nowotny N 2005. Prevalence of neutralizing antibodies to equine rhinitis A and B virus in horses and man. *Veterinary Microbiology* **106**:293–296.

Kriegshäuser G, Kuechler E, Skern T 2009. Aggregation-associated loss of antigenicity observed for denatured virion protein 1 of equine rhinitis A virus in an enzyme-linked immunosorbent assay. *Virus Research* **143**:130–133.

Li F, Drummer HE, Ficorilli N, Studdert MJ, Crabb BS 1997. Identification of noncytopathic equine Rhinovirus 1 as a cause of acute febrile respiratory disease in horses. *Journal of Clinical Microbiology* **35**:937–943.

McGavin MD, Zachary JF 2007. *Pathologic Basis of Veterinary Disease*, 4th edn. Mosby Elsevier, St. Louis, 477.

Mori A, De Benedictis P, Marciano S, *et al.* 2009. Development of a real-time duplex TaqMan-PCR for the detection of equine rhinitis A and B viruses in clinical specimens. *Journal of Virological Methods* **155**:175–181.

Newton JR, Wood JLN, Chanter N 2003. A case control study of factors and infections associated with clinically apparent respiratory disease in UK Thoroughbred racehorses. *Preventive Veterinary Medicine* **60**:107–132.

Plummer G 1962. An equine respiratory virus with enterovirus properties. *Nature* **195**:519–520.

Plummer G 1963. An equine respiratory enterovirus: some biological and physical properties. *Archiv für die Gesamte Virusforschung* **12**:694–700.

Stevenson RA, Hartley CA, Huang JA, Studdert MJ, Crabb BS, Warner S 2003. Mapping epitopes in equine rhinitis A virus VP1 recognized by antibodies elicited in response to infection of the natural host. *Journal of General Virology* **84**:1607–1612.

Stevenson RA, Huang JA, Studdert MJ, Hartley CA 2004. Sialic acid acts as a receptor for equine rhinitis A virus binding and infection. *Journal of General Virology* **85**:2535–2543.

Studdert MJ, Gleeson LJ 1978. Isolation and characterisation of an equine rhinovirus. *Zentralblatt für Veterinärmedizin* **25**:225–237.

Wernery U, Knowles NJ, Hamblin C, *et al.* 2008. Abortions in dromedaries (*Camelus dromedarius*) caused by equine rhinitis A virus. *Journal of General Virology* **89**:660–666.

African horse sickness virus

Aradaib IE 2009. PCR detection of African horse sickness virus serogroup based on genome segment three sequence analysis. *Journal of Virological Methods* **159**:1–5.

Barnard BJ 1993. Circulation of African horsesickness virus in zebra (*Equus burchelli*) in the Kruger National Park, South Africa, as measured by the prevalence of type specific antibodies. *Onderstepoort Journal of Veterinary Research* **60**:111–117.

Brown CC, Meyer RF, Grubman MJ 1994. Presence of African horse sickness virus in equine tissues, as determined by in situ hybridization. *Veterinary Pathology* **31**:689–694.

Calvete C, Estrada R, Miranda MA, *et al.* 2009. Entry of bluetongue vector *Culicoides imicola* into livestock premises in Spain. *Medical and Veterinary Entomology* **23**:202–208.

Chiam R, Sharp E, Maan S, *et al.* 2009. Induction of antibody responses to African horse sickness virus (AHSV) in ponies after vaccination with recombinant modified vaccinia Ankara (MVA). *PLoS One* **4**:e5997.

Clift SJ, Penrith ML 2010. Tissue and cell tropism of African horse sickness virus demonstrated by immunoperoxidase labeling in natural and experimental infection in horses in South Africa. *Veterinary Pathology* **47**:690–697.

Clift SJ, Williams MC, Gerdes T, Smit MM 2009. Standardization and validation of an immunoperoxidase assay for the detection of African horse sickness virus in formalin-fixed, paraffin-embedded tissues. *Journal of Veterinary Diagnostic Investigation* **21**:655–667.

Davies FG, Lund LJ 1974. The application of fluorescent antibody techniques to the virus of African horse sickness. *Research in Veterinary Science* **17**:128–130.

Erasmus BJ 1963. Cultivation of horse sickness virus in tissue culture. *Nature* **200**:716–719.

Erasmus BJ 1964. Some observations on the propagation of horse sickness virus in tissue culture. *Bulletin de l'Office International des Epizooties* **62**:923–928.

Gale P, Brouwer A, Ramnial V, *et al.* 2010. Assessing the impact of climate change on vector-borne viruses in the EU through the elicitation of expert opinion. *Epidemiology and Infection* 138:214–225.

Guthrie AJ, Quan M, Lourens CW, *et al.* 2009. Protective immunization of horses with a recombinant canarypox virus vectored vaccine co-expressing genes encoding the outer capsid proteins of African horse sickness virus. *Vaccine* 27:4434–4438.

Hamblin C, Salt JS, Mellor PS, Graham SD, Smith PR, Wohlsein P 1998. Donkeys as reservoirs of African horse sickness virus. *Archives of Virology Supplement* 14:37–47.

House JA, Lombard M, Dubourget P, House C, Mebus CA 1994. Further studies on the efficacy of an inactivated African horse sickness serotype 4 vaccine. *Vaccine* 12:142–144.

Howell PG, Nurton JP, Nel D, Lourens CW, Guthrie AJ 2008. Prevalence of serotype specific antibody to equine encephalosis virus in Thoroughbred yearlings in South Africa (1999–2004). *Onderstepoort Journal of Veterinary Research* 75:153–161.

Laegreid WW 1994. Diagnosis of African horse sickness. Review. *Comparative Immunology, Microbiology and Infectious Diseases* 17:297–303.

Laegreid WW, Skowronek A, Stone-Marschat M, Burrage T 1993. Characterization of virulence variants of African horse sickness virus. *Virology* 195:836–839.

Mellor PS, Boorman J 1995. The transmission and geographical spread of African horse sickness and bluetongue viruses. *Annals of Tropical Medicine and Parasitology* 89:1–15.

Mellor PS, Hamblin C 2004. African horse sickness. *Veterinary Research* 35:445–466.

Meyden CH van der, Erasmus BJ, Swanepoel R, Prozesky OW 1992. Encephalitis and chorioretinitis associated with neurotropic African horse sickness virus infection in laboratory workers. Part I. Clinical and neurological observations. *South African Medical Journal* 81:451–454.

Portas M, Boinas FS, Oliveira E, Sousa J, Rawlings P 1999. African horse sickness in Portugal: a successful eradication programme. *Epidemiology and Infection* 123:337–346.

Quan M, van Vuuren M, Howell PG, Groenewald D, Guthrie AJ 2008. Molecular epidemiology of the African horse sickness virus S10 gene. *Journal of General Virology* 89:1159–1168.

Rensberg IB van, De Clerk J, Groenewald HB, Botha WS 1981. An outbreak of African horse sickness in dogs. *Journal of the South African Veterinary Association* 52:323–325.

Roth JA, Spickler AR 2003. A survey of vaccines produced for OIE list A diseases in OIE member countries. *Developmental Biology (Basel)* 114:5–25.

Rubio C, Cubillo MA, Hooghuis H, *et al.* 1998. Validation of ELISA for the detection of African horse sickness virus antigens and antibodies. *Archives of Virology Supplement* 14:311–315.

Sánchez-Vizcaíno JM 2004. Control and eradication of African horse sickness with vaccine. Review. *Developmental Biology (Basel)* 119:255–258.

Skowronek AJ, LaFranco L, Stone-Marschat MA, Burrage TG, Rebar AH, Laegreid WW 1995. Clinical pathology and haemostatic abnormalities in experimental African horse sickness. *Veterinary Pathology* 32:112–121.

Teichman BF von, Smit TK 2008. Evaluation of the pathogenicity of African horsesickness (AHS) isolates in vaccinated animals. *Vaccine* 26:5014–5021.

Teichman BF von, Dungu B, Smit TK 2010. *In vivo* cross-protection to African horse sickness Serotypes 5 and 9 after vaccination with Serotypes 8 and 6. *Vaccine* 28:6505–6517.

Equine infectious anaemia virus

Alvarez I, Gutierrez G, Ostlund E, Barrandeguy M, Trono K 2007. Western blot assay using recombinant p26 antigen for detection of equine infectious anemia virus-specific antibodies. *Clinical and Vaccine Immunology* 14:1646–1648.

Brindley MA, Zhang B, Montelaro RC, Maury W 2008. An equine infectious anemia virus variant superinfects cells through novel receptor interactions. *Journal of Virology* 82:9425–9432.

Cappelli K, Capomaccio S, Cook FR, *et al.* 2011. Molecular diagnosis, epidemiology and genetic characterization of novel European field isolates of equine infectious anemia virus. *Journal of Clinical Microbiology* 49:27–33.

Cook SJ, Cook RF, Montelaro RC, Issel CJ 2001. Differential responses of *Equus caballus* and *Equus asinus* to infection with two pathogenic strains of equine infectious anemia virus. *Veterinary Microbiology* 79:93–109.

Craigo JK, Barnes S, Zhang B, *et al.* 2009. An EIAV field isolate reveals much higher levels of subtype variability than currently reported for the equine lentivirus family. *Retrovirology* 6:95.

Cullinane A, Quinlivan M, Nelly M, *et al.* 2007. Diagnosis of equine infectious anaemia during the 2006 outbreak in Ireland. *Veterinary Record* 161:647–652.

Jubb KVF, Kennedy PC, Palmer N 2007. *Pathology of Domestic Animals*, 5th edn. WB Saunders Elsevier, Edinburgh, 3:235–239.

Leroux C, Cadoré J-L, Montelaro RC 2004. Equine infectious anemia virus (EIAV): what has HIV's country cousin got to tell us? *Veterinary Research* 35:485–512.

McGavin MD, Zachary JF 2007. *Pathologic Basis of Veterinary Disease*, 4th edn. Mosby Elsevier, St. Louis, 788.

Mealey RH, Stone DM, Hines MT, *et al.* 2007. Experimental *Rhodococcus equi* and equine infectious anemia virus DNA vaccination in adult and neonatal horses: effect of IL-12, dose, and route. *Vaccine* 25:7582–7597.

Menzies F, Patterson T 2006. Description of the first case of equine infectious anaemia in Northern Ireland. *Veterinary Record* 159:753–754.

Mooney J, Flynn O, Sammin D 2006. Equine infectious anaemia in Ireland: characterisation of the virus. *Veterinary Record* 159:570.

More SJ, Aznar I, Myers T, Leadon DP, Clegg A 2008*a*. An outbreak of equine infectious anaemia in Ireland during 2006: the modes of transmission and spread in the Kildare cluster. *Equine Veterinary Journal* 40:709–711.

More SJ, Aznar I, Bailey DC, *et al.* 2008*b*. An outbreak of equine infectious anaemia in Ireland during 2006: investigation methodology, initial source of infection, diagnosis and clinical presentation, modes of transmission and spread in the Meath cluster. *Equine Veterinary Journal* 40:706–708.

Oaks JL, Long MT, Baszler TV 2004. Leukoencephalitis associated with selective viral replication in the brain of a pony with experimental chronic equine infectious anemia virus infection. *Veterinary Pathology* 41:527–532.

Payne SL, Fuller FJ 2010. Virulence determinants of equine infectious anemia virus. *Current HIV Research* 8:66–72.

Rotavirus

Albert MJ, Unicomb LE, Tzipori SR, Bishop RF 1987. Isolation and serotyping of animal rotaviruses and antigenic comparison with human rotaviruses. Brief report. *Archives of Virology* 93:123–130.

Browning GF, Chalmers RM, Snodgrass DR, *et al.* 1991. The prevalence of enteric pathogens in diarrhoeic Thoroughbred foals in Britain and Ireland. *Equine Veterinary Journal* 23:405–409.

Browning GF, Chalmers RM, Fitzgerald TA, Corley KT, Campbell I, Snodgrass DR 1992. Rotavirus serotype G3 predominates in horses. *Journal of Clinical Microbiology* 30:59–62.

Collins PJ, Cullinane A, Martella V, O'Shea H 2008. Molecular characterization of equine rotavirus in Ireland. *Journal of Clinical Microbiology* 46:3346–3354.

Conner ME, Darlington RW 1980. Rotavirus infection in foals. *American Journal of Veterinary Research* 41:1699–1703.

Elschner M, Prudlo J, Hotzel H, Otto P, Sachse K 2002. Nested reverse transcriptase-polymerase chain reaction for the detection of group A rotaviruses. *Journal of Veterinary Medicine, B. Infectious Diseases and Veterinary Public Health* 49:77–81.

Frederick J, Giguère S, Sanchez LC 2009. Infectious agents detected in the faeces of diarrheic foals: A retrospective study of 233 cases (2003–2008). *Journal of Veterinary Internal Medicine* 23:1254–1260.

Jones DM, Dickson LR, Fu ZF, Wilks CR 1989. Rotaviral diarrhoea and its treatment in a foal. *New Zealand Veterinary Journal* 37:166–168.

Mukherjee A, Dutta D, Ghosh S, *et al.* 2009. Full genomic analysis of a human group A rotavirus G9P[6] strain from Eastern India provides evidence for porcine-to-human interspecies transmission. *Archives of Virology* 154:733–746.

Müller H, Johne R 2007. Rotaviruses: diversity and zoonotic potential – a brief review. *Berliner und Münchener Tierärztliche Wochenschrift* 120:108–112.

Nemoto M, Imagawa H, Tsujimura K, Yamanaka T, Kondo T, Matsumura T 2010. Detection of equine rotavirus by reverse transcription loop-mediated isothermal amplification (RT-LAMP). *Journal of Veterinary Medical Science* 72:823–826.

Rossignol J-F, Abu-Zekry M, Hussein A, Santoro MG 2006. Effect of nitazoxanide for treatment of severe rotavirus diarrhoea: randomised double-blind placebo-controlled trial. *Lancet* 368:124–129.

Steyer A, Poljsak-Prijatelj M, Barlic-Maganja D, Marin J 2008. Human, porcine and bovine rotaviruses in Slovenia: evidence of interspecies transmission and genome reassortment. *Journal of General Virology* 89:1690–1698.

Tzipori S, Walker M 1978. Isolation of rotavirus from foals with diarrhoea. *Australian Journal of Experimental Biology and Medical Science* 56:453–457.

Tzipori SR, Makin TJ, Smith ML 1980. The clinical response of gnotobiotic calves, pigs, and lambs to inoculation with human, calf, pig and foal rotavirus isolates. *Australian Journal of Experimental Biology and Medical Science* 58:309–318.

Tzipori S, Makin T, Smith M, Krautil F 1982. Enteritis in foals induced by rotavirus and enterotoxigenic *Escherichia coli*. *Australian Veterinary Journal* 58:20–23.

Rabies

Blanton JD, Palmer D, Rupprecht CE 2010. Rabies surveillance in the United States during 2009. *Journal of the American Veterinary Medical Association* 237:646–657.

Carrieri ML, Peixoto ZM, Paciencia ML, Kotait I, Germano PM 2006. Laboratory diagnosis of equine rabies and its implications for human postexposure prophylaxis. *Journal of Virological Methods* 138:1–9.

Feder HM, Nelson RS, Cartter ML, Sadre I 1998. Rabies prophylaxis following the feeding of a rabid pony. *Clinical Pediatrics (Philadelphia)* 37:477–481.

Green SL 1997. Rabies. *Veterinary Clinics of North America: Equine Practice* 13:1–11.

Haupt W 1999. Rabies – risk of exposure and current trends in prevention of human cases. *Vaccine* 17:1742–1749.

Hudson LC, Weinstock D, Jordan T, Bold-Fletcher NO 1996. Clinical presentation of experimentally induced rabies in horses. *Zentralblatt für Veterinärmedizin Reihe B* 43:277–285.

Krebs JW, Noll HR, Rupprecht CE, Childs JE 2002. Rabies surveillance in the United States during 2001. *Journal of the American Veterinary Medical Association* 221:1690–1701.

Leung AK, Davies HD, Hon KL 2007. Rabies: epidemiology, pathogenesis, and prophylaxis. *Advances in Therapy* 24:1340–1347.

McCormack JG, Allworth AM 2002. Emerging viral infections in Australia. *Medical Journal of Australia* 177:45–49.

Muirhead TL, McClure JT, Wichtel JJ, *et al.* 2008. The effect of age on serum antibody titres after rabies and influenza vaccination in healthy horses. *Journal of Veterinary Internal Medicine* 22:654–661.

Stein LT, Rech RR, Harrison L, Brown CC 2010. Immunohistochemical study of rabies virus within the central nervous system of domestic and wildlife species. *Veterinary Pathology* 47:630–633.

Wilson PJ, Oertli EH, Hunt PR, Sidwa TJ 2010. Evaluation of a postexposure rabies prophylaxis protocol for domestic animals in Texas: 2000–2009. *Journal of the American Veterinary Medical Association* 237:1395–1401.

Vesicular stomatitis virus

Cantlon JD, Gordy PW, Bowen RA 2000. Immune responses in mice, cattle and horses to a DNA vaccine for vesicular stomatitis. *Vaccine* 18:2368–2374.

Green SL 1993. Vesicular stomatitis in the horse. *Veterinary Clinics of North America: Equine Practice* 9:349–353.

Howerth EW, Mead DG, Mueller PO, Duncan L, Murphy MD, Stallknecht DE 2006. Experimental vesicular stomatitis virus infection in horses: effect of route of inoculation and virus serotype. *Veterinary Pathology* 43:943–955.

Lee HS, Heo EJ, Jeoung HY, et al. 2009. Enzyme-linked immunosorbent assay using glycoprotein and monoclonal antibody for detecting antibodies to vesicular stomatitis virus serotype New Jersey. *Clinical and Vaccine Immunology* 16:667–671.

López-Sánchez A, Guijarro Guijarro B, Hernández Vallejo G 2003. Human repercussions of foot and mouth disease and other similar viral diseases. *Medicina Oral, Patología Oral y Cirugía Bucal* 8:26–32.

McCluskey BJ, Mumford EL 2000. Vesicular stomatitis and other vesicular, erosive, and ulcerative diseases of horses. *Veterinary Clinics of North America: Equine Practice* 16:457–469.

Mumford EL, McCluskey BJ, Traub-Dargatz JL, Schmitt BJ, Salman MD 1998. Public veterinary medicine: public health. Serologic evaluation of vesicular stomatitis virus exposure in horses and cattle in 1996. *Journal of the American Veterinary Medical Association* 213:1265–1269.

Rainwater-Lovett K, Pauszek SJ, Kelley WN, Rodriguez LL 2007. Molecular epidemiology of vesicular stomatitis New Jersey virus from the 2004–2005 US outbreak indicates a common origin with Mexican strains. *Journal of General Virology* 88:2042–2051.

Wilson WC, Letchworth GJ, Jiménez C, et al. 2009. Field evaluation of a multiplex real-time reverse transcription polymerase chain reaction assay for detection of vesicular stomatitis virus. *Journal of Veterinary Diagnostic Investigation* 21:179–186.

Eastern equine encephalomyelitis virus

Adams AP, Aronson JF, Tardif SD, et al. 2008. Common marmosets (*Callithrix jacchus*) as a nonhuman primate model to assess the virulence of eastern equine encephalitis virus strains. *Journal of Virology* 82:9035–9042.

Arrigo NC, Adams AP, Weaver SC 2010. Evolutionary patterns of eastern equine encephalitis virus in North versus South America suggest ecological differences and taxonomic revision. *Journal of Virology* 84:1014–1025.

Brault AC, Powers AM, Chavez CL, et al. 1999. Genetic and antigenic diversity among eastern encephalitis viruses from North, Central, and South America. *American Journal of Tropical Medicine and Hygiene* 61:579–586.

Chénier S, Côté G, Vanderstock J, Macieira S, Laperle A, Hélie P 2010. An eastern equine encephalomyelitis (EEE) outbreak in Quebec in the fall of 2008. *Canadian Veterinary Journal* 51:1011–1015.

Fine DL, Roberts BA, Teehee ML, et al. 2007. Venezuelan equine encephalitis virus vaccine candidate (V3526) safety, immunogenicity and efficacy in horses. *Vaccine* 25:1868–1876.

Holmes MA, Townsend HGG, Kohler AK, et al. 2006. Immune responses to commercial equine vaccines against equine herpesvirus-1, equine influenza virus, eastern equine encephalomyelitis, and tetanus. *Veterinary Immunology and Immunopathology* 111:67–80.

Johnston RE, Peters CJ 1996. Alphaviruses. In: Fields BN, Knipe DM, Howley PM (eds). *Fields Virology*, 3rd edn. Lippincott-Raven, Philadelphia, 843–898.

Lambert AJ, Martin DA, Lanciotti RS 2003. Detection of North American eastern and western equine encephalitis viruses by nucleic acid amplification assays. *Journal of Clinical Microbiology* 41:379–385.

Larkin M 2010. High prevalence of EEE in Michigan. *Journal of the American Veterinary Medical Association* 237:1001.

Linssen B, Kinney RM, Aguilar P, et al. 2000. Development of reverse transcription-PCR assays specific for detection of equine encephalitis viruses. *Journal of Clinical Microbiology* 38:1527–1535.

McLean RG, Frier G, Parham GL, et al. 1985. Investigations of the vertebrate hosts of eastern equine encephalitis during an epizootic in Michigan, 1980. *American Journal of Tropical Medicine and Hygiene* 34:1190–1202.

Peters CJ, Dalrymple JM 1990. Alphaviruses. In: Fields BN, Knipe DM (eds). *Virology*, 2nd edition. Raven Press, New York.

Poonacha KB, Gregory CR, Vickers ML 1998. Intestinal lesions in a horse associated with eastern equine encephalomyelitis virus infection. *Veterinary Pathology* 35:535–538.

Roehrig JT 1993. Immunogens of encephalitis viruses. *Veterinary Microbiology* 37:273–284.

Sabattini MS, Daffner JF, Monath TP, et al. 1991. Localized eastern equine encephalitis in Santiago del Estero Province, Argentina, without human infection. *Medicina (Buenos Aires)* 51:3–8.

Schmitt SM, Cooley TM, Fitzgerald SD, et al. 2007. An outbreak of eastern equine encephalitis virus in free-ranging white-tailed deer in Michigan. *Journal of Wildlife Diseases* 43:635–644.

Scott TW, Weaver SC 1989. Eastern equine encephalomyelitis virus: epidemiology and evolution of mosquito transmission. *Advances in Virus Research* 37:277–328.

Vanderwagen LC, Pearson JL, Franti CE, Tamm EL, Riemann HP, Behymer DE 1975. A field study of persistence of antibodies in California horses vaccinated against western, eastern, and Venezuelan equine encephalitis. *American Journal of Veterinary Research* 36:1567–1571.

Walton TE, Jochim MM, Barber TL, Thompson LH 1989. Cross-protective immunity between equine encephalomyelitis viruses in equids. *American Journal of Veterinary Research* 50:1442–1446.

Weaver SC, Scott TW, Rico-Hesse R 1991. Molecular evolution of eastern equine encephalomyelitis virus in North America. *Virology* 182:774–784.

Western equine encephalomyelitis virus

Adams AP, Aronson JF, Tardif SD, et al. 2008. Common marmosets (*Callithrix jacchus*) as a nonhuman primate model to assess the virulence of eastern equine encephalitis virus strains. *Journal of Virology* 82:9035–9042.

Aviles G, Bianchi TI, Daffner JF, Sabattini MS 1993. Post-epizootic activity of western equine encephalitis virus in Argentina. *La Revista Argentina de Microbiología* 25:88–99.

Barabé ND, Rayner GA, Christopher ME, Nagata LP, Wu JQ 2007. Single-dose, fast-acting vaccine candidate against western equine encephalitis virus completely protects mice from intranasal challenge with different strains of the virus. *Vaccine* 25:6271–6276.

Bianchi TI, Avilés G, Sabattini MS 1997. Biological characteristics of an enzootic subtype of western equine encephalomyelitis virus from Argentina. *Acta Virologica* 41:13–20.

Calisher CH, Emerson JK, Muth DJ, Lazuick JS, Monath TP 1983. Serodiagnosis of western equine encephalitis virus infections: relationships of antibody titre and test to observed onset of clinical illness. *Journal of the American Veterinary Medical Association* 183:438–440.

Calisher CH, Mahmud MI, el-Kafrawi AO, Emerson JK, Muth DJ 1986. Rapid and specific serodiagnosis of western equine encephalitis virus infection in horses. *American Journal of Veterinary Research* 47:1296–1299.

Fine DL, Roberts BA, Teehee ML, et al. 2007. Venezuelan equine encephalitis virus vaccine candidate (V3526) safety, immunogenicity and efficacy in horses. *Vaccine* 25:1868–1876.

Forrester NL, Kenney JL, Deardorff E, Wang E, Weaver SC 2008. Western equine encephalitis submergence: lack of evidence for a decline in virus virulence. *Virology* 380:170–172.

Iversson LB, Silva RA, da Rosa AP, Barros VL 1993. Circulation of eastern equine encephalitis, western equine encephalitis, Ilhéus, Maguari and Tacaiuma viruses in equines of the Brazilian Pantanal, South America. *Revista do Instituto de Medicina Tropical de São Paulo* 35:355–359.

Janousek TE, Kramer WL 1998. Surveillance for arthropod-borne viral activity in Nebraska, 1994–1995. *Journal of Medical Entomology* 35:758–762.

Johnston RE, Peters CJ 1996. Alphaviruses. In: Fields BN, Knipe DM, Howley PM (eds). *Fields Virology*, 3rd edition. Lippincott-Raven, Philadelphia, 843–898.

Jubb KVF, Kennedy PC, Palmer N 2007. *Pathology of Domestic Animals*, 5th edn. WB Saunders Elsevier, Edinburgh, 1:423–424.

Karabatsos N, Lewis AL, Calisher CH, Hunt AR, Roehrig JT 1988. Identification of Highlands J virus from a Florida horse. *American Journal of Tropical Medicine and Hygiene* 39:603–606.

Lambert AJ, Martin DA, Lanciotti RS 2003. Detection of North American eastern and western equine encephalitis viruses by nucleic acid amplification assays. *Journal of Clinical Microbiology* 41:379–385.

Linssen B, Kinney RM, Aguilar P, et al. 2000. Development of reverse transcription-PCR assays specific for detection of equine encephalitis viruses. *Journal of Clinical Microbiology* 38:1527–1535.

Potter ME, Currier RW, Pearson JE, Harris JC, Parker RL 1977. Western equine encephalomyelitis in horses in the Northern Red River Valley, 1975. *Journal of the American Veterinary Medical Association* 170:1396–1399.

Roehrig JT 1993. Immunogens of encephalitis viruses. *Veterinary Microbiology* 37:273–284.

Sellers RF, Maarouf AR 1988. Impact of climate on western equine encephalitis in Manitoba, Minnesota and North Dakota, 1980–1983. *Epidemiology and Infection* 101:511–535.

Waldridge BM, Wenzel JG, Ellis AC, et al. 2003. Serologic responses to eastern and western equine encephalomyelitis vaccination in previously vaccinated horses. *Veterinary Therapeutics* 4:242–248.

Walton TE, Jochim MM, Barber TL, Thompson LH 1989. Cross-protective immunity between equine encephalomyelitis viruses in equids. *American Journal of Veterinary Research* 50:1442–1446.

Zacks MA, Paessler S 2010. Encephalitic alphaviruses. *Veterinary Microbiology* 140:281–286.

Venezuelan equine encephalomyelitis virus

Anishchenko M, Bowen RA, Paessler S, Austgen L, Greene IP, Weaver SC 2006. Venezuelan encephalitis emergence mediated by a phylogenetically predicted viral mutation. *Proceedings of the National Academy of Sciences USA* 103:4994–4999.

Atasheva S, Garmashova N, Frolov I, Frolova E 2008. Venezuelan equine encephalitis virus capsid protein inhibits nuclear import in mammalian but not in mosquito cells. *Journal of Virology* 82:4028–4041.

Baker EF Jr, Sasso DR, Maness K, Prichard WD, Parker RL 1978. Venezuelan equine encephalomyelitis vaccine (strain TC-83): a field study. *American Journal of Veterinary Research* 39:1627–1631.

Calisher CH, Sasso DR, Sather GE 1973. Possible evidence for interference with Venezuelan equine encephalitis virus vaccination of equines by pre-existing antibody to eastern or western equine encephalitis virus, or both. *Applied Microbiology* 26:485–488.

Deardorff ER, Forrester NL, Travassos-da-Rosa AP, et al. 2009. Experimental infection of potential reservoir hosts with Venezuelan equine encephalitis virus, Mexico. *Emerging Infectious Diseases* 15:519–525.

Ferguson JA, Reeves WC, Milby MM, Hardy JL 1978. Study of homologous and heterologous antibody response in California horses vaccinated with attenuated Venezuelan equine encephalomyelitis vaccine (strain TC-83). *American Journal of Veterinary Research* 39:371–376.

Fine DL, Roberts BA, Teehee ML, et al. 2007. Venezuelan equine encephalitis virus vaccine candidate (V3526) safety, immunogenicity and efficacy in horses. *Vaccine* 25:1868–1876.

Gibbs EP 1976. Equine viral encephalitis. Review. *Equine Veterinary Journal* 8:66–71.

Greene IP, Paessler S, Austgen L, et al. 2005. Envelope glycoprotein mutations mediate equine amplification and virulence of epizootic Venezuelan equine encephalitis virus. *Journal of Virology* 79:9128–9133.

Johnson KM, Martin DH 1974. Venezuelan equine encephalitis. *Advances in Veterinary Science and Comparative Medicine* 18:79–116.

Jubb KVF, Kennedy PC, Palmer N 2007. *Pathology of Domestic Animals*, 5th edn. WB Saunders Elsevier, Edinburgh, 1:423–424.

Linssen B, Kinney RM, Aguilar P, *et al.* 2000. Development of reverse transcription-PCR assays specific for detection of equine encephalitis viruses. *Journal of Clinical Microbiology* 38:1527–1535.

Navarro JC, Medina G, Vasquez C, *et al.* 2005. Postepizootic persistence of Venezuelan equine encephalitis virus, Venezuela. *Emerging Infectious Diseases* 11:1907–1915.

Ni H, Yun NE, Zacks MA, *et al.* 2007. Recombinant alphaviruses are safe and useful serological diagnostic tools. *American Journal of Tropical Medicine and Hygiene* 76:774–781.

Regenmortel MHV van, Fauquet CM, Bishop DHL, *et al.* 2000. *Virus Taxonomy: Classification and Nomenclature of Viruses*. Academic Press, San Diego, 879–889.

Roehrig JT 1993. Immunogens of encephalitis viruses. *Veterinary Microbiology* 37:273–284.

Sharma A, Maheshwari RK 2009. Oligonucleotide array analysis of Toll-like receptors and associated signalling genes in Venezuelan equine encephalitis virus-infected mouse brain. *Journal of General Virology* 90:1836–1847.

Walton TE, Alvarez O jr, Buckwalter RM, Johnson KM 1973. Experimental infection of horses with enzootic and epizootic strains of Venezuelan equine encephalomyelitis virus. *Journal of Infectious Diseases* 128:271–282.

Wang E, Bowen RA, Medina G, *et al.*, Cysticercosis Working Group in Peru 2001. Virulence and viraemia characteristics of 1992 epizootic subtype IC Venezuelan equine encephalitis viruses and closely related enzootic subtype ID strains. *American Journal of Tropical Medicine and Hygiene* 65:64–69.

Weaver SC, Salas R, Rico-Hesse R, *et al.* 1996. Re-emergence of epidemic Venezuelan equine encephalomyelitis in South America. VEE study group. *Lancet* 348:436–440.

Weaver SC, Ferro C, Barrera R, Boshell J, Navarro J-C 2004*a*. Venezuelan equine encephalitis. *Annual Review of Entomology* 49:141–174.

Weaver SC, Anishchenko M, Bowen R, *et al.* 2004*b*. Genetic determinants of Venezuelan equine encephalitis emergence. Review. *Archives of Virology Supplement* 18:43–64.

Getah virus and Ross River virus: Ross River virus and Sagiyama virus

Brown CM, Timoney PJ 1998. Getah virus infection of Indian horses. *Tropical Animal Health and Production* 30:241–252.

El-Hage CM, McCluskey MJ, Azuolas JK 2008. Disease suspected to be caused by Ross River virus infection of horses. *Australian Veterinary Journal* 86:367–370.

Fukunaga Y, Kumanomido T, Kamada M 2000. Getah virus as an equine pathogen. Review. *Veterinary Clinics of North America: Equine Practice* 16:605–617.

Imagawa H, Ando Y, Kamada M, *et al.* 1981. Sero-epizootiological survey of Getah virus infection in light horses in Japan. *Japanese Journal of Veterinary Science* 43:797–802.

Jones A, Lowry K, Aaskov JG, Holmes EC, Kitchen A 2010. Molecular evolutionary dynamics of Ross River virus and implications for vaccine efficacy. *Journal of General Virology* 91:182–188.

Kay BH, Pollitt CC, Fanning ID, Hall RA 1987. The experimental infection of horses with Murray Valley encephalitis and Ross River viruses. *Australian Veterinary Journal* 64:52–55.

Kumanomido T, Kamada M, Wada R, Kenemaru T, Sugiura T, Akiyama Y 1988. Pathogenicity for horses of original Sagiyama virus, a member of the Getah virus group. *Veterinary Microbiology* 17:367–373.

Marchette NJ, Reednick A, Garcia R, MacVean DW 1978. Alphaviruses in penninsular Malaysia. 1. Virus isolations and animal serology. *South East Asian Journal of Tropical Medicine and Public Health* 9:317–329.

Matsamura A, Goto H, Shimizu K, *et al.* 1982. Prevalence and distribution of antibodies to Getah and Japanese encephalitis viruses in horses raised in Hokkaido. *Japanese Journal of Veterinary Science* 44:967–970.

Sentsui H, Kono Y 1980. An epidemic of Getah virus infection among racehorses: isolation of the virus. *Research in Veterinary Science* 29:157–161.

Studdert MJ, Azuolas JK, Vasey JR, Hall RA, Ficorilli N, Huang JA 2003. Polymerase chain reaction tests for the identification of Ross River, Kunjin and Murray Valley encephalitis virus infections in horses. *Australian Veterinary Journal* 81:76–80.

Wekesa SN, Inoshima Y, Murakami K, Sentsui H 2001. Genomic analysis of some Japanese isolates of Getah virus. *Veterinary Microbiology* 83:137–146.

CHAPTER 3 PROTOZOAL DISEASES

Klossiella equi

Anderson WI, Picut CA 1988. *Klossiella equi* induced tubular nephrosis and interstitial nephritis in a pony. *Journal of Comparative Pathology* 98:363–366.

Karanja DN, Ngatia TA, Wandera JG 1995. Donkey Klossiellosis in Kenya. *Veterinary Parasitology* 59:1–5.

Marcato PS 1977. Glomerulonefrite diffusa associata a Klossiellosi in un cavallo. *Atti della Societa Italiana della Scienze Veterinarie* 31:691–692.

Reinemeyer CR, Jacobs RM, Spurlock GN 1983. A coccidial sporocyst in equine urine. *Journal of the American Veterinary Medical Association* 182:1250–1251.

Reppas GP, Collins GH 1995. *Klossiella equi* infection in horses; sporocyst stage identified in urine. *Australian Veterinary Journal* 72:316–318.

Suedmeyer WK, Restis E, Beerntsen BT 2006. *Klossiella equi* infection in a Hartmann's mountain zebra (*Equus zebra hartmannae*). *Journal of Zoo and Wildlife Medicine* 37:420–423.

Equine protozoal myeloencephalitis

Cohen ND, Mackay RJ, Toby E, *et al*. 2007. A multicenter case-control study of risk factors for equine protozoal myeloencephalitis. *Journal of the American Veterinary Medical Association* 231:1857–1863.

Elitsur E, Marsh AE, Reed SM, *et al*. 2007. Early migration of *Sarcocystis neurona* in ponies fed sporocysts. *Journal of Parasitology* 93:1222–1225.

Ellison S, Witonsky S 2009. Evidence that antibodies against recombinant SnSAG1 of *Sarcocystis neurona* merozoites are involved in infection and immunity in equine protozoal myeloencephalitis. *Canadian Journal of Veterinary Research* 73:176–183.

Fayer R, Mayhew IG, Baird JD, *et al*. 1990. Epidemiology of equine protozoal myeloencephalitis in North America based on histologically confirmed cases. *Journal of Veterinary Internal Medicine* 4:54–57.

Finno CJ, Aleman M, Pusterla N 2007. Equine protozoal myeloencephalitis associated with neosporosis in 3 horses. *Journal of Veterinary Internal Medicine* 21:1405–1408.

Furr M, MacKay R, Granstrom D, Schott H 2nd, Andrews F 2002. Clinical diagnosis of equine protozoal myeloencephalitis (EPM). *Journal of Veterinary Internal Medicine* 16:618–621.

Furr M, Howe D, Reed S, Yeargan M 2011. Antibody coefficients for the diagnosis of equine protozoal myeloencephalitis. *Journal of Veterinary Internal Medicine* 25:138–142.

Granstrom DE, MacPherson JM, Gajadhar AA, Dubey JP, Tramontin R, Stamper S 1994. Differentiation of *Sarcocystis neurona* from eight related coccidia by random amplified polymorphic DNA assay. *Molecular and Cellular Probes* 8:353–356.

Johnson AL 2008. Which is the most sensitive and specific commercial test to diagnose *Sarcocystis neurona* infection (equine protozoal myeloencephalitis) in horses? *Equine Veterinary Education* 20:166–168.

Jubb KVF, Kennedy PC, Palmer N 2007. *Pathology of Domestic Animals*, 5th edn. WB Saunders Elsevier, Edinburgh, 1:435.

MacKay RJ, Tanhauser ST, Gillis KD, Mayhew IG, Kennedy TJ 2008. Effect of intermittent oral administration of ponazuril on experimental *Sarcocystis neurona* infection of horses. *American Journal of Veterinary Research* 69:396–402.

MacKay RJS, Davis SW, Dubey JP 1992. Equine protozoal myeloencephalitis. *Compendium on Continuing Education for the Practicing Veterinarian* 14:1359–1366.

Marsh A, Barr B, Madigan J, Lakritz J, Nordhausen R, Conrad PA 1996. Neosporosis as a cause of equine protozoal myeloencephalitis. *Journal of the American Veterinary Medical Association* 209:1907–1913.

Morley PS, Traub-Dargatz JL, Benedict KM, Saville WJ, Voelker LD, Wagner BA 2008. Risk factors for owner-reported occurrence of equine protozoal myeloencephalitis in the US equine population. *Journal of Veterinary Internal Medicine* 22:616–629.

Mullaney T, Murphy AJ, Kiupel M, Bell JA, Rossano MG, Mansfield LS 2005. Evidence to support horses as natural intermediate hosts for *Sarcocystis neurona*. *Veterinary Parasitology* 133:27–36.

Packham A, Conrad P, Wilson W, *et al*. 2002. Qualitative evaluation of selective tests for detection of *Neospora hughesi* antibodies in serum and cerebrospinal fluid of experimentally infected horses. *Journal of Parasitology* 88:1239–1246.

Rossano MG, Kaneene JB, Schott HC 2nd, Sheline KD, Mansfield LS 2003. Assessing the agreement of Western blot test results for paired serum and cerebrospinal fluid samples from horses tested for antibodies to *Sarcocystis neurona*. *Veterinary Parasitology* 115:233–238.

Rossano MG, Schott HC 2nd, Murphy AJ, *et al*. 2005. Parasitemia in an immunocompetent horse experimentally challenged with *Sarcocystis neurona* sporocysts. *Veterinary Parasitology* 127:3–8.

Saville WJ, Stich RW, Reed SM, *et al*. 2001. Utilization of stress in the development of an equine model for equine protozoal myeloencephalitis. *Veterinary Parasitology* 95:211–222.

Sellon DC, Knowles DP, Greiner EC, *et al*. 2004. Infection of immunodeficient horses with *Sarcocystis neurona* does not result in neurologic disease. *Clinical and Diagnostic Laboratory Immunology* 11:1134–1139.

Sundar N, Asmundsson IM, Thomas NJ, Samuel MD, Dubey JP, Rosenthal BM 2008. Modest genetic differentiation among North American populations of *Sarcocystis neurona* may reflect expansion in its geographic range. *Veterinary Parasitology* 152:8–15.

Witonsky SG, Ellison S, Yang J, *et al*. 2008. Horses experimentally infected with *Sarcocystis neurona* develop altered immune responses *in vitro*. *Journal of Parasitology* 94:1047–1054.

Wobeser BK, Godson DL, Rejmanek D, Dowling P 2009. Equine protozoal myeloencephalitis caused by *Neospora hughesi* in an adult horse in Saskatchewan. *Canadian Veterinary Journal* 50:851–853.

Yeargan MR, Howe DK 2011. Improved detection of equine antibodies against *Sarcocystis neurona* using polyvalent ELISAs based on the parasite SnSAG surface antigens. *Veterinary Parasitology* 176:16–22.

Cryptosporidiosis

Atwill ER, McDougald NK, Perea L 2000. Cross-sectional study of faecal shedding of *Giardia duodenalis* and *Cryptosporidium parvum* among packstock in the Sierra Nevada Range. *Equine Veterinary Journal* 32:247–252.

Bakheit MA, Torra D, Palomino LA, *et al*. 2008. Sensitive and specific detection of *Cryptosporidium* species in PCR-negative samples by loop-mediated isothermal DNA amplification and confirmation of generated LAMP products by sequencing. *Veterinary Parasitology* 158:11–22.

Burton AJ, Nydam DV, Dearen TK, Mitchell K, Bowman DD, Xiao L 2010. The prevalence of *Cryptosporidium*, and identification of the *Cryptosporidium* horse genotype in foals in New York State. *Veterinary Parasitology* 174:139–144.

Chalmers RM, Grinberg A 2005. Significance of *Cryptosporidium parvum* in horses. *Veterinary Record* 156:688.

Chalmers RM, Thomas AL, Butler BA, Davies Morel MCG 2005. Identification of *Cryptosporidium parvum* genotype 2 in domestic horses. *Veterinary Record* 156:49–50.

Cohen ND, Snowden K 1997. Cryptosporidial diarrhea in foals. *Compendium on Continuing Education for the Practicing Veterinarian* 18:298–306.

Dupont HI, Chappell CL, Sterling CR, Okhuysen PC, Rose JB, Jakubowski W 1995. The infectivity of *Cryptosporidium parvum* in healthy volunteers. *New England Journal of Medicine* 332:855–859.

Fayer R, Morgan U, Upton SJ 2000. Epidemiology of *Cryptosporidium* transmission, detection and identification. *International Journal of Parasitology* 30:1305–1322.

Gajadhar AA, Caron JP, Allen JR 1985. Cryptosporidiosis in two foals. *Canadian Veterinary Journal* 26:132–134.

Grinberg A, Pomroy WE, Carslake HB, Shi Y, Gibson IR, Drayton BM 2009. A study of neonatal cryptosporidiosis of foals in New Zealand. *New Zealand Veterinary Journal* 57:284–289.

Grinberg A, Learmonth J, Kwan E, et al. 2008. Genetic diversity and zoonotic potential of *Cryptosporidium parvum* causing foal diarrhea. *Journal of Clinical Microbiology* 46:2396–2398.

Hunter PR, Hughes LS, Woodhouse S, et al. 2004. Sporadic cryptosporidiosis case–control study with genotyping. *Emerging Infectious Diseases* 10:1241–1249.

Netherwood T, Wood JL, Townsend HG, Mumford JA, Chanter N 1996. Foal diarrhoea between 1991 and 1994 in the United Kingdom associated with *Clostridium perfringens*, rotavirus, *Strongyloides westeri*, and *Cryptosporidium* spp. *Epidemiology and Infection* 117:375–383.

Smith RP, Chalmers RM, Mueller-Doblies D, et al. 2010. Investigation of farms linked to human patients with cryptosporidiosis in England and Wales. *Preventive Veterinary Medicine* 94:9–17.

Veronesi F, Passamonti F, Cacciò S, Diaferia M, Piergili Fioretti D 2010. Epidemiological survey on equine cryptosporidium and giardia infections in Italy and molecular characterization of isolates. *Zoonoses and Public Health* 57:510–517.

Xiao L, Herd RP 1994. Epidemiology of equine *Cryptosporidium* and *Giardia* infections. *Equine Veterinary Journal* 26:14–17.

Eimeria leuckarti

Barker IK, Remmer O 1972. The endogenous development of *Eimeria leuckarti* in ponies. *Journal of Parasitology* 58:112–122.

De Souza PN, Bomfim TC, Huber F, Abboud LC, Gomes RS 2009. Natural infection by *Cryptosporidium* sp., *Giardia* sp., and *Eimeria leuckarti* in three groups of equines with different handlings in Rio de Janeiro, Brazil. *Veterinary Parasitology* 160:327–333.

Hirayama K, Okamoto M, Sako T, et al. 2002. *Eimeria* organisms develop in the epithelial cells of equine small intestine. *Veterinary Pathology* 39:505–508.

Lyons ET, Tolliver SC 2004. Prevalence of parasite eggs (*Strongyloides westeri*, *Parascaris equorum*, and *strongyles*) and oocysts (*Eimeria leuckarti*) in the feces of Thoroughbred foals on 14 farms in central Kentucky in 2003. *Parasitology Research* 92:400–404.

Lyons ET, Tolliver SC, Rathgeber RA, Collins SS 2007. Parasite field study in central Kentucky on thoroughbred foals (born in 2004) treated with pyrantel tartrate daily and other parasiticides periodically. *Parasitology Research* 100:473–478.

Soulsby EJL 1968. *Helminths, Arthropods & Protozoa of Domesticated Animals*. Baillière, Tindall and Cassell, London.

Babesiosis/Piroplasmosis

Bhoora R, Franssen L, Oosthuizen MC, et al. 2009. Sequence heterogeneity in the 18S rRNA gene within *Theileria equi* and *Babesia caballi* from horses in South Africa. *Veterinary Parasitology* 159:112–120.

Bhoora R, Quan M, Franssen L, et al. 2010. Development and evaluation of real-time PCR assays for the quantitative detection of *Babesia caballi* and *Theileria equi* infections in horses from South Africa. *Veterinary Parasitology* 168:201–211.

Brüning A 1996. Equine piroplasmosis an update on diagnosis, treatment and prevention. *British Veterinary Journal* 152:139–151.

Butler CM, Gils JAM van, Kolk JH van der 2005. Acute infection with *B. caballi* in a Dutch Standardbred foal after visiting a stud in Normandy (France). *Tijdschrift voor Diergeneeskunde* 130:726–731.

Butler CM, Nijhof AM, Kolk JH van der, et al. 2008. Repeated high dose imidocarb dipropionate treatment did not eliminate *Babesia caballi* from naturally infected horses as determined by PCR-reverse line blot hybridization. *Veterinary Parasitology* 151:320–322.

Caccio S, Camma C, Onuma M, Severini C 2000. The beta-tubulin gene of *Babesia* and *Theileria* parasites is an informative marker for species discrimination. *International Journal of Parasitology* 30:1181–1185.

Frerichs WM, Holbrook AA, Johnson AJ 1969. Equine piroplasmosis: complement-fixation titers of horses infected with *Babesia caballi*. *American Journal of Veterinary Research* 30:697–702.

Fritz D 2010. A PCR study of piroplasms in 166 dogs and 111 horses in France (March 2006 to March 2008). *Parasitology Research* 106:1339–1342.

Jaffer O, Abdishakur F, Hakimuddin F, Riya A, Wernery U, Schuster RK 2010. A comparative study of serological tests and PCR for the diagnosis of equine piroplasmosis. *Parasitology Research* 106:709–713.

Kerber CE, Labruna MB, Ferreira F, De Waal DT, Knowles DP, Gennari SM 2009. Prevalence of equine piroplasmosis and its association with tick infestation in the State of São Paulo, Brazil. *Revista Brasileira de Parasitologia Veterinária* 18:1–8.

Kim CM, Blanco LBC, Alhassan A, Iseki H, Yokoyama N, Xuan X, Igarashi I 2008. Diagnostic real-time PCR assay for the quantitative detection of *Theileria equi* from equine blood samples. *Veterinary Parasitology* 151:158–163.

Krause PJ, Telford S 3rd, Spielman A, et al. 1996. Comparison of PCR with blood smear and inoculation of small animals for diagnosis of *Babesia microti* parasitemia. *Journal of Clinical Microbiology* 34:2791–2794.

Lewis BD, Penzhorn BL, Volkmann DH 1999. Could treatment of pregnant mares prevent abortions due to equine piroplasmosis? *Journal of the South African Veterinary Association* 70:90–91.

Meyer C, Guthrie AJ, Stevens KB 2005. Clinical and clinicopathological changes in 6 healthy ponies following intramuscular administration of multiple doses of imidocarb dipropionate. *Journal of the South African Veterinary Association* 76:26–32.

Moretti A, Mangili V, Salvatori R, *et al.* 2010. Prevalence and diagnosis of *Babesia* and *Theileria* infections in horses in Italy: a preliminary study. *Veterinary Journal* 184:346–350.

Nagore D, Garcia-Sanmartin J, Garcia-Perez AL, Juste RA, Hurtado A 2004. Detection and identification of equine *Theileria* and *Babesia* species by reverse line blotting: epidemiological survey and phylogenetic analysis. *Veterinary Parasitology* 123:41–54.

Persing DH, Conrad PA 1995. Babesiosis: new insights from phylogenetic analysis. *Infectious Agents and Disease* 4:182–195.

Pitel PH, Pronost S, Scrive T, Léon A, Richard E, Fortier G 2010. Molecular detection of *Theileria equi* and *Babesia caballi* in the bone marrow of asymptomatic horses. *Veterinary Parasitology* 170:182–184.

Schwint ON, Ueti MW, Palmer GH, *et al.* 2009. Imidocarb dipropionate clears persistent *Babesia caballi* infection with elimination of transmission potential. *Antimicrobial Agents and Chemotherapy* 53:4327–4332.

Sigg L, Gerber V, Gottstein B, Doherr MG, Frey CF 2010. Seroprevalence of *Babesia caballi* and *Theileria equi* in the Swiss horse population. *Parasitology International* 59:313–317.

Uilenberg G 2006. Babesia – A historical overview. *Veterinary Parasitology* 138:3–10.

Vial HJ, Gorenflot A 2006. Chemotherapy against babesiosis. *Veterinary Parasitology* 138:147–160.

Waal DT de 1992. Equine piroplasmosis: a review. *British Veterinary Journal* 148:6–14.

Weiland G 1986. Species-specific serodiagnosis of equine piroplasma infections by means of complement fixation test (CFT), immunofluorescence (IIF), and enzyme-linked immunosorbent assay (ELISA). *Veterinary Parasitology* 20:43–48.

Giardia duodenalis

Atwill ER, McDougald NK, Perea L 2000. Cross-sectional study of faecal shedding of *Giardia duodenalis* and *Cryptosporidium parvum* among packstock in the Sierra Nevada Range. *Equine Veterinary Journal* 32:247–252.

Bemrick WJ 1968. *Giardia* in North American horses. *Veterinary Medicine & Small Animal Clinician* 63:163–165.

Kirkpatrick CE, Skand DL 1985. Giardiasis in a horse. *Journal of the American Veterinary Medical Association* 187:163–164.

Manahan FF 1970. Diarrhoea in horses with particular reference to a chronic diarrhoea syndrome. *Australian Veterinary Journal* 46:231–234.

Soulsby EJL 1968. *Helminths, Arthropods & Protozoa of Domesticated Animals.* Baillière, Tindall and Cassell, London.

Traub R, Wade S, Read C, Thompson A, Mohammed H 2005. Molecular characterization of potentially zoonotic isolates of *Giardia duodenalis* in horses. *Veterinary Parasitology* 130:317–321.

Wienecka J, Olding-Stenkvist E, Schröder H, Huldt G 1989. Detection of *Giardia* antigen in stool samples by a semi-quantitative enzyme immunoassay (EIA) test. *Scandinavian Journal of Infectious Diseases* 21:443–448.

Xiao L, Herd RP 1994. Epidemiology of equine *Cryptosporidium* and *Giardia* infections. *Equine Veterinary Journal* 26:14–17.

Trypanosomosis

Assefa E, Abebe G 2001. Drug-resistant *Trypanosoma congolense* in naturally infected donkeys in north Omo Zone, southern Ethiopia. *Veterinary Parasitology* 99:261–271.

Barrowman PR 1976. Experimental intraspinal *Trypanosoma equiperdum* infection in a horse. *Onderstepoort Journal of Veterinary Research* 43:201–202.

Berlin D, Loeb E, Baneth G 2009. Disseminated central nervous system disease caused by *Trypanosoma evansi* in a horse. *Veterinary Parasitology* 161:316–319.

Brun R, Hecker H, Lun Z-R 1998. *Trypanosoma evansi* and *T. equiperdum*: distribution, biology, treatment and phylogenetic relationship. *Veterinary Parasitology* 79:95–107.

Camargo RE, Uzcanga GL, Bubis J 2004. Isolation of two antigens from *Trypanosoma evansi* that are partially responsible for its cross-reactivity with *Trypanosoma vivax*. *Veterinary Parasitology* 123:67–81.

Claes F, Büscher P, Touratier L, Goddeeris BM 2005. *Trypanosoma equiperdum*: master of disguise or historical mistake? Review. *Trends in Parasitology* 21:316–321.

Faye D, Pereira de Almeida PJL, Goossens B, *et al.* 2001. Prevalence and incidence of trypanosomosis in horses and donkeys in the Gambia. *Veterinary Parasitology* 101:101–114.

Gillingwater K, Büscher P, Brun R 2007. Establishment of a panel of reference *Trypanosoma evansi* and *Trypanosoma equiperdum* strains for drug screening. *Veterinary Parasitology* 148:114–121.

Hagos A, Goddeeris BM, Yilkal K, *et al.* 2010. Efficacy of Cymelarsan and Diminasan against *Trypanosoma equiperdum* infections in mice and horses. *Veterinary Parasitology* 171:200–206.

Katz J, Dewald R, Nicholson J 2000. Procedurally similar competitive immunoassay systems for the serodiagnosis of *Babesia equi*, *Babesia caballi*, *Trypanosoma equiperdum*, and *Burkholderia mallei* infection in horses. *Journal of Veterinary Diagnostic Investigation* 12:46–50.

Kaur R, Gupta VK, Dhariwal AC, Jain DC, Shiv L 2007. A rare case of trypanosomiasis in a two month old infant in Mumbai, India. *Journal of Communicable Diseases* 39:71–74.

Kumba FF, Claasen B, Petrus P 2002. Apparent prevalence of dourine in the Khomas region of Namibia. *Onderstepoort Journal of Veterinary Research* 69:295–298.

Laha R, Sasmal NK 2009. Detection of *Trypanosoma evansi* infection in clinically ill cattle, buffaloes, and horses using various diagnostic tests. *Epidemiology and Infection* 137:1583–1585.

Lai DH, Hashimi H, Lun ZR, Ayala FJ, Lukes J 2008. Adaptations of *Trypanosoma brucei* to gradual loss of kinetoplast DNA: *Trypanosoma equiperdum* and *Trypanosoma evansi* are petite mutants of *T. brucei*. *Proceedings of the National Academy of Sciences of the USA* 105:1999–2004.

Lemos KR, Marques LC, Deaquino LP, Alessi AC, Machado RZ 2007. Immunohistochemical characterization of mononuclear cells and MHC II expression in the brain of horses with experimental chronic *Trypanosoma evansi* infection. *Revista Brasileira de Parasitologia Veterinária* 16:186–192.

Lemos KR, Marques LC, Aquino LP, Alessi AC, Zacarias RZ 2008. Astrocytic and microglial response and histopathological changes in the brain of horses with experimental chronic *Trypanosoma evansi* infection. *Revista do Instituto de Medicina Tropical de São Paulo* 50:243–249.

Menezes VT de, Queiroz AO, Gomes MA, Marques MA, Jansen AM 2004. *Trypanosoma evansi* in inbred and Swiss-Webster mice: distinct aspects of pathogenesis. *Parasitology Research* 94:193–200.

Metcalf ES 2001. The role of international transport of equine semen on disease transmission. Review. *Animal Reproduction Science* 68:229–237.

Rodrigues A, Fighera RA, Souza TM, Schild AL, Barros CS 2009. Neuropathology of naturally occurring *Trypanosoma evansi* infection of horses. *Veterinary Pathology* 46:251–258.

Tamarit A, Gutierrez C, Arroyo R, *et al.* 2010. *Trypanosoma evansi* infection in mainland Spain. *Veterinary Parasitology* 167:74–76.

Tuntasuvan D, Jarabrum W, Viseshakul N, *et al.* 2003. Chemotherapy of surra in horses and mules with diminazene aceturate. *Veterinary Parasitology* 110:227–233.

Uzcanga G, Mendoza M, Aso PM, Bubis J 2002. Purification of a 64 kDa antigen from *Trypanosoma evansi* that exhibits cross-reactivity with *Trypanosoma vivax*. *Parasitology* 124:287–299.

Watier-Grillot S 2008. Outbreak of animal trypanosomiasis (*T. evansi*) in the Aveyron department of France: risk for implantation of an animal disease with zoonotic potential. *Médecine Tropicale (Marseilles)* 68:468–470.

Watson EA 1915. Dourine and the complement fixation test. *Parasitology* 8:156–183.

Wernery U, Zachariah R, Mumford JA, Luckins T 2001. Preliminary evaluation of diagnostic tests using horses experimentally infected with *Trypanosoma evansi*. *Veterinary Journal* 161:287–300.

CHAPTER 4 FUNGAL DISEASES

Invasive mycoses

Andrew SE, Nguyen A, Jones GL, Brooks DE 2003. Seasonal effects on the aerobic bacterial and fungal conjunctival flora of normal thoroughbred brood mares in Florida. *Veterinary Ophthalmology* 6:45–50.

Brooks M, Royse C, Eisen D, Sparks P, Bhagwat K, Royse A 2011. An accidental mass. *Lancet* 377:1806.

Bruijn CM de, Wijnberg ID 2004. Potential role of *Candida* species in antibiotic-associated diarrhoea in a foal. *Veterinary Record* 155:26–28.

Chaffin MK, Schumacher J, McMullan WC 1995. Cutaneous pythiosis in the horse. Review. *Veterinary Clinics of North America: Equine Practice* 11:91–103.

Chermette R, Ferreiro L, Guillot J 2008. Dermatophytoses in animals. Review. *Mycopathologia* 166:385–405.

Church S, Wyn-Jones G, Parks AH, Ritchie HE 1986. Treatment of guttural pouch mycosis. *Equine Veterinary Journal* 18:362–365.

Dagenais TR, Keller NP 2009. Pathogenesis of *Aspergillus fumigatus* in invasive aspergillosis. Review. *Clinical Microbiology Reviews* 22:447–465.

Davis FW, Legendre AM 1994. Successful treatment of guttural pouch mycosis with itraconazole and topical enilconazole in a horse. *Journal of Veterinary Internal Medicine* 8:304–305.

Dixon PM, McGorum BC, Railton DI, *et al.* 2001. Laryngeal paralysis: a study of 375 cases in a mixed-breed population of horses. *Equine Veterinary Journal* 33:452–458.

Freeman DE 2006. Long-term follow-up on a large number of horses that underwent transarterial coil embolisation (TCE) for guttural pouch mycosis (GPM). *Equine Veterinary Journal* 38:271. Comment on *Equine Veterinary Journal* 2005; 37:430–434.

Gemensky-Metzler AJ, Wilkie DA, Kowalski JJ, Schmall LM, Willis AM, Yamagata M 2005. Changes in bacterial and fungal ocular flora of clinically normal horses following experimental application of topical antimicrobial or antimicrobial-corticosteroid ophthalmic preparations. *American Journal of Veterinary Research* 66:800–811.

Greet TR 1987. Outcome of treatment in 35 cases of guttural pouch mycosis. *Equine Veterinary Journal* 19:483–487.

Guillot J, Sarfati J, Ribot X, Jensen HE, Latgé JP 1997. Detection of antibodies to *Aspergillus fumigatus* in serum of horses with mycosis of the auditory tube diverticulum (guttural pouch). *American Journal of Veterinary Research* 58:1364–1366.

Hatziolos BC, Sass B, Albert TF, Stevenson MC 1975. Ocular changes in a horse with gutturomycosis. *Journal of the American Veterinary Medical Association* 167:51–54.

King JM, Kavanaugh JF, Bentinck-Smith J 1962. Diabetes mellitus with pituitary neoplasms in a horse and a dog. *Cornell Veterinarian* 52:133–145.

Kipar A, Frese K 1993. Hypoglossal neuritis with associated lingual hemiplegia secondary to guttural pouch mycosis. *Veterinary Pathology* 30:574–576.

Kosuge J, Goto Y, Shinjo T, Anzai T, Takatori K 2000. Detection of *Emericella nidulans* from bedding materials in horse breeding environment and its significance as a causative agent of guttural pouch mycosis in horses. *Nippon Ishinkin Gakkai Zasshi* 41:251–256.

Lane JG, Mair TS 1987. Observations on headshaking in the horse. *Equine Veterinary Journal* 19:331–336.

Lepage OM, Piccot-Crézollet C 2005. Transarterial coil embolisation in 31 horses (1999–2002) with guttural pouch mycosis: a 2-year follow-up. *Equine Veterinary Journal* 37:430–434.

Lepage OM, Perron MF, Cadoré JL 2004. The mystery of fungal infection in the guttural pouches. Review. *Veterinary Journal* 168:60–64.

Ludwig A, Gatineau S, Reynaud MC, Cadoré JL, Bourdoiseau G 2005. Fungal isolation and identification in 21 cases of guttural pouch mycosis in horses (1998–2002). *Veterinary Journal* 169:457–461.

Lund A, Deboer DJ 2008. Immunoprophylaxis of dermatophytosis in animals. *Mycopathologia* 166:407–424.

McLaughlin BG, O'Brien JL 1986. Guttural pouch mycosis and mycotic encephalitis in a horse. *Canadian Veterinary Journal* 27:109–111.

Millar H 2006. Guttural pouch mycosis in a 6-month-old filly. *Canadian Veterinary Journal* 47:259–261.

Nieuwstadt RA van, Kalsbeek HC 1994. Air sac mycosis: topical treatment using enilconazole administered via indwelling catheter. *Tijdschrift voor Diergeneeskunde* 119:3–5.

Patterson TF 2005. Advances and challenges in management of invasive mycoses. *Lancet* 366:1013–1025.

Sharma R, Hoog S de, Presber W, Gräser Y 2007. A virulent genotype of *Microsporum canis* is responsible for the majority of human infections. *Journal of Medical Microbiology* 56:1377–1385.

Sweeney CR, Freeman DE, Sweeney RW, Rubin JL, Maxson AD 1993. Hemorrhage into the guttural pouch (auditory tube diverticulum) associated with rupture of the longus capitis muscle in three horses. *Journal of the American Veterinary Medical Association* 202:1129–1131.

Thirion-Delalande C, Guillot J, Jensen HE, Crespeau FL, Bernex F 2005. Disseminated acute concomitant aspergillosis and mucormycosis in a pony. *Journal of Veterinary Medicine, A. Physiology, Pathology and Clinical Medicine* 52:121–124.

Walmsley JP 1988. A case of atlanto-occipital arthropathy following guttural pouch mycosis in a horse. The use of radioisotope bone scanning as an aid to diagnosis. *Equine Veterinary Journal* 20:219–220.

Equine histoplasmosis

Al-Ani FK 1999. Epizootic lymphangitis in horses: a review of the literature. *Revue Scientifique et Technique (Paris)* 18:691–699.

Ameni G 2006a. Epidemiology of equine histoplasmosis (epizootic lymphangitis) in carthorses in Ethiopia. *Veterinary Journal* 172:160–165.

Ameni G 2006b. Preliminary trial on the reproducibility of epizootic lymphangitis through experimental infection of two horses. *Veterinary Journal* 172:553–555.

Ameni G, Terefe W, Hailu A 2006. Histofarcin test for the diagnosis of epizootic lymphangitis in Ethiopia: development, optimisation and validation in the field. *Veterinary Journal* 171:358–362.

Cornick JL 1990. Diagnosis and treatment of pulmonary histoplasmosis in a horse. *Cornell Veterinarian* 80:97–103.

Fawi MT 1969. Fluorescent antibody test for the serodiagnosis of *Histoplasma farciminosum* infections in equidae. *British Veterinary Journal* 125:231–234.

Gabal MA, Mohammed KA 1985. Use of enzyme-linked immunosorbent assay for the diagnosis of equine *Histoplasmosis farciminosi* (epizootic lymphangitis). *Mycopathologia* 91:35–37.

Gugnani HC 2000. Histoplasmosis in Africa: a review. *Indian Journal of Chest Diseases and Allied Science* 42:271–277.

Hall AD 1979. An equine abortion due to histoplasmosis. *Veterinary Medicine & Small Animal Clinician* 74:200–201.

Jubb KVF, Kennedy PC, Palmer N 2007. *Pathology of Domestic Animals*, 5th edn. WB Saunders Elsevier, Edinburgh, 3:101–102.

Kasuga T, White TJ, Koenig G, et al. 2003. Phylogeography of the fungal pathogen *Histoplasma capsulatum*. *Molecular Ecology* 12:3383–3401.

Katayama Y, Kuwano A, Yoshihara T 2001. Histoplasmosis in the lung of a race horse with yersiniosis. *Journal of Veterinary Medical Science* 63:1229–1231.

Kauffman CA 2009. Histoplasmosis. *Clinical Chest Medicine* 30:217–225.

Miller RM, Dresher LK 1981. Equine ulcerative lymphangitis caused by *Pasteurella hemolytica* (2 case reports). *Veterinary Medicine & Small Animal Clinician* 76:1335–1338.

Nunes J, Mackie JT, Kiupel M 2006. Equine histoplasmosis presenting as a tumor in the abdominal cavity. *Journal of Veterinary Diagnostic Investigation* 18:508–510.

Randall CC, Orr MF, Schell FG 1951. Detection by tissue culture of an organism resembling *Histoplasma capsulatum* in an apparently healthy horse. *Proceedings of the Society of Experimental Biology and Medicine* 78:447–450.

Rezabek GB, Donahue JM, Giles RC, et al. 1993. Histoplasmosis in horses. *Journal of Comparative Pathology* 109:47–55.

Richter M, Hauser B, Kaps S, Spiess BM 2003. Keratitis due to *Histoplasma* spp. in a horse. *Veterinary Ophthalmology* 6:99–103.

Scantlebury C 2008. Epizootic lymphangitis in working equines: it's not just about the horse. *Proceedings of the 47th BEVA Congress*, 10th–13th September 2008 Liverpool:311–312.

CHAPTER 5 ECTOPARASITICAL DISEASES

Gasterophilus spp.

Bezdekova B, Jahn P, Vyskocil M 2007. Pathomorphological study on gastroduodenal ulceration in horses: localisation of lesions. *Acta Veterinaria Hungarica* 55:241–249.

Coles GC, Hillyer MH, Taylor FGR, Parker LD 1998. Activity of moxidectin against bots and lungworm in equids. *Veterinary Record* 143:169–170.

Dart AJ, Hutchins DR, Begg AP 1987. Suppurative splenitis and peritonitis in a horse after gastric ulceration caused by larvae of *Gasterophilus intestinalis*. *Australian Veterinary Journal* 64:155–158.

Kolk JH van der, Sloet van Oldruitenborgh-Oosterbaan MM, Gruys E 1989. Bilateral pleuritis following esophageal fistula in a horse as a complication of a *Gasterophilus* infection. *Tijdschrift voor Diergeneeskunde* 114:769–774.

Lapointe JM, Céleste C, Villeneuve A 2003. Septic peritonitis due to colonic perforation associated with aberrant migration of a *Gasterophilus intestinalis* larva in a horse. *Veterinary Pathology* 40:338–339.

Lyons ET, Swerczek TW, Tolliver SC, Bair HD, Drudge JH, Ennis LE 2000. Prevalence of selected species of internal parasites in equids at necropsy in central Kentucky (1995–1999). *Veterinary Parasitology* **92**:51–62.

Pawlas-Opiela M, Wojciech Ł, Sołtysiak Z, Otranto D, Ugorski M 2010. Molecular comparison of *Gasterophilus intestinalis* and *Gasterophilus nasalis* from two distinct areas of Poland and Italy based on cox1 sequence analysis. *Veterinary Parasitology* **169**:219–221.

Roelfstra L, Deeg CA, Hauck SM, *et al.* 2009. Protein expression profile of *Gasterophilus intestinalis* larvae causing horse gastric myiasis and characterization of horse immune reaction. *Parasites and Vectors* **2**:6.

Roelfstra L, Vlimant M, Betschart B, Pfister K, Diehl PA 2010. Light and electron microscopy studies of the midgut and salivary glands of second and third instars of the horse stomach bot, *Gasterophilus intestinalis*. *Medical and Veterinary Entomology* **24**:236–249.

Sánchez-Andrade R, Cortiñas FJ, Francisco I, *et al.* 2010. A novel second instar *Gasterophilus* excretory/secretory antigen-based ELISA for the diagnosis of gasterophilosis in grazing horses. *Veterinary Parasitology* **171**:314–320.

Smith MA, McGarry JW, Kelly DF, Proudman CJ 2005. *Gasterophilus pecorum* in the soft palate of a British pony. *Veterinary Record* **156**:283–284.

Soulsby EJL 1968. *Helminths, Arthropods & Protozoa of Domesticated Animals*. Baillière, Tindall and Cassell, London.

Mites

Bates PG 1999. Inter- and intra-specific variation within the genus *Psoroptes* (Acari: Psoroptidae). Review. *Veterinary Parasitology* **83**:201–217.

Cremers HJ 1985. The incidence of *Chorioptes bovis* (Acarina: Psoroptidae) on the feet of horses, sheep, and goats in the Netherlands. *Veterinary Quarterly* **7**:283–289.

Essig A, Rinder H, Gothe R, Zahler M 1999. Genetic differentiation of mites of the genus Chorioptes (Acari: Psoroptidae). *Experimental and Applied Acarology* **23**:309–318.

Fain A 1975. New taxa in Psoroptinae. Hypothesis on the origin of the group (Acarina, Sarcoptiformes, Psoroptidae). *Acta Zoologica et Pathologica Antverpiensia* **61**:57–84.

Osman SA, Hanafy A, Amer SE 2006. Clinical and therapeutic studies on mange in horses. *Veterinary Parasitology* **141**:191–195.

Paterson S, Coumbe K 2009. An open study to evaluate topical treatment of equine chorioptic mange with shampooing and lime sulphur solution. *Veterinary Dermatology* **20**:623–629.

Rendle DI, Cottle HJ, Love S, Hughes KJ 2007. Comparative study of doramectin and fipronil in the treatment of equine chorioptic mange. *Veterinary Record* **161**:335–338.

Rüfenacht S, Roosje PJ, Sager H, *et al.* 2011. Combined moxidectin and environmental therapy do not eliminate *Chorioptes bovis* infestation in heavily feathered horses. *Veterinary Dermatology* **22**:17–23.

Soulsby EJL 1968. *Helminths, Arthropods & Protozoa of Domesticated Animals*. Baillière, Tindall and Cassell, London.

Ural K, Ulutas B, Kar S 2008. Eprinomectin treatment of psoroptic mange in hunter/jumper and dressage horses: a prospective, randomized, double-blinded, placebo-controlled clinical trial. *Veterinary Parasitology* **156**:353–357.

Lice

Larsen KS, Eydal M, Mencke N, Sigurdsson H 2005. Infestation of *Werneckiella equi* on Icelandic horses, characteristics of predilection sites and lice dermatitis. *Parasitology Research* **96**:398–401.

Mencke N, Larsen KS, Eydal M, Sigurethsson H 2005. Dermatological and parasitological evaluation of infestations with chewing lice (*Werneckiella equi*) on horses and treatment using imidacloprid. *Parasitology Research* **97**:7–12.

Soulsby EJL 1968. *Helminths, Arthropods & Protozoa of Domesticated Animals*. Baillière, Tindall and Cassell, London.

CHAPTER 6 HELMINTIC DISEASES

Fasciola hepatica

Alasaad S, Li QY, Lin RQ, *et al.* 2008. Genetic variability among *Fasciola hepatica* samples from different host species and geographical localities in Spain revealed by the novel SRAP marker. *Parasitology Research* **103**:181–186.

Alves RM, Rensburg LJ van, Wyk JA van 1988. *Fasciola* in horses in the Republic of South Africa: a single natural case of *Fasciola hepatica* and the failure to infest ten horses with *F. hepatica* or *F. gigantica*. *Onderstepoort Journal of Veterinary Research* **55**:157–163.

Epe C, Coati N, Schnieder T 2004. Results of parasitological examinations of faecal samples from horses, ruminants, pigs, dogs, cats, hedgehogs, and rabbits between 1998 and 2002. *Deutsche Tierärztliche Wochenschrift* **111**:243–247.

Gorman T, Aballay J, Fredes F, Silva M, Aguillón JC, Alcaíno HA 1997. Immunodiagnosis of fasciolosis in horses and pigs using western blots. *International Journal of Parasitology* **27**:1429–1432.

Haridy FM, Morsy GH, Abdou NE, Morsy TA 2007. Zoonotic fascioliasis in donkeys: ELISA (Fges) and postmortum examination in the Zoo, Giza, Egypt. *Journal of the Egyptian Society of Parasitology* **37**:1101–1110.

Keiser J, Utzinger J 2009. Food-borne trematodiases. *Clinical and Microbiology Reviews* **22**:466–483.

Nansen P, Andersen S, Hesselholt M 1975. Experimental infection of the horse with *Fasciola hepatica*. *Experimental Parasitology* **37**:15–19.

Owen JM 1977. Liver fluke infection in horses and ponies. *Equine Veterinary Journal* **9**:29–31.

Rubilar L, Cabreira A, Giacaman L 1988. Treatment of *Fasciola hepatica* infection in horses with triclabendazole. *Veterinary Record* **123**:320–321.

Soulé C, Boulard C, Levieux D, Barnouin J, Plateau E 1989. Experimental equine fascioliasis: evolution of serologic, enzymatic, and parasitic parameters. *Annales de Recherches Vétérinaires* **20**:295–307.

Soulsby EJL 1968. *Helminths, Arthropods & Protozoa of Domesticated Animals*. Baillière, Tindall and Cassell, London.

Valero MA, Mas-Coma S 2000. Comparative infectivity of *Fasciola hepatica* metacercariae from isolates of the main and secondary reservoir animal host species in the Bolivian Altiplano high human endemic region. *Folia Parasitologica (Praha)* **47**:17–22.

Valero MA, Perez-Crespo I, Periago MV, Khoubbane M, Mas-Coma S 2009. Fluke egg characteristics for the diagnosis of human and animal fascioliasis by *Fasciola hepatica* and *F. gigantica*. *Acta Tropica* **111**:150–159.

Anoplocephala spp.

Abbott JB, Mellor DJ, Barrett EJ, Proudman CJ, Love S 2008. Serological changes observed in horses infected with *Anoplocephala perfoliata* after treatment with praziquantel and natural reinfection. *Veterinary Record* **162**:50–53.

Beroza GA, Barclay WP, Phillips TN, Foerner JJ, Donawick WJ 1983. Cecal perforation and peritonitis associated with *Anoplocephala perfoliata* infection in three horses. *Journal of the American Veterinary Medical Association* **183**:804–806.

Cosgrove JS, Sheeran JJ, Sainty TJ 1986. Intussusception associated with infection with *Anoplocephala perfoliata* in a two-year-old Thoroughbred. *Irish Veterinary Journal* **40**:35–36.

Edwards GB 1986. Surgical management of intussusception in the horse. *Equine Veterinary Journal* **18**:313–321.

French DD, Chapman MR, Klei TR 1994. Effects of treatment with ivermectin for five years on the prevalence of *Anoplocephala perfoliata* in three Louisiana pony herds. *Veterinary Record* **135**:63–65.

Lyons ET, Swerczek TW, Tolliver SC, Bair HD, Drudge JH, Ennis LE 2000. Prevalence of selected species of internal parasites in equids at necropsy in central Kentucky (1995–1999). *Veterinary Parasitology* **92**:51–62.

Pavone S, Veronesi F, Piergili Fioretti D, Mandara MT 2010. Pathological changes caused by *Anoplocephala perfoliata* in the equine ileocecal junction. *Veterinary Research Communications* **34**(Supplement 1):S53–S56.

Proudman CJ, Edwards GB 1992. Validation of a centrifugation/flotation technique for the diagnosis of equine cestodiasis. *Veterinary Record* **131**:71–72.

Proudman CJ, Holdstock NB 2000. Investigation of an outbreak of tapeworm-associated colic in a training yard. *Equine Veterinary Journal Supplement* **32**:37–41.

Proudman CJ, French DD, Trees AJ 1998. Tapeworm infection is a significant risk factor for spasmodic colic and ileal impaction colic in the horse. *Equine Veterinary Journal* **30**:194–199.

Rehbein S, Lindner T, Visser M, Winter R 2011. Evaluation of a double centrifugation technique for the detection of *Anoplocephala* eggs in horse faeces. *Journal of Helminthology* **85**:409–414.

Reinemeyer CR, Nielsen MK 2009. Parasitism and colic. *Veterinary Clinics of North America: Equine Practice* **25**:233–245.

Skotarek SL, Colwell DD, Goater CP 2010. Evaluation of diagnostic techniques for *Anoplocephala perfoliata* in horses from Alberta, Canada. *Veterinary Parasitology* **172**:249–255.

Soulsby EJL 1968. *Helminths, Arthropods & Protozoa of Domesticated Animals*. Baillière, Tindall and Cassell, London.

Traversa D, Fichi G, Campigli M, *et al.* 2008. A comparison of coprological, serological, and molecular methods for the diagnosis of horse infection with *Anoplocephala perfoliata* (Cestoda, Cyclophyllidea). *Veterinary Parasitology* **152**:271–277.

Echinococcus equinus

Acosta-Jamett G, Cleaveland S, Cunningham AA, Bronsvoort BM, Craig PS 2010. *Echinococcus granulosus* infection in humans and livestock in the Coquimbo region, north-central Chile. *Veterinary Parasitology* **169**:102–110.

Blutke A, Hamel D, Hüttner M, *et al.* 2010. Cystic echinococcosis due to *Echinococcus equinus* in a horse from southern Germany. *Journal of Veterinary Diagnostic Investigation* **22**:458–462.

Carmena D, Sánchez-Serrano LP, Barbero-Martínez I 2008. *Echinococcus granulosus* infection in Spain. *Zoonoses and Public Health* **55**:156–165.

Cook BR 1989. The epidemiology of *Echinococcus granulosus* in Great Britain. V. The status of subspecies of *Echinococcus granulosus* in Great Britain. *Annals of Tropical Medicine and Parasitology* **83**:51–61.

Nakao M, McManus DP, Schantz PM, Craig PS, Ito A 2007. A molecular phylogeny of the genus *Echinococcus* inferred from complete mitochondrial genomes. *Parasitology* **134**:713–722.

Romig T, Dinkel A, Mackenstedt U 2006. The present situation of echinococcosis in Europe. Review. *Parasitology International* **55** (Supplement):S187–S191.

Soulsby EJL 1968. *Helminths, Arthropods & Protozoa of Domesticated Animals*. Baillière, Tindall and Cassell, London.

Varcasia A, Garippa G, Pipia AP, *et al.* 2008. Cystic echinococcosis in equids in Italy. *Parasitology Research* **102**:815–818.

Strongyloides westeri

Araujo JM, Araújo JV, Braga FR, Carvalho RO 2010. *In vitro* predatory activity of nematophagous fungi and after passing through gastrointestinal tract of equine on infective larvae of *Strongyloides westeri*. *Parasitology Research* **107**:103–108.

Brown CA, MacKay RJ, Chandra S, Davenport D, Lyons ET 1997. Overwhelming strongyloidosis in a foal. *Journal of the American Veterinary Medical Association* **211**:333–334.

Dewes HF 1972. *Strongyloides westeri* and *Corynebacterium equi* in foals. *New Zealand Veterinary Journal* **20**:82.

Dewes HF 1989. The association between weather, frenzied behaviour, percutaneous invasion by *Strongyloides westeri* larvae and *Rhodococcus equi* disease in foals. *New Zealand Veterinary Journal* **37**:69–73.

Dewes HF, Townsend KG 1990. Further observations on *Strongyloides westeri* dermatitis: recovery of larvae from soil and bedding, and survival in treated sites. *New Zealand Veterinary Journal* **38**:34–37.

Drudge JH, Lyons ET, Tolliver SC 1982. Controlled tests of pastes of dichlorvos and thiabendazole against induced *Strongyloides westeri* infections in pony foals in 1973–1974. *American Journal of Veterinary Research* 43:1675–1677.

Ludwig KG, Craig TM, Bowen JM, Ansari MM, Ley WB 1983. Efficacy of ivermectin in controlling *Strongyloides westeri* infections in foals. *American Journal of Veterinary Research* 44:314–316.

Lyons ET, Drudge JH, Tolliver SC 1973. On the life cycle of *Strongyloides westeri* in the equine. *Journal of Parasitology* 59:780–787.

Lyons ET, Tolliver SC, Drudge JH, Granstrom DE, Collins SS 1993. Natural infections of *Strongyloides westeri*: prevalence in horse foals on several farms in central Kentucky in 1992. *Veterinary Parasitology* 50:101–107.

Lyons ET, Tolliver SC, Rathgeber RA, Collins SS 2007. Parasite field study in central Kentucky on thoroughbred foals (born in 2004) treated with pyrantel tartrate daily and other parasiticides periodically. *Parasitology Research* 100:473–478.

Mirck MH, Meurs GK van 1982. The efficacy of ivermectin against *Strongyloides westeri* in foals. *Veterinary Quarterly* 4:89–91.

Netherwood T, Wood JL, Townsend HG, Mumford JA, Chanter N 1996. Foal diarrhoea between 1991 and 1994 in the United Kingdom associated with *Clostridium perfringens*, rotavirus, *Strongyloides westeri*, and *Cryptosporidium* spp. *Epidemiology and Infection* 117:375–383.

Russell AMF 1948. The development of helminthiasis in Thoroughbred foals. *Journal of Comparative Pathology and Therapeutics* 58:107–127.

Soulsby EJL 1968. *Helminths, Arthropods & Protozoa of Domesticated Animals*. Baillière, Tindall and Cassell, London.

Halicephalobus gingivalis

Anderson RC, Linder KE, Peregrine AS 1998. *Halicephalobus gingivalis* (Stefanski, 1954) from a fatal infection in a horse in Ontario, Canada with comments on the validity of *H. deletrix* and a review of the genus. *Parasite* 5:255–261.

Boswinkel M, Neyens IJ, Sloet van Oldruitenborgh-Oosterbaan MM 2006. *Halicephalobus gingivalis* infection in a 5-year-old Tinker gelding. *Tijdschrift voor Diergeneeskunde* 131:74–80.

Bryant UK, Lyons ET, Bain FT, Hong CB 2006. *Halicephalobus gingivalis*-associated meningoencephalitis in a Thoroughbred foal. *Journal of Veterinary Diagnostic Investigation* 18:612–615.

Cantile C, Rossi G, Braca G, Vitali CG, Taccini E, Renzoni G 1997. A horse with *Halicephalobus deletrix* encephalitis in Italy. *European Journal of Veterinary Pathology* 3:29–33.

Ferguson R, van Dreumel T, Keystone JS, *et al.* 2008. Unsuccessful treatment of a horse with mandibular granulomatous osteomyelitis due to *Halicephalobus gingivalis*. *Canadian Veterinary Journal* 49:1099–1103.

Gardiner CH, Koh DS, Cardella TA 1981. Micronema in man: third fatal infection. *American Journal of Tropical Medicine and Hygiene* 30:586–589.

Kinde H, Mathews M, Ash L, St Leger J 2000. *Halicephalobus gingivalis* (*H. deletrix*) infection in two horses in Southern California. *Journal of Veterinary Diagnostic Investigation* 12:162–165.

Muller S, Grzybowski M, Sager H, Bornand V, Brehm W 2008. A nodular granulomatous posthitis caused by *Halicephalobus* sp. in a horse. *Veterinary Dermatology* 19:44–48.

Nadler SA, Carreno RA, Adams BJ, Kinde H, Baldwin JG, Mundo-Ocampo M 2003. Molecular phylogenetics and diagnosis of soil and clinical isolates of *Halicephalobus gingivalis* (Nematoda: Cephalobina: Panagrolaimoidea), an opportunistic pathogen of horses. *International Journal of Parasitology* 33:1115–1125.

Pearce SG, Bouré LP, Taylor JA, Peregrine AS 2001. Treatment of a granuloma caused by *Halicephalobus gingivalis* in a horse. *Journal of the American Veterinary Medical Association* 219:1735–1738, 1708.

Shibahara T, Takai H, Shimizu C, Ishikawa Y, Kadota K 2002. Equine renal granuloma caused by *Halicephalobus* species. *Veterinary Record* 151:672–674.

Wilkins PA, Wacholder S, Nolan TJ, *et al.* 2001. Evidence for transmission of *Halicephalobus deletrix* (*H. gingivalis*) from dam to foal. *Journal of Veterinary Internal Medicine* 15:412–417.

Strongylus spp.

Bauer C, Cirak VY, Hermosilla C, Okoro H 1998. Efficacy of a 2 per cent moxidectin gel against gastrointestinal parasites of ponies. *Veterinary Record* 143:558–561.

Bonneau S, Maynard L, Tomczuk K, Kok D, Eun HM 2009. Anthelmintic efficacies of a tablet formula of ivermectin-praziquantel on horses experimentally infected with three *Strongylus* species. *Parasitology Research* 105:817–823.

Chapman MR, Hutchinson GW, Cenac MJ, Klei TR 1994. *In vitro* culture of equine strongylidae to the fourth larval stage in a cell-free medium. *Journal of Parasitology* 80:225–231.

Cohen ND, Loy JK, Lay JC, Craig TM, McMullan WC 1992. Eosinophilic gastroenteritis with encapsulated nematodes in a horse. *Journal of the American Veterinary Medical Association* 200:1518–1520.

Costa AJ, Barbosa OF, Moraes FR, *et al.* 1998. Comparative efficacy evaluation of moxidectin gel and ivermectin paste against internal parasites of equines in Brazil. *Veterinary Parasitology* 80:29–36.

DeLay J, Peregrine AS, Parsons DA 2001. Verminous arteritis in a 3-month-old thoroughbred foal. *Canadian Veterinary Journal* 42:289–291.

Hubert JD, Seahorn TL, Klei TR, Hosgood G, Horohov DW, Moore RM 2004. Clinical signs and hematologic, cytokine, and plasma nitric oxide alterations in response to *Strongylus vulgaris* infection in helminth-naïve ponies. *Canadian Journal of Veterinary Research* 68:193–200.

Lester GD, Bolton JR, Cambridge H, Thurgate S 1989. The effect of *Strongylus vulgaris* larvae on equine intestinal myoelectrical activity. *Equine Veterinary Journal Supplement* 7:8–13.

Lyons ET, Swerczek TW, Tolliver SC, Bair HD, Drudge JH, Ennis LE 2000. Prevalence of selected species of internal parasites in equids at necropsy in central Kentucky (1995–1999). *Veterinary Parasitology* 92:51–62.

McClure JR, Chapman MR, Klei TR 1994. Production and characterization of monospecific adult worm infections of *Strongylus vulgaris* and *Strongylus edentatus* in ponies. *Veterinary Parasitology* 51:249–254.

Mobarak MS, Ryan MF 1998. An immunohistochemical investigation of the adult stage of the equine parasite *Strongylus vulgaris*. *Journal of Helminthology* 72:159–166.

Mobarak MS, Ryan MF 1999. Ultrastructural aspects of feeding and secretion-excretion by the equine parasite *Strongylus vulgaris*. *Journal of Helminthology* 73:147–155.

Monahan CM, Taylor HW, Chapman MR, Klei TR 1994. Experimental immunization of ponies with *Strongylus vulgaris* radiation-attenuated larvae or crude soluble somatic extracts from larval or adult stages. *Journal of Parasitology* 80:911–923.

Monahan CM, Chapman MR, Taylor HW, French DD, Klei TR 1996. Comparison of moxidectin oral gel and ivermectin oral paste against a spectrum of internal parasites of ponies with special attention to encysted cyathostome larvae. *Veterinary Parasitology* 63:225–235.

Morgan SJ, Stromberg PC, Storts RW, Sowa BA, Lay JC 1991. Histology and morphometry of *Strongylus vulgaris*-mediated equine mesenteric arteritis. *Journal of Comparative Pathology* 104:89–99.

Nielsen MK, Peterson DS, Monrad J, Thamsborg SM, Olsen SN, Kaplan RM 2008. Detection and semi-quantification of *Strongylus vulgaris* DNA in equine faeces by real-time quantitative PCR. *International Journal of Parasitology* 38:443–453.

Rao UR, Chapman MR, Singh RN, Mehta K, Klei TR 1999. Transglutaminase activity in equine strongyles and its potential role in growth and development. *Parasite* 6:131–139.

Reinemeyer CR, Nielsen MK 2009. Parasitism and colic. *Veterinary Clinics of North America: Equine Practice* 25:233–245.

Rötting AK, Freeman DE, Constable PD, *et al.* 2008. The effects of *Strongylus vulgaris* parasitism on eosinophil distribution and accumulation in equine large intestinal mucosa. *Equine Veterinary Journal* 40:379–384.

Soulsby EJL 1968. *Helminths, Arthropods & Protozoa of Domesticated Animals*. Baillière, Tindall and Cassell, London.

Stancampiano L, Mughini Gras L, Poglayen G 2010. Spatial niche competition among helminth parasites in horse's large intestine. *Veterinary Parasitology* 170:88–95.

Swiderski CE, Klei TR, Folsom RW, *et al.* 1999. Vaccination against *Strongylus vulgaris* in ponies: comparison of the humoral and cytokine responses of vaccinates and nonvaccinates. *Advances in Veterinary Medicine* 41:389–404.

Traversa D, Iorio R, Klei TR, *et al.* 2007. New method for simultaneous species-specific identification of equine strongyles (Nematoda, Strongylida) by reverse line blot hybridization. *Journal of Clinical Microbiology* 45:2937–2942.

Cyathostomum spp.

Corning S 2009. Equine cyathostomins: a review of biology, clinical significance and therapy. *Parasites and Vectors* 2 (Suppl 2):S1.

Deprez P, Vercruysse J 2003. Treatment and follow-up of clinical cyathostominosis in horses. *Journal of Veterinary Medicine A: Physiology, Pathology and Clinical Medicine* 50:527–529.

Dowdall SM, Proudman CJ, Klei TR, Mair T, Matthews JB 2004. Characterisation of IgG(T) serum antibody responses to two larval antigen complexes in horses naturally- or experimentally-infected with cyathostomins. *International Journal of Parasitology* 34:101–108.

Hodgkinson JE, Lichtenfels JR, Mair TS, *et al.* 2003. A PCR-ELISA for the identification of cyathostomin fourth-stage larvae from clinical cases of larval cyathostominosis. *International Journal of Parasitology* 33:1427–1435.

Kaplan RM 2002. Anthelmintic resistance in nematodes of horses. Review. *Veterinary Research* 33:491–507.

Lichtenfels JR, Gibbons LM, Krecek RC 2002. Recommended terminology and advances in the systematics of the Cyathostominea (Nematoda: Strongyloidea) of horses. *Veterinary Parasitology* 107:337–342.

Love S, Murphy D, Mellor D 1999. Pathogenicity of cyathostome infection. Review. *Veterinary Parasitology* 85:113–121.

Lyons ET, Drudge JH, Tolliver SC 2000. Larval cyathostomiasis. *Veterinary Clinics of North America: Equine Practice* 16:501–513.

Mair TS, Sutton DG, Love S 2000. Caecocaecal and caecocolic intussusceptions associated with larval cyathostomosis in four young horses. *Equine Veterinary Journal Supplement* 32:77–80.

Matthews JB, Johnson DR, Lazari O, Craig R, Matthews KR 2008. Identification of a LIM domain-containing gene in the Cyathostominae. *Veterinary Parasitology* 154:82–93.

McWilliam HE, Nisbet AJ, Dowdall SM, Hodgkinson JE, Matthews JB 2010. Identification and characterisation of an immunodiagnostic marker for cyathostomin developing stage larvae. *International Journal of Parasitology* 40:265–275.

Samson-Himmelstjerna G von, Fritzen B, Demeler J, *et al.* 2007. Cases of reduced cyathostomin egg-reappearance period and failure of *Parascaris equorum* egg count reduction following ivermectin treatment as well as survey on pyrantel efficacy on German horse farms. *Veterinary Parasitology* 144:74–80.

Soulsby EJL 1968. *Helminths, Arthropods & Protozoa of Domesticated Animals*. Baillière, Tindall and Cassell, London.

Steinbach T, Bauer C, Sasse H, *et al.* 2006. Small strongyle infection: consequences of larvicidal treatment of horses with fenbendazole and moxidectin. *Veterinary Parasitology* 139:115–131.

Traversa D, Iorio R, Klei TR, *et al.* 2007. New method for simultaneous species-specific identification of equine strongyles (Nematoda, Strongylida) by reverse line blot hybridization. *Journal of Clinical Microbiology* 45:2937–2942.

Dictyocaulus arnfieldi

Britt DP, Preston JM 1985. Efficacy of ivermectin against *Dictyocaulus arnfieldi* in ponies. *Veterinary Record* 116:343–345.

Clayton HM, Duncan JL 1981. Natural infection with *Dictyocaulus arnfieldi* in pony and donkey foals. *Research in Veterinary Science* 31:278–280.

Coles GC, Hillyer MH, Taylor FGR, Parker LD 1998. Activity of moxidectin against bots and lungworm in equids. *Veterinary Record* 143:169–170.

Epe C, Bienioschek S, Rehbein S, Schnieder T 1995. Comparative RAPD-PCR analysis of lungworms (*Dictyocaulidae*) from fallow deer, cattle, sheep, and horses. *Zentralblatt für Veterinärmedizin Reihe B* 42:187–191.

Lyons ET, Tolliver SC, Drudge JH, Swerczek TW, Crowe MW 1985. Lungworms (*Dictyocaulus arnfieldi*): prevalence in live equids in Kentucky. *American Journal of Veterinary Research* 46:921–923.

Soulsby EJL 1968. *Helminths, Arthropods & Protozoa of Domesticated Animals*. Baillière, Tindall and Cassell, London.

Urch DL, Allen WR 1980. Studies on fenbendazole for treating lung and intestinal parasites in horses and donkeys. *Equine Veterinary Journal* 12:74–77.

Parelaphostrongylus tenuis

Anderson RC 2000. The superfamily *Metastrongyloidea*. In: Anderson RC (ed). *Nematode Parasites of Vertebrates, Their Development and Transmission*, 2nd edn. CABI Publishing, Oxon, 129–172.

Lester G 1992. Parasitic encephalomyelitis in horses. *Compendium on Continuing Education of the Practicing Veterinarian* 14:1624–1630.

Reinstein SL, Lucio-Forster A, Bowman DD, *et al*. 2010. Surgical extraction of an intraocular infection of *Parelaphostrongylus tenuis* in a horse. *Journal of the American Veterinary Medical Association* 237:196–199.

Soulsby EJL 1968. *Helminths, Arthropods & Protozoa of Domesticated Animals*. Baillière, Tindall and Cassell, London.

Tanabe M, Kelly R, de Lahunta A, Duffy MS, Wade SE, Divers TJ 2007. Verminous encephalitis in a horse produced by nematodes in the family *Protostrongylidae*. *Veterinary Pathology* 44:119–122.

Parascaris equorum

Austin SM, DiPietro JA, Foreman JH 1990. *Parascaris equorum* infections in horses. *Compendium of Continuing Education for the Practicing Veterinarian* 12:1110–1119.

Boersema JH, Eysker M, Nas JWM 2002. Apparent resistance of *Parascaris equorum* to macrocyclic lactones. *Veterinary Record* 150:279–281.

Clayton HM 1986. Ascarids. Recent advances. *Veterinary Clinics of North America: Equine Practice* 2:313–328.

Cribb NC, Coté NM, Bouré LP, Peregrine AS 2006. Acute small intestinal obstruction associated with *Parascaris equorum* infection in young horses: 25 cases (1985–2004). *New Zealand Veterinary Journal* 54:338–343.

Hébert L, Cauchard J, Doligez P, Quitard L, Laugier C, Petry S 2010. Viability of *Rhodococcus equi* and *Parascaris equorum* eggs exposed to high temperatures. *Current Microbiology* 60:38–41.

Lyons ET, Swerczek TW, Tolliver SC, Bair HD, Drudge JH, Ennis LE 2000. Prevalence of selected species of internal parasites in equids at necropsy in central Kentucky (1995–1999). *Veterinary Parasitology* 92:51–62.

Lyons ET, Tolliver SC, Rathgeber RA, Collins SS 2007. Parasite field study in central Kentucky on thoroughbred foals (born in 2004) treated with pyrantel tartrate daily and other parasiticides periodically. *Parasitology Research* 100:473–478.

Reinemeyer CR, Prado JC, Nichols EC, Marchiondo AA 2010. Efficacy of pyrantel pamoate against a macrocyclic lactone-resistant isolate of *Parascaris equorum* in horses. *Veterinary Parasitology* 171:111–115.

Samson-Himmelstjerna G von, Fritzen B, Demeler J, *et al*. 2007. Cases of reduced cyathostomin egg-reappearance period and failure of *Parascaris equorum* egg count reduction following ivermectin treatment as well as survey on pyrantel efficacy on German horse farms. *Veterinary Parasitology* 144:74–80.

Schougaard H, Nielsen MK 2007. Apparent ivermectin resistance of *Parascaris equorum* in foals in Denmark. *Veterinary Record* 160:439–440.

Soulsby EJL 1968. *Helminths, Arthropods & Protozoa of Domesticated Animals*. Baillière, Tindall and Cassell, London.

Southwood LL, Ragle CA, Snyder JR, Hendrickson DA 1996. Surgical treatment of ascarid impactions in horses and foals. *Proceedings of the 42nd Annual Convention of the American Association of Equine Practitioners* 258–261.

Oxyuris equi

Bauer C, Cirak VY, Hermosilla C, Okoro H 1998. Efficacy of a 2 per cent moxidectin gel against gastrointestinal parasites of ponies. *Veterinary Record* 143:558–561.

Braga FR, Araújo JV, Silva AR, *et al*. 2010. *Duddingtonia flagrans*, *Monacrosporium thaumasium*, and *Pochonia chlamydosporia* as possible biological control agents of *Oxyuris equi* and *Austroxyuris finlaysoni*. *Journal of Helminthology* 84:21–25.

Chapman MR, French DD, Klei TR 2002. Gastrointestinal helminths of ponies in Louisiana: a comparison of species currently prevalent with those present 20 years ago. *Journal of Parasitology* 88:1130–1134.

Klei TR, Rehbein S, Visser M, *et al*. 2001. Re-evaluation of ivermectin efficacy against equine gastrointestinal parasites. *Veterinary Parasitology* 98:315–320.

Monahan CM, Chapman MR, Taylor HW, French DD, Klei TR 1996. Comparison of moxidectin oral gel and ivermectin oral paste against a spectrum of internal parasites of ponies with special attention to encysted cyathostome larvae. *Veterinary Parasitology* 63:225–235.

Reinemeyer CR, Prado JC, Nichols EC, Marchiondo AA 2010. Efficacy of pyrantel pamoate and ivermectin paste formulations against naturally acquired *Oxyuris equi* infections in horses. *Veterinary Parasitology* 171:106–110.

Soulsby EJL 1968. *Helminths, Arthropods & Protozoa of Domesticated Animals*. Baillière, Tindall and Cassell, London.

Tolliver SC, Swerczek TW, Lyons ET 1999. Recovery of *Oxyuris equi* eggs from hemomelasma ilei lesions on ileal serosa of a Thoroughbred yearling filly. *Veterinary Parasitology* 80:353–357.

Torbert BJ, Klei TR, Lichtenfels JR, Chapman MR 1986. A survey in Louisiana of intestinal helminths of ponies with little exposure to anthelmintics. *Journal of Parasitology* 72:926–930.

Probstmayria vivipara

Malan FS, Reinecke RK, Scialdo RC 1981. Anthelmintic efficacy fenbendazole paste in equines. *Journal of the South African Veterinary Association* 52:127–130.

Mfitilodze MW, Hutchinson GW 1989. Prevalence and intensity of non-strongyle intestinal parasites of horses in northern Queensland. *Australian Veterinary Journal* 66:23–26.

Smith HJ 1979. *Probstmayria vivipara* pinworms in ponies. *Canadian Journal of Comparative Medicine* 43:341–342.

Soulsby EJL 1968. *Helminths, Arthropods & Protozoa of Domesticated Animals*. Baillière, Tindall and Cassell, London.

Tolliver SC, Lyons ET, Drudge JH 1987. Prevalence of internal parasites in horses in critical tests of activity of parasiticides over a 28-year period (1956–1983) in Kentucky. *Veterinary Parasitology* 23:273–284.

Thelazia lacrymalis

Collobert C, Bernard N, Lamidey C 1995. Prevalence of *Onchocerca species* and *Thelazia lacrimalis* in horses examined post mortem in Normandy. *Veterinary Record* 136:463–465.

Dongus H, Beelitz P, Schöl H 2003. Embryogenesis and the first-stage larva of *Thelazia lacrymalis*. *Journal of Helminthology* 77:227–233.

Lyons ET, Drudge JH, Tolliver SC 1981. Apparent inactivity of several antiparasitic compounds against the eyeworm *Thelazia lacrymalis* in equids. *American Journal of Veterinary Research* 42:1046–1047.

Lyons ET, Swerczek TW, Tolliver SC, Bair HD, Drudge JH, Ennis LE 2000. Prevalence of selected species of internal parasites in equids at necropsy in central Kentucky (1995–1999). *Veterinary Parasitology* 92:51–62.

Soulsby EJL 1968. *Helminths, Arthropods & Protozoa of Domesticated Animals*. Baillière, Tindall and Cassell, London.

Traversa D, Otranto D, Iorio R, Giangaspero A 2005. Molecular characterization of *Thelazia lacrymalis* (Nematoda, Spirurida) affecting equids: a tool for vector identification. *Molecular and Cell Probes* 19:245–249.

Setaria equina

Campbell WC 1982. Efficacy of the avermectins against filarial parasites: a short review. *Veterinary Research Communications* 5:251–262.

Chirgwin SR, Porthouse KH, Nowling JM, Klei TR 2002. The filarial endosymbiont *Wolbachia* sp. is absent from *Setaria equina*. *Journal of Parasitology* 88:1248–1250.

El-Shahawi GA, Abdel-Latif M, Saad AH, Bahgat M 2010. *Setaria equina*: *in vivo* effect of diethylcarbamazine citrate on microfilariae in albino rats. *Experimental Parasitology* 126:603–610.

Hornok S, Genchi C, Bazzocchi C, Fok E, Farkas R 2007. Prevalence of *Setaria equina* microfilaraemia in horses in Hungary. *Veterinary Record* 161:814–816.

Jubb KVF, Kennedy PC, Palmer N 2007. *Pathology of Domestic Animals*, 5th edn. WB Saunders Elsevier, Edinburgh, 2:293.

Lyons ET, Tolliver SC, Drudge JH, Swerczek TW, Crowe MW 1983. Parasites in Kentucky Thoroughbreds at necropsy: emphasis on stomach worms and tapeworms. *American Journal of Veterinary Research* 44:839–844.

Oge S, Oge H, Yildirim A, Kircali F 2003. *Setaria equina* infection of Turkish equines: estimates of prevalence based on necropsy and the detection of microfilaraemia. *Annals of Tropical Medicine and Parasitology* 97:403–409.

Soulsby EJL 1968. *Helminths, Arthropods & Protozoa of Domesticated Animals*. Baillière, Tindall and Cassell, London.

Stolk WA, Vlas SJ de, Habbema JDF 2005. Anti-*Wolbachia* treatment for lymphatic filariasis. *Lancet* 365:2067–2068.

Taylor MJ, Makunde WH, McGarry HF, Turner JD, Mand S, Hoerauf A 2005. Macrofilaricidal activity after doxycycline treatment of *Wuchereria bancrofti*: a double-blind, randomised placebo-controlled trial. *Lancet* 365:2116–2121.

Yeargan MR, Lyons ET, Kania SA, *et al*. 2009. Incidental isolation of *Setaria equina* microfilariae in preparations of equine peripheral blood mononuclear cells. *Veterinary Parasitology* 161:142–145.

APPENDICES

Appendix 3 Clinical Pathology

Coles EH 1986. *Veterinary Clinical Pathology*, 4th edn. WB Saunders, London.

Cowell RL, Tyler RD 2002. *Diagnostic Cytology and Hematology of the Horse*, 2nd edn. Mosby, St. Louis.

Franken P, Wensing T, Schotman AJH 1982. The bone marrow of the horse. I. The techniques of sampling and examination and values of normal warm-blooded horses. *Zentralblatt für Veterinärmedizin Reihe A* 29:16–22.

Hoogmoed L van, Snyder JR, Christopher M, Vatistas N 1996. Peritoneal fluid analysis in peripartum mares. *Journal of the American Veterinary Medical Association* 209:1280–1282.

Junqueira LC, Carneiro J 1980. *Basic Histology*, 3rd edn. Lange Medical Publications, Los Altos.

Taylor FGR, Hillyer MH 1997. *Diagnostic Techniques in Equine Medicine*. WB Saunders, London.

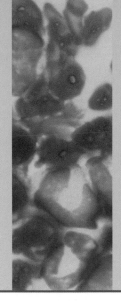

Index